Healthcare Community Synergism between Patients, Practitioners, and Researchers

Valerie C. Bryan
Florida Atlantic University, USA

Jennifer Lynne Bird
Florida Atlantic University, USA

A volume in the Advances in Medical Diagnosis, Treatment, and Care (AMDTC) Book Series

Medical Information Science Reference
An Imprint of IGI Global

Published in the United States of America by
Medical Information Science Reference (an imprint of IGI Global)
701 E. Chocolate Avenue
Hershey PA, USA 17033
Tel: 717-533-8845
Fax: 717-533-8661
E-mail: cust@igi-global.com
Web site: http://www.igi-global.com

Library of Congress Cataloging-in-Publication Data

Names: Bryan, Valerie C., editor. | Bird, Jennifer Lynne, editor.
Title: Healthcare community synergism between patients, practitioners, and researchers / Valerie C. Bryan and Jennifer Lynne Bird, editors.
Description: Hershey PA : Medical Information Science Reference, [2017] | Includes bibliographical references and index.
Identifiers: LCCN 2016017558| ISBN 9781522506409 (hardcover) | ISBN 9781522506416 (ebook)
Subjects: | MESH: Health Promotion | Community Networks | Health Education | Health Knowledge, Attitudes, Practice
Classification: LCC R727.4 | NLM WA 590 | DDC 615.5071--dc23 LC record available at https://lccn.loc.gov/2016017558

This book is published in the IGI Global book series Advances in Medical Diagnosis, Treatment, and Care (AMDTC) (ISSN: Pending; eISSN: Pending)

British Cataloguing in Publication Data
A Cataloguing in Publication record for this book is available from the British Library.

For electronic access to this publication, please contact: eresources@igi-global.com.

Advances in Medical Diagnosis, Treatment, and Care (AMDTC) Book Series

ISSN: Pending
EISSN: Pending

Mission

Advancements in medicine have prolonged the life expectancy of individuals all over the world. Once life-threatening conditions have become significantly easier to treat and even cure in many cases. Continued research in the medical field will further improve the quality of life, longevity, and wellbeing of individuals.

The **Advances in Medical Diagnosis, Treatment, and Care (AMDTC)** book series seeks to highlight publications on innovative treatment methodologies, diagnosis tools and techniques, and best practices for patient care. Comprised of comprehensive resources aimed to assist professionals in the medical field apply the latest innovations in the identification and management of medical conditions as well as patient care and interaction, the books within the AMDTC series are relevant to the research and practical needs of medical practitioners, researchers, students, and hospital administrators.

Coverage

- Experimental Medicine
- Medical Procedures
- Disease Management
- Disease Prevention
- Emergency Medicine
- Patient-Centered Care
- Chronic Conditions
- Cancer Treatment
- Medical Testing
- Alternative Medicine

IGI Global is currently accepting manuscripts for publication within this series. To submit a proposal for a volume in this series, please contact our Acquisition Editors at Acquisitions@igi-global.com or visit: http://www.igi-global.com/publish/.

The Advances in Medical Diagnosis, Treatment, and Care (AMDTC) Book Series (ISSN Pending) is published by IGI Global, 701 E. Chocolate Avenue, Hershey, PA 17033-1240, USA, www.igi-global.com. This series is composed of titles available for purchase individually; each title is edited to be contextually exclusive from any other title within the series. For pricing and ordering information please visit http://www.igi-global.com/book-series/advances-medical-diagnosis-treatment-care/129618. Postmaster: Send all address changes to above address.

Titles in this Series

For a list of additional titles in this series, please visit: www.igi-global.com

Promoting Patient Engagement and Participation for Effective Healthcare Reform
Guendalina Graffigna (Catholic University of the Sacred Heart of Milan, Italy)
Medical Information Science Reference • copyright 2016 • 357pp • H/C (ISBN: 9781466699922) • US $220.00 (our price)

Effective Methods for Modern Healthcare Service Quality and Evaluation
Panagiotis Manolitzas (Technical University of Crete, Greece) Evangelos Grigoroudis (Technical University of Crete, Greece) Nikolaos Matsatsinis (Technical University of Crete, Greece) and Denis Yannacopoulos (Piraeus University of Applied Sciences, Greece)
Medical Information Science Reference • copyright 2016 • 315pp • H/C (ISBN: 9781466699618) • US $190.00 (our price)

Handbook of Research on Trends in the Diagnosis and Treatment of Chronic Conditions
Dimitrios I. Fotiadis (University of Ioannina, Greece)
Medical Information Science Reference • copyright 2016 • 659pp • H/C (ISBN: 9781466688285) • US $385.00 (our price)

Editorial Advisory Board

Table of Contents

Detailed Table of Contents

India, one of the oldest civilizations and second most populous country is ethnically, linguistically, geographically, religious, and demographically diverse is poorly ranked due to complex public healthcare system, which suffers from insufficient funding, poor management. Poor health intertwined with poverty, affordability, accessibility, burden of infectious and non-communicable affecting lives of most Indians. Healthcare ecosystems are complex and still evolving, investments in service delivery system, infrastructure, and technology, are still being experimented and explored. India's booming population; increasing purchasing power; rising awareness of personal health and hygiene; and significant growth in infectious, chronic degenerative, and lifestyle diseases are driving the growing market. In this chapter we will explore accessible and affordable healthcare system, state of public healthcare, healthcare reforms, governance (Constitutional Provisions, Law, and Policy framework) in healthcare delivery, and Opportunity offered by market drivers.

In this chapter, we explore the neuroscience of grief and grieving. Even though the cognitive portion of the initiation into loss implores us to see a correlation between what is expected of us and the concept of reality as we move toward the outcome, the brain is meaning-driven, attempting to match new information with prior understanding. And as neural connections continue to develop and change throughout grief and grieving the "emotional monster" may not be capable of being quieted through support, whether professional or personal. The resistance from a cognitive approach is taken over by our effort to tame that "emotional monster" and images and feelings that are unique to the loss process stunt the capability of the brain to provide rational thinking. We end by picturing how our relentless search began, as we are in awe of what we intuitively know to be true, and that we are not fixed in toxicity, but can change the most challenging neurological situation. Our search was to understand the process of cognition as we move through grief and grieving. We wrote this chapter hoping it would shed a well-lit conversation on the most difficult time we will experience in our lives, the initiation into loss. The light shines on the neuroscience of this journey – as it would not honor 'self' if we did not look at 'self 'in a wholesome way. We frame this chapter through four focus lenses: self and self-discovery focus; emotion focus; social context and role identity focus; and cognitive focus.

Preface

Dear Reader,

We asked for stories, and received them. The authors who contributed chapters to this book shared their stories with the hope of inspiring you as the reader of this book to write your own story and share it with a trusted medical professional the next time you feel either physical or emotional pain. All of us will be patients, or in need of medical care for someone we love, at some point in our lives. When you are a patient it becomes easy to feel scared and uncomfortable with the surroundings and the nomenclature of the medical care system. Through some of the chapters we hope you see the need to become more engaged in your care and advocate for yourself or your family member with your own questions, concerns, and observations.

Medical professionals can best help you if they know the entire story. Despite the complexities the current medical practitioner deals with daily, his or her goal is the same as yours—for you or your loved one to become healthy. Your experience during your treatment will be enhanced if you become a collaborator with your medical practitioners. Ask questions, Write things down. Do your own research. Share concerns. Be your own advocate and/or for that of your loved one.

DISCLAIMER

The strategies and treatments discussed by the authors in this book do not take the place of a visit with a medical professional such as a physician, physical therapist, psychiatrist, nutritionist, or other trained specialist. As the editors of this publication, we do not advocate attempting any treatment plan on your own. We encourage you to feel inspired by the stories the authors share, but please consult a medical professional if you are experiencing physical or emotional pain. Just as it takes a village to teach a child, it may take a community of healthcare professionals and yourself to treat you or your loved one.

THIS BOOK'S PURPOSE

This book has the overall objective of connecting the fields of education and medicine to demonstrate effective collaborations among patients, practitioners, and researchers. *The Expanded Chronic Care Model: Integrating Population Health Promotion* (Barr et al, 2001) suggests that the health of a population for prevention and management of chronic disease requires a more collaborative approach for the people and their communities to be healthy. The health of the community, the individual, and the health system must work in a synergistic fashion for the positive results.

Figure 1. The Expanded Chronic Care Model: Integrating population health promotion
Created by: Victoria Barr, Sylvia Robinson, Brenda Marin-Link, Lisa Underhill, Anita Dotts, & Darlene Ravensdale (2002). Adapted from Glasgow, R., Orleans, C., Wagner, E., Curry, S., Solberg, L. (2001). "Does the Chronic Care Model also serve as a template for improving prevention?, The Milbank Quarterly, 79(4), and World Health Organization, Health and Welfare Canada and Canadian Public Health Association (1986), Ottawa Charter of Health Promotion.

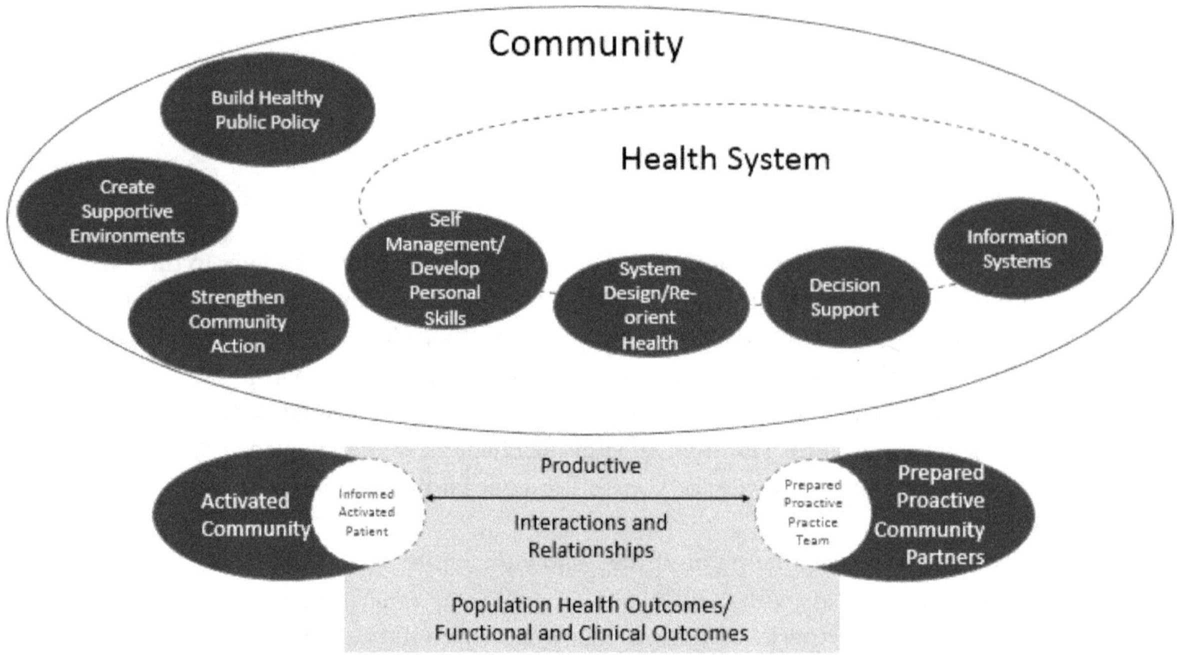

The Ottawa Charter for Health Promotion refers to five action areas:

- Develop personal skills,
- Re-orient health services,
- Build healthy public policy,
- Create supportive environments,
- Strengthen community action (Barr et al, 2003, p. 77).

In many of the chapters that will follow you will see evidence of how programs and services are being developed to help people develop life skills in health management that can affect both the individual and the community. You will also see evidence of health systems advocating for more "health" research and less "illness" research. Partnering between people to people and agency to agency as advocates are evident in many of the chapters; building supportive healthcare environments and healthy communities are also evident throughout the book.

The goal is to foster individual responsibility for health while addressing underlying social determinants of health such as poverty, lack of access to health care, and other societal issues, even addressing the view of some health professionals regarding patients as "non-compliant". Communities that are composed of people with the triple jeopardy of minority status, poverty, and communication barriers are also referred to in some of the chapters.

Table 1. Comparison of the Chronic Care Model with the Expanded Chronic Care Model

COMPONENTS OF THE CHRONIC CARE MODEL		COMPONENTS OF THE EXPANDED CHRONIC CARE MODEL		EXAMPLES
Health System - Organization of Healthcare	Program planning that includes measurable goals for better care of chronic illness			
Self-Management Support	Emphasis on the importance of the central role that patients have in managing their own care	Self-Management / Develop Personal Skills	Enhancing skills and capacities for personal health and wellness	• Smoking prevention and cessation programs • Seniors' walking programs
Decision Support	Integration of evidence-based guidelines into daily clinical practice	Decision Support	Integration of strategies for facilitating the community's abilities to stay healthy	• Development of health promotion and prevention "best practice" guidelines
Delivery System Design	Focus on teamwork and an expanded scope of practice to support chronic care	Delivery System Design / Re-orient Health Services	Expansion of mandate to support individuals and communities in a more holistic way	• Advocacy on behalf of (and with) vulnerable populations • Emphasis in quality improvement on health and quality of life outcomes, not just clinical outcomes
Clinical Information Systems	Developing information systems based on patient populations to provide relevant client data	Information Systems	Creation of broadly based information systems to include community data beyond the healthcare system	• Use of broad community needs assessments that take into account: • poverty rates • availability of public transportation • violent crime rate
Community Resources and Policies	Developing partnerships with community organizations that support and meet patients' needs	Build Healthy Public Policy	Development and implementation of policies designed to improve population health	• Advocating for / developing: • smoking bylaws • walking trails • reductions in the price of whole wheat flour
		Create Supportive Environments	Generating living and employment conditions that are safe, stimulating, satisfying and enjoyable	• Maintaining older people in their homes for as long as possible • Work towards the development of well-lit streets and bicycle paths
		Strengthen Community Action	Working with community groups to set priorities and achieve goals that enhance the health of the community	• Supporting the community in addressing the need for safe, affordable housing

Courtesy of Barr, V.J., Robinson, S., Marin-Link, B. Underhill, A.D., Ravensdale, D., & Salivares, S. (2003). The expanded chronic care model: an integration of concepts and strategies from population health promotion and the chronic care model. *Hospital Quarterly, 7*(1), p. 79)

Research leads to new treatments in the field of medicine. Medical practitioners can combine objective research data with subjective patient narratives to design treatment plans that will best help the patient. The patient will also need to become an active participant in the process by complying with the treatment plan and providing feedback to the medical practitioner. What worked and what didn't work can lead to additional reflection and research. Synergy exists when the combined effect of the collaboration becomes greater than what an individual could do alone. This positive interdependence means that everyone works together to accomplish a common goal. In designing a city, city planners may use community synergism so residents have a happy, healthy place to live. The healthier your community, the more likely its inhabitants will be as well.

In the medical field, community synergism exists when all members of a medical team, the researchers in the field, as well as the patient and the patient's family, work together so patients have a happy, healthy treatment experience. This book's title, *Healthcare Community Synergism Between Patients, Practitioners, and Researchers* reflects this theme and features chapters from educators, patients, and members of the medical community that illustrate powerful narratives of synergy.

DESCRIPTION OF BOOK CHAPTERS

We now present a brief overview of each of the chapters before you turn the pages and experience them. We grouped chapters with similar themes together, so if you read the book in order it will have a flow to it. If you prefer to jump in anywhere and begin reading, you will still learn an amazing amount of information from each author. We feel grateful to all of the authors for sharing their stories, and writing from every person in this book enhanced the quality of the publication. Another moment of synergy occurred when this diverse group of authors contributed their chapters to *Healthcare Community Synergism between Patients, Practitioners, and Researchers* so we could achieve our shared goal of educating and helping others.

In Chapter 1, *Writing Healing Narratives,* Jennifer Lynne Bird connects the emerging field of health coaching with the practice of journal writing to illustrate the power of using writing to help people heal.

In Chapter 2, *Synergism through Therapeutic Visual Arts,* Susannah Brown and Ashley Hartman discuss the value of art therapy and illustrate the benefits of art for patients.

In Chapter 3, *Heartmath: A University Initiative,* Beth M. King, Charlotte D. Barry, Jo Ann M. Bamdas, Kimberly Bronner and Karethy A. Edwards introduce a new program and explain how the program enhances resilience as well as coping skills.

In Chapter 4, *A Need for Greater Collaboration: Initiatives to Improve Transitions of Care,* Mariette Sourial, Jo Ann M. Bamdas, Angelica Constanzo, and Marina E. Ishak explain how a team approach to medical care can optimize patient care while lowering hospital readmission rates.

In Chapter 5, *Humane Education: A Call to Action for Elementary School Students,* Cassandra M. Kenski and Jaclyn Falcone describe the implementation of a humane education curriculum that teaches students not only about caring for animals while also developing more humane character traits.

In Chapter 6, *Preparing Future Physicians to Adapt to the Changing Health Care System: Promoting Humanism through Curricular Design,* Joanna Lauren Drowos and Sarah K. Wood describe a medical school program which creates stronger connections between medical students and their patients and promotes comprehensive care.

In Chapter 7, *Mental Illness, Youth, and Applicable Lessons from Residential Treatment Centers,* Krista Allison and Chris Allison increase awareness of mental illness and provide resources for comprehensive and holistic care.

In Chapter 8, *Culture of Learning Cities: Connecting Leisure and Health for Lifelong Learning,* Ebbin Dotson, Dan K. Hibbler, and Leodis Scott address the health of communities and discuss the implementation of solutions that increase both the environment of cities and the health of the cities' residents.

In Chapter 9, *The Role of Self-Efficacy and Aging in Managing Disease,* Debra N. Weiss-Randall presents a self-management program which improves patients' quality of life using an integrative approach.

In Chapter 10, *Stress and Its Relationship to Leadership and a Healthy Workplace Culture,* David B. Ross, Julie A. Exposito, and Tom Kennedy discuss how stress management can be improved for organizations so the organizations can be driven by effective leaders.

In Chapter 11, *Framework of Indian Healthcare System and its Challenges: An Insight,* Prashant Mehta explores the healthcare system along with possible reforms and opportunities.

In Chapter 12, *Incognito: The Neuroscience of Grief and Grieving,* Linda Marie Ellington and Valerie C. Bryan explore the difference between what society expects of someone who is grieving and the complex feelings of people who have experienced grief.

We enjoyed compiling the chapters for this book and hope they inspire you to be an advocate for your health as well as the health of your loved ones.

REFERENCES

Barr, V. J., Robinson, S., Marin-Link, B., Underhill, A. D., Ravensdale, D., & Salivares, S. (2003). The expanded chronic care model: An integration of concepts and strategies from population health promotion and the chronic care model. *Hospital Quarterly*, *7*(1), 77. PMID:14674182

Acknowledgment

From Jennifer Lynne Bird:

Whenever I write a thank you page, I always hope I don't forget anyone! Thanks to the entire team of people who made this project possible.

Thanks to our editor at IGI, Courtney Tychinski, and the rest of the publishing team who helped with this book. My co-editor Valerie Bryan and I have edited previous publications with IGI and it was wonderful to return for this one. Thanks also to all the authors of chapters in this book for sharing your research and stories. We would also like to share our gratitude for the Editorial Board, the dream team of intelligent and creative reviewers who never hesitated to help us with whatever needed to be done.

Every day I feel blessed to belong to my amazing family who supports my dreams and makes me feel I can do anything. Much love to Dann Bird, Diane McLoughlin, Susie DeBeck, Bill DeBeck, Robin Perry, David Bird, Patricia Bird, Melissa Bird, Derek Bird, Gabrielle Bird, Marsha Bird, Sandy Bridges, Joanna Claridge, Mike Bridges, Carl Claridge, Erica Younkvich, Daniel Younkvich, Margaret Earl, Tim Earl, Michael Schafer, Cher Schafer, Benjamin Schafer, Crystal Schafer, Arthur Bruggisser, Brian Bruggisser, Amanda Bruggisser, Lucy Bird, Andy Bird, and all the new kids in the family!

I am writing these words now because of the support from all my friends, colleagues, and students throughout the years. The names are too numerous to mention in this space, but please know that I thank you for being part of my life and appreciate the role each one of you played in my journey throughout the years.

And to Marilyn Kepler Bird, I know somehow you can read these words. Thanks for being my guardian angel and the reason I ventured into the medical field.

From Valerie C. Bryan:

My first thank you is to Jennifer Lynne Bird who was always present to keep the book rolling alone. She did a superb job of organizing and shepherding the book forward despite all the initial obstacles we were both encountering. We were both aware when we started this book that the topic meant a great deal to both of us—we both were passionate about the topic. What we were not aware of was the chapters would come alive to us individually as we engaged in this adventure. Thank you, Courtney Tychinski, for keeping us on target despite the numerous obstacles.

Our authors and ourselves were 'living' what we were writing about: the *healing narratives*; *coping skills*; the *role of collaboration*; varied forms of dealing with *others, ourselves and even animals;* new training of health professionals regarding *how to promote comprehensive and holistic care; self-management* and the role it plays; and last, but certainly not least, *death and grief of loss.* Because of this, I especially want to thank all of our superb authors and our remarkable editing team. Many of us have experienced health issues and stress for ourselves or our loved ones, loss of a loved one or loss of a career or a way of life. We have each found a way as we were writing, to learn more about how to cope and collaborate with our health professionals and how to encourage them to do the same with us. Specifically, to the authors—thank you for finding the time to put your heart and scholarship on each page. It is evident that you are each unique in your contributions.

I want to thank my department for allowing me to do labors of love as part of my scholarship. I want to thank my family for supporting me even though the effort took me away from them and their health issues, and even my own health issues, at times. I want to also acknowledge the passing of a great doctoral student during the writing of this book, that would have loved to add chapters and chapters to the book, of good and bad, based on her experience with cancer and the health care system and the role of a community in addressing illnesses. She inspired me every day as I wrote. I also have to acknowledge that my Dad who continues to inspire me *to write and lead from the heart.* Thanks, Dad, for that lesson.

Chapter 1
Writing Healing Narratives

Jennifer Lynne Bird
Florida Atlantic University, USA

ABSTRACT

People, especially hospital patients, want someone to know their stories. Teachers in English classrooms rely on narratives to learn their students' stories. Since learning patients' narratives is an emerging trend in the field of physical therapy as well as other medical practice, this chapter makes connections between writing, health coaching, and physical therapy to illustrate the value of narratives for patients not only in physical therapy, but also in other fields of medicine. Health coaching is a relatively new addition to the medical field that encourages patients to share their stories and set goals for themselves in addition to the goals set for them by their medical team. This chapter uses a multigenre format which discusses writing theory while simultaneously demonstrating an innovative narrative.

I JUST WANT YOU TO KNOW WHO I AM

In this narrative, the practice of writing meets the practice of medicine. The story begins with a conversation about multigenre writing, since this chapter unfolds in a nontraditional format not typically seen in academic publications. Then you will read a story that immerses you into the world of an English professor/health coach/Stephen Minister, since while I play three distinct professional roles during any given week, the roles intertwine in a beautiful mosaic that enables me to use writing to help people heal. After the story, you will read additional ideas on writing, medicine, and spirituality, which will provide additional illumination of how the puzzle pieces of this narrative fit together. Finally, I introduce the acronym MICE and explain how it can be used in the medical community to provide additional hope and healing for patients.

This section's title, *I Just Want You to Know Who I Am*, is a line from the song *Iris* by the Goo Goo Dolls. It also describes how patients feel when seeking help: They want someone to know their stories. When seeking medical treatment, a patient wants to feel like his or her story is being heard and the medical provider sees a person and not just a name on a chart. Rankin (2015b) advises that despite demands from a sometimes frustrating medical system, those practicing medicine need to take the time to look their patients in the eyes and not stand with a hand on the door to the exam room because, "just

DOI: 10.4018/978-1-5225-0640-9.ch001

as healers must stand up and reclaim the lineage of their professions, patients must reclaim their own power, standing up with their autonomy, their intuition, their willingness to question and participate in changing the system from within, and their vote. It all starts with change at the level of the healer-patient relationship" (p. 238). This narrative will explore the value of writing and how writing can be applied to the field of medicine to help people heal. Whether a patient talks to a health coach, receives prayers from a Stephen Minister, or writes in a journal, the important thing is that the patient feels the story is heard.

While a story can be spoken, writing enables the author to capture additional details of a narrative. Pennebaker (1997) theorized from his research as a psychologist, "if my experience was any indication, writing about upsetting issues must work in ways similar to talking about them" (p. 30). Any patient who has ever walked out of a doctor's office with the realization of forgetting an important question can benefit from writing notes to remember experiences. Brown (2015) summarizes, "Pennebaker's research, combined with what I've learned in my own work, has convinced me that even brief engagements with writing can lead to significant results" (p. 88). Patients therefore do not have to write a long narrative for their medical practitioners or themselves; a short series of notes or freewriting of a few sentences can be enough to share the story.

Journal writing may be relatively new to the medical field, but for years English teachers have used journal writing in their classrooms. Anderson and MacCurdy (2000) advise English teachers, "we are, however, arguing what we know to be true – stories about painful, traumatic events in the lives of students do appear in our classrooms, they have always appeared, and they will continue to appear, not because we want or don't want them to, but because writing is quite simply the medium in which, for many people, the deepest, most effective, and most profound healing can take place" (pp. 8-9). Writing in journals gives students a space to explore their thoughts and feelings. While some students do choose to write about painful events, students can also choose to write in their journals about other topics, such as their feelings about an inspirational quote. By writing, students transfer emotions out of their heads and onto the page. Gruwell (2007), whose students became known as the Freedom Writers, states, "I, like my students, realized that it would take more than just writing to feel better – but at least it was a start" (p. 148). The purpose of journal writing is for students to trust themselves and their first impressions while they write narratives. As Goldberg (1990) states, "trusting your own mind is essential for writing. Words come out of the mind" (p. 1). Students have a short amount of time, such as five or ten minutes, to write their first impression on a topic. The time limit is to capture the writer's first impression about an idea before self-criticism can create any doubt or second guessing.

Journal writing helps students find their writing voice. Lamott (1994) discusses her own experiences and shares, "so I sit for a moment and then say a small prayer – please help me get out of the way so I can write what needs to be written" (p. 117). Writing what needs to be written serves as a form of self-expression that leads to the discovery of writing voice. English teachers know that no matter what the story is now, students always have the power to rewrite their narratives. As Cameron (1998) states, "when we just let ourselves write, we get it 'right'" (p. 8). If we find the courage to write our stories and trust our writing voices, we write a new narrative.

A SHORT SYNOPSIS OF HEALTH COACHING

Health coaching is still new to the field of medicine; consequently, research studying the benefits of health coaching is only emerging as of this writing. While health coaches have training in the field of psychology, they are not psychologists. While psychology encourages patients to look backward and health coaching encourages patients to look forward, both fields share the common thread of narratives providing connections. According to Caldwell, Grey, and Wolever (2013), "the major tenets of the health coaching process are patient-centeredness and patient-control focused around patient-originated health goals that guide the work within a supportive coaching partnership" (p. 48). The health coach works with the patient to explore the patient's attitude about change. What are the factors causing the patient to not be motivated to take care of his or her health, not think the treatment plan is important, not feel confidence in completing the treatment plan, or not feel ready to express why changing is not a priority? The health coach does not tell the patient what to do, but asks open ended questions while the patient finds his or her own answers. Defined by Smith, Lake, Simmons, Perlman, Wroth, and Wolever (2013) as "through techniques sourced from humanistic and positive psychology, solution-focused and mindfulness-based therapies, and leadership coaching, Integrative Health Coaching (IHC) provides a mechanism to empower patients through various stages of learning and change" (p. 66). The health coach partners with the physical therapist and any other member of the patient's medical team to not only help the patient comply with goals set by the medical team, but also any personal goals the patient may have which align with the treatment goals.

A SHORT SYNOPSIS OF STEPHEN MINISTRY

Helping people through their experiences is a role of not only health coaches, but also Stephen Ministers. Haugk (2000) provides the definition as, "Stephen Ministers are lay Christians carefully recruited, selected, trained, commissioned, and supervised for lay caring ministry" (p. 17). Both roles are similar yet different. Health coaches use the same skills as Stephen Ministers of reflective listening, maintaining boundaries, encouraging people to express their feelings, asking open ended questions to lead to solutions, and providing a supportive presence. However, they differ in that health coaches encourage people to set goals to improve their health while Stephen Ministers provide prayers. Prayers can provide comfort to patients as they heal. Alexander (2012) demonstrates belief in the science of medicine because "I'm still a scientist. I'm still a doctor, and as such I have two essential duties: to honor truth and to help heal" (p. 171). Alexander (2014), however, also argues, "the fact is, science and faith, the two ways of knowing the world that have defined our culture, are much, much more entwined than we tend to think they are" (p. 63). While patients do need all the advantages of modern medicine, if saying a prayer or writing in a journal helps a patient feel better, such techniques effectively supplement their medical treatment.

MULTIGENRE NARRATIVES

Multigenre writing provides authors the opportunity to tell their narratives using creative and unique perspectives. The practice of multigenre writing originated in the field of English Education, where Romano (2008) provides the definition as, "instead of producing one long expository paper, students wrote about their topics in many genres. Although each piece was self-contained, making a point of its own, taken together, all the writing created a unified whole. I called the assignment a multigenre research paper" (p. 180). Multigenre writing helps writers surprise the reader and let creativity shine through traditional reporting of research. Romano (2004) elaborates, "it isn't simply one expository or narrative monolog. In multigenre papers, writers put together information from many perspectives, angles, and voices" (p. 34). Of course, as with all research papers, all the facts reported in a multigenre paper must be accurate. The most important thing with multigenre writing, however, becomes for the author to use the research to tell a compelling story.

Multigenre writing means looking at a topic from multiple perspectives, with narratives becoming the driving force. As Romano (2013) explains, "while expository forms like clear explanations, succinct position statements, and tight arguments surely have a place in multigenre papers, genres of narrative thinking carry the cognitive load" (p. 20). Multigenre writing opens up additional dimensions for research by giving the author of a multigenre paper the opportunity to present findings using innovative formats such as artwork, creative writing, and fictionalized interpretations of stories. For example, in the practice of both health coaching and Stephen Ministry, specific accounts of patient conversations cannot be repeated in order to protect confidentiality. Consequently, sometimes the best method to present facts is by using fiction. The essence of the story remains true, but details have been changed to maintain confidentiality for participants. Romano (2000) advises teachers, "whether your students are doing secondary research and writing multigenre papers out of that or whether they are exploring aspects of their lives, urge them to use the techniques of fiction" (p. 72). Fictionalized experiences protect details confidential to people involved in the narrative while retaining the emotional truth of a story. It becomes possible for readers to feel what the author felt without needing to know names or identifying details of other participants in the story. Romano (1995) believes, "by creating fictional dreams peopled with fully realized characters driven by tension amid enough detail of setting to create atmosphere, students can create truths that show what they know" (p. 8). Fiction frees the writer of having to remember factual details, or in this case, allows for the reader to gain a better comprehension of health coaching without the author compromising confidential information unable to be shared in a publication. The goal becomes to tell a captivating story while simultaneously honoring the lives of the patients who made the story possible.

I previously edited a collection of chapters applying multigenre writing to medicine. Three colleagues and I wrote a chapter about multigenre medicine (Bird, Wanner, Urenda, and Perry, 2015) and the entire book I edited encouraged medical practitioners and patients to share their stories using creative methods (Bird, 2015). The current narrative you are reading continues the tradition. First, you will read a story showing the theory in practice. The story will then be followed by a series of end notes explaining a rationale for the events in the narrative.

Helldorfer and Moss (2007) believe, "in health care, we have a distinct mission to relieve suffering and restore hope" (p. 213). Helping a patient with the awareness that just because pain exists now doesn't mean it will exist in the future can provide a patient with hope and courage to rewrite an existing narrative. Adams (1990) describes the writing as healing process as journal therapy and explains, "when you move your negative emotions out of your body through exercise or writing, they aren't lurking around to cause tension or disease via tight muscles, stiff necks, headaches, ulcers, or heart attacks" (p. 39). She continues, "if there is one inviolate rule of journal writing, it is that there are simply no rules. Writing naturally means that you do what works for you and that you don't worry about what you're not doing in the journal" (p. 42). Therefore, writing can not only relieve emotional pain, but physical pain as well. Obviously, if a patient experiences pain, no amount of journal writing will take the place of a treatment plan prescribed by a medical practitioner. However, writing can be used in conjunction with the treatment plan to enhance patient healing. Zimmermann (2002) believes, "by giving voice to fears, anger, and despair, by letting go of old dreams and hopes, our self-healing powers come into play" (p.

18). Writing can help us figure out what concerns us so we can help heal ourselves; we can then share our concerns with medical professionals so they can use that information to design a treatment plan that will best help us continue to heal.

All of this background provides support of why you will read fictionalized narratives of a health coach's factual experiences. The fictional stories have their foundation in factual truth. Health coaches adhere to a code of ethics and must honor confidentiality to provide patients with a safe place to share their stories. Creating that safe space includes not sharing any real patient stories in a publication. To protect confidentiality, no real names of patients are used in the following narrative. All patients described are composites of several patients, and no patient described is based on the experiences of a single real person to add an additional layer of confidentiality. Patients are named after characters in works of literature. Furthermore, additional details have also been fictionalized so there is no possibility of a single patient being identified. Think of the patients in this narrative as fictional characters. While their stories were inspired by real patients, the important thing for you as a reader is to experience what the health coach felt when learning the patient narratives, and all the emotions are true. When writing fiction from the factual experiences in his life, O'Brien (1990) explains, "I want you to feel what I felt. I want you to know why story-truth is truer sometimes than happening truth" (p. 179). Goldberg (2000) concurs, "sometimes the more fictional a writer becomes, the closer he actually gets to dead center. Fiction lets us unhinge from the facts and unleashes the soul of a thing" (p. 129). All of the patients received total knee arthroplasty (TKA) surgery and spoke to the health coach while in a hospital inpatient orthopedic setting. In addition to speaking with a health coach, the patients all received treatments from a physical therapist and an occupational therapist, as well as hospital care from nurses and physicians. The narrative is told in the first person "I" from the perspective of the health coach who is also an English professor and Stephen Minister.

HEALTH COACHING NARRATIVES

I sling my lanyard with my ID badge around my neck and pick up the list of patients I am scheduled to visit today, as I look forward to another day of health coaching and helping people. A gift card I received from my family enabled me to afford a stack of composition books for hospital patients. Every patient did not receive a journal due to the fact that some patients experienced surgical complications that made neither coaching nor writing possible for them. When patients in the hospital received a journal, there was a note on it that read as follows:

This is your journal!

Use it to...

1. *Write questions for your medical team.*
2. *Write a list of your goals.*
3. *Freewrite about anything on your mind.*
4. *Draw pictures.*
5. *Annotate medical advice so you remember.*

I refer to my first patient of the day as Newland, named after the indecisive character in the novel *The Age of Innocence*. On the one hand, this Newland loves being surrounded by the constant visitors to his room; on the other hand, he is tired and in pain. Overall, Newland is at peace with his life and very optimistic. He is telling jokes with the physical therapist and occupational therapist who are in the room when I arrive and I notice his great sense of humor. I appreciate the support for health coaching from all the members of the medical team. The physical therapist and occupational therapist tell Newland they think it would be good for him to talk to me before they leave to help another patient.

"What are you looking forward to the most when you go home?" I ask. Questions like this motivate patients to envision their lives after the hospital.

"Outdoors. My bike. My boat. My dog. Being pain free when going on a drive." He smiles and describes a beautiful scene of going for a drive, which I hope comes true for him after he leaves the hospital.

"Sometimes it's the little things we miss most." I try to add meaning while reflecting one of his statements. Newland changes the direction of the conversation.

"I'm happy, but exhausted. I love all my visitors, but they won't leave." He leans back against his pillows, signaling he would like to rest. Health coaching conversations in the hospital are usually short, since patients are on medication and need their rest between physical and occupational therapy treatment sessions. I have learned to make the most of the short time I have. We talk about ideas of how he could get some rest without being rude to his guests. As a health coach in a hospital, I have to accept that patients are in my life for only the duration of their short hospital stays; therefore, I do not have the opportunity to know the next chapters they write in their stories.

I then stop by to check on the writing of my second patient of the day. I call her Edna, after the main character in the novel *The Awakening*, because, like her literary namesake, she is quiet and reluctant to talk about her feelings. I'm hoping that the composition notebook I gave her will encourage her to write what she is feeling. Edna was excited to write in her journal. I knock on the door and push it open. A nurse is in the room with Edna.

"These notebooks are a great idea," Edna says. The nurse smiles. Typically patients open up more when I am the only person in the room with them, but Edna keeps on talking. "I have no pain today."

"That's great news." I look at the journal buried under a book, a food tray, and other items on the table next to her and know she won't be reading her writing to me. That's okay; I've learned from the college students I teach and a large amount of research that it is the act of writing that helps people, regardless of whether or not the writing is shared. Writing in a journal gives patients such as Edna the opportunity to explore their thoughts on paper without worrying about staying awake to talk to a visitor in their hospital rooms.

"I need some rest," Edna says, but she is smiling and seems happy as she says it. "I'm excited to write more."

"Writing can help you remember things," I tell her. "Sometimes you think of your best questions after your medical team leaves the room." I notice the nurse nod in agreement while I mentally reprimand myself, because I've just lapsed into teaching, and health coaches are supposed to listen, not teach.

"Very true," Edna picks up on my thread of conversation anyway. "Oh. I'm starting to feel some pain now." That's my cue to leave as the nurse takes over Edna's care. I wonder how much she can focus on her future goals while she is in pain. Even if she's not sharing her feelings with me verbally, at least she is writing them in her journal. The nurse stops me before I go into the next patient's room and tells me the journals are a great idea.

My third patient of the day earns the name Jay. I name him after the title character in the novel *The Great Gatsby*, because he is overall doing well but more interested in talking about other people instead of himself. His wife, who I name Daisy after Gatsby's great love, hovers over him like a bird that doesn't know where to land.

"This machine is making too much noise," Daisy remarks as she reaches for one of the machines.

"Let me get a nurse," I quickly tell her, not knowing much about the machine in question but suspecting that unplugging it would be bad. After the situation is resolved, I evaluate my options. The purpose of health coaching is to have individual conversations with people; family members, as well meaning as they are, can easily redirect a conversation.

"Will I ever leave this hospital?" Jay asks. I can still encourage him on his healing journey and talk to his wife about practicing self-care so she can better take care of him once he returns home from the hospital. I switch from a coaching role to that of motivational speaker and notice that Daisy has been writing in the journal. I am reminded that the hospital patients are receiving care from all the medical professionals, but who is taking care of the caregivers?

"I gave her the journal," Jay explains.

"That's fine." I look at Daisy, wondering if she needs coaching more than her husband the hospital patient.

"Take care of yourself so you can better take care of him," I tell her.

"I will," Daisy promises, but she is already reaching for Jay's pillows. This wasn't a coaching session, but hopefully I helped both Daisy and Jay. All I can do is my best, I tell myself. The good news about seeing patients one right after another is that I can't dwell too much on one conversation. I need to practice mindfulness and focus on each patient in the moment, not think about the ones I spoke to earlier or the ones I am going to speak to later.

"Get out of my room! Go away!" That is my introduction to my fourth patient of the day, who earns the name Rebecca. The main character in the novel *Rebecca* remains a mystery, and the mystery I need to solve immediately is why Rebecca has never met me, yet doesn't like me. "I can't watch my favorite singer in peace!" Rebecca yells, and slumps against the pillow angrily. I glance at the television screen and see a singer typically more popular with the college students I teach than members of Rebecca's older generation, and remind myself of the advice I tell my college students when I teach a reading diagnosis class. Interest + Area of Need = Effective Assessment. I assess I am not going to have an effective coaching session at this moment in time, especially when I see Rebecca is not alone in the room. Her daughter is there with her.

"She's in pain. Please leave," Rebecca's daughter orders. Concern of family members is understandable; anytime my grandma had surgery, my mom insisted on staying in the hospital room with her even after visiting hours.

"I'll be back," I tell Rebecca, leaving her to her concert. A physical therapist and occupational therapist who heard the exchange with Rebecca smile at me encouragingly. Don't let it get to you, I tell myself. As I walk past the patient admitting desk, the kind receptionist who I see multiple times a day asks me how much I've walked today. Thanks to my iPhone app, I already know that by the end of the day I will walk six miles and climb ten flights of stairs. I'm grateful a colleague advised me to wear comfortable shoes as I go to the cafeteria for a free cup of coffee I won't finish because it takes too long to drink and I want to return to my patients. I stop by the documentation room, greet the physical therapists and occupational therapists who are there, and quickly write my notes for the patients I have seen so far. The team is listening to a mix CD I made during a team development workshop, and I realize I am not just helping patients while I am here, but also my colleagues. By the time I don't finish my coffee and do finish my notes, Rebecca's television concert has ended and I try talking to her again.

One of the physical therapists is in the room helping Rebecca and suggests we work together. While the physical therapist teaches Rebecca exercises, I ask her to visualize her ideal health. Her focus remains in the present, not in the future. She visualizes a peaceful scene while completing the exercises the physical therapist gives her. While health coaching encourages the setting of long term goals in timeframes of three to six months in the future, Rebecca can only visualize one moment to the next. For her, that is what she needs. She mentions her love of antiques. My dad has been known to keep things for years and now has an impressive collection of antiques. I found the opening I needed to get her to trust me and talk. Once the physical therapist leaves, Rebecca glares at me.

"I'm glad my daughter left. A three day hospital stay means a three day vacation from family. Where are my glasses? Have you seen my toothbrush?" Confusion has taken over her. The ethics of doing what is best for a patient overrules any additional coaching, so it's time for me to leave and let her sleep.

My fifth patient of the day wants to talk about Shakespeare instead of his health goals. I assign him the name Cyrano, after the title character in *Cyrano de Bergerac,* who is poetic when speaking.

"Have you read this book?" Cyrano asks, holding up a popular contemporary novel.

"I have," I confirm. "My students like it too."

"You're a professor!" Cyrano claps his hands. "I always believe reading and writing have value. What's your favorite Shakespeare play? If I tell you a quote from a Shakespeare play, can you identify it? My son in high school needs to learn more quotes and appreciate the value of reading!" He is not doing it intentionally, but he is trying to distract me. This could easily turn into a conversation about literature, which I love, but that would put the focus on me and not on Cyrano.

"How would you compare your journey to the journey of a literary character?" I ask. While, as health coaches, we do self-manage our own thoughts and feelings, we are only human and sometimes patients learn parts of our stories. And just as English teachers discuss poems in the literature we teach, health coaches often use metaphors to reflect part of the stories they hear. In Cyrano's case, he compared himself to various characters in a Shakespeare play. He was on a quest just like they were, and his quest was to heal from his surgery. By the time I leave, I'm pleased with the session, and happy Cyrano now sees himself as the hero of his life story, just like his favorite Shakespeare characters.

"Please pray with me," instructs my sixth patient of the day, a happy and peaceful woman I refer to as Nora Elizabeth, a combination of two character names from the play *A Doll's House* and the novel *Pride and Prejudice*. Both literary characters are strong heroines, and I soon learn Nora Elizabeth has more strength than both of her literary namesakes combined. I find my dual roles as Stephen Minister and health coach emerging as I hold her hand and pray. Often when people pray, they don't know the words to say and that's okay. Word choice doesn't matter as much as the intent of the message; the same can be said for writing. I have learned to trust my heart with both prayer and writing and try not to overthink the words of my prayer. "That was beautiful," Elizabeth wipes away a tear.

"How are you feeling?" I ask, knowing that one of the physical therapists told me she experienced complications during her surgery.

"What happens when we die?" Nora Elizabeth asks. I pause before answering. While she had complications during her surgery, they were not life threatening, but sometimes medical experiences cause patients to reflect on their lives.

"What do you think happens when we die?" I turn her question back to her, using another health coaching strategy of exploring what the patients feel instead of asking as experts answering all their questions. Both health coaches and Stephen Ministers guide others to find their own answers. Unlike teaching, we don't direct others what to do. In both of my roles, reflective listening and being present for another person becomes essential. I believe Heaven is a beautiful place with peace and love and happiness, where I will be reunited with everyone in my family who died, but I don't want to tell her what to believe if she has a different opinion. Nora Elizabeth starts telling me about a book she read where the author had a near death experience.

"I'm scared," she admits.

"It's okay to feel that way," I assure her. "What are you looking forward to the most when you go home?" I ask, bringing my day full circle by asking my last patient of the day the same question I asked the first.

"Watching football. Eating chocolate. Can we pray again?" Nora Elizabeth reaches for my hand. While we are praying, Nora Elizabeth's doctor arrives. He bows his head and remains silent as I finish the prayer.

"Spirituality has value. It helps patients," the doctor remarks. Since patients have limited time with their doctors, I always leave the room when a doctor arrives. I never want patients to miss a moment of discussing their medical care. Nora Elizabeth's story will become another one to which I will never know the sequel. Spirituality is one of the dimensions of health explored by health coaches and it was the one that Nora Elizabeth wanted to discuss the most during my coaching session with her.

Before I conclude my day at the hospital, I leave the orthopedic wing of the hospital where I visited my six patients because I am asked to visit an oncology patient coping with a cancer diagnosis. I try to offer some comfort to a shocked patient immediately after the cancer treatment didn't work and there are no more medical options. For this patient, there is no setting of long term goals but reflecting on the question: What do you need to do to feel at peace with the time you have left? Health coaches don't usually make visits to the emergency room, but I am asked to sit with a patient's family until they can receive an update on their loved one's condition from someone on the medical team. Mixed with the tragedy of sad diagnoses are the triumphs, as I walk through the hospital hallways and witness a physical therapist and occupational therapist help a patient walk again against the odds. The best moments are the ones talking to patients, learning their narratives, and know that for a short moment in time, my life story intersected with theirs and I hopefully helped make a difference in their lives by being there.

END NOTES FOR PATIENT NARRATIVES

These notes focus primarily on the role of using health coaching with physical therapy patients since that is the setting where I worked as a health coach, but health coaching can also be used with cardiac patients, oncology patients, or even healthy patients who desire lifestyle changes. Some health coaches have medical backgrounds; for example, many health coaches are nurses. But other health coaches bring our own unique knowledge to the field and offer different perspectives. My area of expertise is writing, so I am able to use that skill to help patients heal. Regardless of background, all health coaches need to receive specific training in order to practice. The goal of using journaling as a health coach is not for the writing to result in publication, but to provide patients with another way to think about their progress. Germer (2009) discusses the value of journals and writes, "journaling is an opportunity to monitor habit change, to troubleshoot, and, most important, to notice new ways you might be responding to problems in your life" (p. 241). Journals can be used for recording narratives, tracking pain, setting goals, and celebrating the small victories in life. Neff (2011) believes in the power of gratitude journals and states, "after a relatively short time, keeping a gratitude journal can make a substantial contribution to your level of happiness" (p. 279). Writing in journals can contribute to the positive outlook that helps people heal. It reminds patients to take their recovery process during physical therapy one day and one step at a time, because small steps can lead to big changes.

Journal writing can also provide accountability for achieving goals. Lea Michele (2015) explains, "this might be a way for you to hold yourself accountable for achieving everything you want. Keeping a journal and asking yourself hard questions about what you really want to get out of your life is the best way, in my experience, to actually help you achieve your dreams" (p. 11). Displaying the list of goals in a prominent place is another way of remaining accountable and providing inspiration during the healing journey.

While Romano (1987) is describing a writing conference in an English classroom instead of a health coaching session, the same goal of establishing a safe environment applies to both a student in an English classroom and a patient in a health coaching session because, "once a comfortable, reassuring atmosphere is established, the conference proceeds. How it proceeds depends upon many things: where the student is in the writing process, what her attitude is toward the work, what problem is foremost in her mind at the moment, how far she has moved or been nudged in previous conferences. The teacher must listen and take cues from the student" (p. 87). The same description applies to health coaching, as the health coach must listen and take cues from the patient before proceeding with the conversation.

Health coaching is not therapy but shares similarities with solution-oriented brief therapy (SBT) in psychology. As Weiner-Davis (1995) describes, "the secret to its brevity is that, instead of taking a long introspective journey into the past, SBT helps people to envision a positive future and to identify fail-safe strategies for getting there" (p. 18). In her practice, she found that people often know what they need to do but need someone to ask them the right questions to help them get there. The difference is that psychologists use narratives to help patients understand the past, whereas health coaches use narratives to help patients set goals for the future. In narrative therapy, White and Epston (1990) explain, "stories are full of gaps which persons must fill in order for the story to be performed. These gaps recruit the lived experience and the imagination of persons. With every performance, persons are reauthoring their lives" (p. 13). And in that reauthoring of a story, a sense of gratitude emerges for all that was learned as the journey unfolded. Madigan (2011) draws a parallel between narratives used in literature and narratives told in therapy settings by stating, "if there was to be any interest and/or consistency between narrative therapy theory, practice, and research, the task of any research would be akin to that of the literary critic, insofar as cultural behavior can be treated only as a text that requires interpretation" (p. 140). English teachers encourage students to interpret the texts they read. Similarly, medical practitioners can help patients interpret the stories they tell themselves. The only difference is that the endings of classic works of literature will never change. People's lives, however, are not a book that has already been written; their lives contain unwritten pages waiting to be filled with new stories. Charon (2006) discusses narrative medicine and argues, "by virtue of being trained in the style appropriate to the genre of the chart, doctors learn to suppress their own authorial voice, their own I" (p. 142). Conversely, narrative medicine encourages medical practitioners to see each patient as living a story, not as only a name on a chart and a list of notes. Narratives enable individuals to use the theory of literary analysis to interpret their own lives just as they would interpret a work of classic literature. White (2011) observes, "the ideas of narrative practice are now being used within organizational consultancy, coaching, and work communities" (p. 164). Health coaches listen more than they talk, which opens the door for patients to reflect on their narratives and think how minor differences, like a change in routine for the day, can lead to major behavior change.

Most caregivers find joy and purpose in helping others. As Carter (2015) describes it, "it's the person. It isn't about the prestige or even the helping nature of our work. It's about the meaning we personally find in it and express through it, and the effort and commitment we give to it" (p. 241). Health coaches, physical therapists, and their medical colleagues may only have one chance to make a difference in a patient's life. While the patient must be the one to literally or metaphorically pick up the pen and do the work, it becomes comforting to be surrounded by members of the medical team who will remain a supportive presence. Brown (2015) writes, "when we decide to own our stories and live our truth, we bring our light to the darkness" (p. 75). By learning the stories of others, we continue to write our own.

CONNECTING WRITING PRACTICE TO MEDICINE

If students in an English class have the power to rewrite their narratives, so do patients in a hospital or clinic. Goldberg (1986) discusses that when writing, writers need to trust their first impressions and not censor their thoughts because "to do writing practice means to deal ultimately with your whole life" (p. 3). To deal with your life means to be honest with yourself. As Heard (1995) explains, "in writing, I try to tell the truth" (p. 119). Writers write about an event, but then choose how to interpret their narrative when rereading their stories. An interpretation can range from positive feelings of acknowledging the story happened and moving forward, to negative feelings of remaining stuck in the story. Regardless of the writer's attitude, he or she must own the story and write honestly, even if no one sees the story but the writer. Lamott (1994) elaborates, "you set out to tell a story of some sort, to tell the truth as you feel it, because something is calling you to do so" (p. 31). When writers write the truth, it leads to awareness of the stories they tell themselves. Because each person views a story through the lens of experience, while a story may seem true to the author, a person's subjective interpretation may differ from objective facts.

Seeing thoughts and feelings on paper serves the dual purpose of gaining clarity and releasing feelings. Brown (2015) believes, "writing can be an extremely powerful tool for uncovering the story we're making up" (p. 218). Sometimes we believe a story to be true because we are emotionally connected to it, but writing can help us uncover the facts and strip a story down to its basic essence so we see if the story is really factually true or emotionally what we perceive to be true. For example, the objective truth of a situation is that a patient looks up her symptoms on a website. The subjective truth, filtered through the lens of emotion, is that the patient thinks something is seriously wrong with her, and that is the story she tells herself. When transferring her thoughts from mind to paper, however, the patient realizes there could be other interpretations of the story, such as perhaps the website contained out of date information or she was inaccurate in her self-diagnosis. Rereading the story after writing it may motivate the patient to reach out to her doctor to get an expert's opinion about her symptoms. Cameron (1998) states, "I write to tell myself the truth, the whole truth, and nothing but the truth. I write, not to make art, but to make sense" (p. 109). By trusting our first impressions when writing, we learn the truth of what is in our hearts and minds and what we may need to address before we can move forward with our stories. When people own their stories, they tend to feel happier and more in control of their lives. Brown (2010) believes, "the willingness to tell our stories, feel the pain of others, and stay genuinely connected in this disconnected world is not something we can do halfheartedly" (p. 21). No matter what has happened to us in the past, each day brings a new opportunity to write a new chapter in a life story.

Using the theory of writing can benefit the practice of medicine. In addition to helping clinicians learn their patients' stories, writing can empower patients to take control of their own stories. Statistics and objective data serve as a cornerstone of medical practice. Wheelan (2013) argues, "statistics is more important than ever before because we have more meaningful opportunities to make use of data" (p. 255). Nevertheless, statistics do not capture a patient's entire story. In her medical practice, Rankin (2013) tells her patients that in addition to receiving care from medical providers, they need to do their part in their own healing because "you need radical self-care, not just in your health habits, but in the rest of your life" (p. 163). Writing can encourage patients to process their emotions, help patients set goals for their healing, record symptoms and identify activities that cause pain that can help physical therapists, physicians, or other medical practitioners implement the most effective treatment plan and help people write the next chapters in their healing journeys.

Medical practitioners such as health coaches or physical therapists can use conversation or writing to help people rewrite their stories and create a next new chapter of health and hope. Tindle (2013) reports, "even the brightest bulbs sometimes flicker. Being an optimist doesn't necessarily mean you're the brightest bulb on the Christmas tree. It means you keep your bulb burning brightly and steadily enough to light up your own path – and maybe the path of others – to better physical, mental, and spiritual health" (p. 72). Rankin (2013) adds, "if you're a pessimist prone to unhappiness, don't despair. According to happiness researchers, things like optimism and happiness can be learned, and you can enjoy the physical and mental health benefits as a result" (p. 138). When people own their stories, they tend to feel happier and more in control of their lives. Brown (2012) explains, "we must also remember that our worthiness, that core belief that we are enough, comes only when we live inside our story" (p. 132). Writing and speaking our stories helps us own them.

If the stories we tell ourselves create stress, it becomes time to change them and use writing to craft a new narrative. Enayati (2015) feels perspective can alleviate the stress people experience since "we may have a story of stress that does not serve us, but we have the power to choose our perceptions, to choose different stories, more aligned with reality, that do serve us better. We can choose a narrative that helps reframe the stressors that besiege and overwhelm us as catalysts that become our strengths and guides" (p. 32). The stories people tell about themselves can influence their health, especially if the topic of the narrative is a stressful life. People can often be their own worst critics. Patients in pain may find themselves stuck in their stories, blaming themselves for what caused their current condition, and making themselves feel worse. Brown (2015) explains, "there's growing empirical evidence that not owning and integrating our stories affects not just our emotional health but also our physical well-being" (p. 67). It therefore becomes important to not only own our stories, but demonstrate self-compassion for ourselves and our narratives.

INTERPRETING AND OWNING STORIES

We can't change a story but can change how we interpret it. Too often, people become too busy living a story to truly observe it. Writing allows for the story to be relived and reinterpreted. This changes our perspective of a narrative. When things don't happen the way we want them to happen, it becomes essential to own the story and practice self-compassion. Handler (2013) states, "you've started to accept that your story is part of you" (p. 225). Sometimes people can mentally beat themselves up and relieve the story, thinking what could have, should have, or would have been different if only another outcome occurred. Once again, writing can help. Conner (2008) believes, "writing can't change the story, but it can change how you think about it. It can change how you feel about it. It can change what it means to you" (p. 122). Writing about an experience helps us relive it and see it from a new perspective with the benefit of reflecting on our learning experience. Perhaps meaning can be found in the madness and a new goal can emerge. Beck (2008) reminds people that it is never too late to make changes in life because, "if you feel stuck in your present life, if you feel no enthusiasm for anything, if you think you have no purpose or that you lost that purpose somewhere along the way, I guarantee you are living in a dungeon made of stories – and that none of those limiting stories are true" (p. 53). Through the lens of self-compassion and kindness, we prevent our stories from limiting us as we learn from them, readjust our plans, and keep moving forward.

Some people find strength from spirituality. Hale (2013) believes, "just like a puzzle, it takes time for all of the pieces in your life to come together" (p. 142). It can be disappointing when a story doesn't have the ending you want, but that means it becomes time to write another story and have faith in the new narrative. Arterburn (2011) concurs, "You lack a unifying understanding of why all these unrelated pieces are hanging together in your life. If so, the choice to serve may be the choice that puts it all together for you" (p. 370). People in various health professions often end up where they are because of their own personal experiences. Often people who have experienced physical or emotional pain in their own lives find careers in healing professions because they want to help others through similar experiences. Once we write new chapters in our own stories, we can turn around and help others on their healing journeys. Beck (2012) describes this as, "if you are currently on your highest life purpose, comfortably back from your personal hell and sure of your navigational skills, then for God's sake, begin guiding the rest of us" (pp. 280-281). Regardless of our spiritual beliefs, we can all benefit from being kind to ourselves.

When we write, our words on the page capture who we are. We need to trust our words. Too often, the self-censor wonders what other people will think. Quindlen (2004) advises journalism students, "but still I urge them to write, uncompensated, even if they have no plans to become writers, for one reason only, and that is to know themselves, for now and for later. Their written words are their personal histories, as they have been mine" (p. 233). But it always remains our choice whether or not to share our writing with anyone. All writers have written words that no one ever sees, that are hidden in a storage box or ripped up and destroyed. Because, in those instances, keeping the writing private is what the writer needs. But sharing the writing can also be beneficial. Writing gives others a glimpse into our hopes, dreams, and personalities. It can give medical professionals insights into how we feel so they can design a treatment plan that can help us. It helps friends, acquaintances, or even strangers who are experiencing similar events in their lives to find strength in our stories. In order to share our stories, we need to stop the self-censor, trust ourselves, and just write. As Goldberg (2007) writes, "let your mind first believe you are dedicated, that you sincerely want the truth, are willing to take what comes through. Keep moving the pen. Keep practicing" (p. 4). If we get out of our own way, the stories will unfold on the page. And our words can lead us to the answers we need. Not only can our words lead us to the answers we need, but they can also help us heal both physically and emotionally.

In writing a paragraph such as this one, it becomes easy to try to think of the perfect lead or the exact choice of words to convey an idea. The best method, however, is to just write. The ideas will follow and connect as the words flow. Zimmermann (2002) believes, "writing about the same thing repeatedly from slightly different angles is a healthy part of the process. You create new dimensions. You gain distance and clarity" (p. 27). Thanks to the magic of editing and revision, writers can rearrange words into different combinations, but the original intent of the writing, the heart of the piece, often appears in the very first draft. Some call it intuition, others call it purpose, but we trust the writing to lead us where we need to go. If we wrestle too much with words, the message we really want to say gets lost along the way. What stories do we choose to tell ourselves and how do we interpret them? Begin by capturing the inspirations and first impressions in an initial piece of writing. There is time later for interpretation and revision. Medical professionals can also help patients not only revise their thoughts, such as turning a negative perspective into a positive one.

By rereading previous writing and interpreting the narrative thread that runs through our stories, we rewrite our narratives. Clandinin and Connelly (2000) believe, "as narrative inquirers we work within the space not only with our participants but also with ourselves. Working in this space means that we become visible with our own lived and told stories" (pp. 61-62). This means researchers conducting a narrative inquiry can use the first person "I" when writing about an event and place themselves in the story as well as reporting the stories of others. The combination of actively telling the stories of others while reflecting on their own stories enables researchers to relate to the story themselves and encourage others to relate to the story in the sharing of personal narratives. Connelly and Clandinin (1988) elaborate, "this ongoing reflection-on-action on a daily basis begins to provide insight into personal knowledge when you reread entries over several days and weeks. What connecting threads are apparent over time? Are there events or ideas that recur?" (p. 35). From this perspective, one narrative can be placed in a larger context to show how the puzzle pieces of life fit together. When stories are shared, sometimes they become open to interpretation. Gilbert (2015) recalls a time when a reader misinterpreted the words she wrote and elaborates, "whatever her emotional motive, though, she had embroidered herself into my story and erased my actual narrative in the process. Strange as it seems, I submit that it was her absolute right to do this. I submit that this woman has the God-given right to misread my book however she wants to misread it. Once my book entered her hands, after all, everything about it belonged to her, and never again to me" (p. 125). Works of literature will always have a variety of perspectives and opinions. The same applies to people's personal narratives as well.

THE PROCESS OF WRITING NARRATIVES

Advice that follows is designed for patients interested in using writing while in an inpatient or outpatient setting, as well as for medical professionals interested in knowing more about the healing benefits of learning patients' narratives. So, if you are a patient who has a hospital stay for a surgery, a series of physical therapy treatments for an injury, or questions for your medical provider, consider writing your narrative in a journal. If you are a medical practitioner, consider using writing as a supplement to traditional objective clinical measures. Writing our narratives and sharing them leads to numerous potential opportunities for healing.

To begin, writing doesn't have to be kept in a journal or be a long narrative. Transferring thoughts from the mind to the page becomes the most important thing, especially for hospital patients who may not have a lot of time to write because they are taking pain medication or need to rest. Also keep in mind that no English teacher is going to grade this writing, so it doesn't matter if there are incomplete thoughts, grammar mistakes, or no clear structure to the writing. The important thing is to accept yourself as you are and don't judge yourself or your writing. Cameron (1998) explains, "we can either demand that we write well or we can settle more comfortably into writing down what seems to want to come through us – good, bad, or indifferent" (p. 11). Another key component of writing narratives is to trust the writing process of what Romano (1987) refers to as "percolating, drafting, revising, editing, and publication" (p. 55).

Percolating: Thinking about ideas to possibly put on paper. Goldberg (2000) discusses the value of trusting first impressions as "our ideas and intentions can mask and cover up a story; there is a life force that will declare itself if you let it. Get out of the way" (p. 42). The truest impression of what a person thinks is usually the first impression before the writer has time to second guess thoughts and question the words.

Drafting: Capturing a vision on paper, and continuing to follow initial ideas. Writing can help the writer sort through emotions and discover insights. Health coaching accomplishes the same thing, but often people remember something more when they write it down instead of trying to memorize the information. Goldberg (1990) describes this as, "we are going to write down what we think. Right or wrong doesn't matter. We are standing up and saying who we are" (p. 139). Hence, writing benefits the writer.

Revising: Reframing ideas to allow for new perspective. Goldberg (1986) elaborates, "so while we are busy writing, all the burning life we are eager to express should come out of a place of peace" (p. 167). Writing can create such peace; the writer releases worry and stress onto the page. Rereading the words provides the opportunity to gain a new perspective.

Editing: Cleaning up a piece of writing in preparation to share with an audience. While some writing is for the writer's eyes only, in the medical field sharing writing with a trusted medical professional can bring additional healing benefits. Goldberg (2013) advises writers, "you have to find the entry into what you know inside, the way to bring it out so people will listen" (p. 26). Writing down a list of symptoms and bringing it to the attention of the physical therapist or physician can help the clinician see patterns and obtain additional insights about a patient's health to adjust the treatment plan if necessary.

Publishing: Trusting someone else enough to share the written words. As Goldberg (2007) states, "it's your call, when you write. Trust the urge inside you to lead you to the right choice" (p. 165). If we trust our words, writing will lead us where we need to go. And with the support of a strong medical team, writing becomes an additional resource in the healing process.

Some patients may not want to write but may prefer to draw instead. Heart maps ask the author to draw a heart on a sheet of paper and inside the heart write the names of beloved people, places, and things. Heard (1999) instructs, "if it's something that you really care about then it belongs in your heart map. Only you can decide what should be in your heart map" (p. 109). In heart maps, the common thread is that the designer loves each item in it. Heard (1995) writes, "the seemingly random observations I make or the subjects I choose to write about are like the branches of a tree whose roots reach down to the depths of myself and reveal my obsessions" (pp. 69-70). Heart maps can reveal the designer's values (Figure 1). Health coaches can also use heart maps to ask patients to provide a vision of what they truly value.

MICE

When people align their goals with their vision and values, they become more likely to enact change in their lives. Change begins with four components: motivation, importance, confidence, and expression. I use the acronym MICE to refer to these components. By using both conversational methods such as motivational interviewing and writing strategies such as expressive writing, health coaches can help patients identify the stories they are telling themselves. Rankin (2015a) argues, "it's not life's stressors

Figure 1. Heart map designed by the author

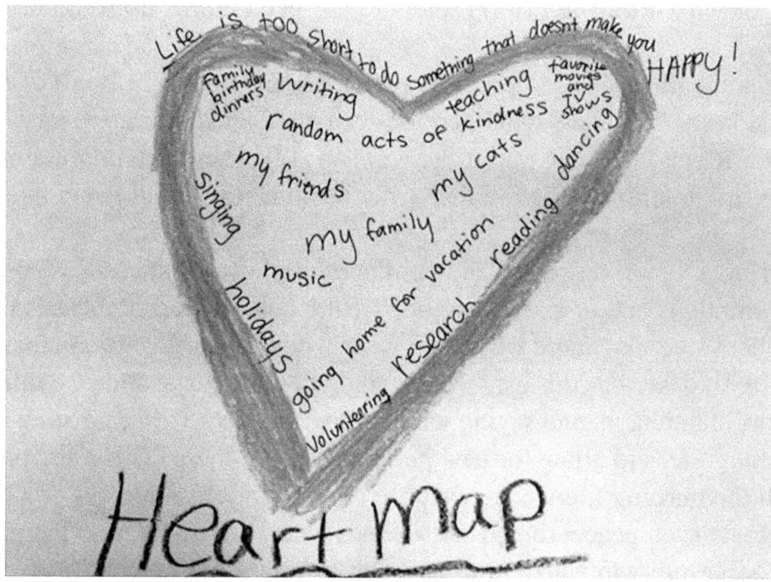

per se that make us sick and miserable. It's the stories we make up about these events, which translate into negative beliefs that activate chronic repetitive stress responses, shorten our life expectancy, and lead us into despair" (pp. 37-38). Conversely, Rankin (2015b) believes, "when the mind heals from loneliness, anxiety, fear, depression, resentment, anger, and negative beliefs about health and life, at least a percentage of the time, the health of the body follows suit" (p. 204). As far as implications for your life, you do not have to be a patient to practice the components of MICE which will help you the next time you set a goal that requires sustained behavior change.

Part I: Motivation

Motivation manifests as two types, extrinsic and intrinsic. In other words, what inspires you to do something? External or internal factors? Does a student write a research paper to earn a specific grade or for the love of the topic? Does a patient complete exercises to earn a compliment from a physical therapist or for a personal desire to heal? One of the foundations of health coaching is the field of motivational interviewing. Caldwell, Gray, and Wolever (2013) explain, "while some professionals are actually using the terms health coaching and MI synonymously, this analysis suggests there are overlapping but also distinct elements to health coaching" (p. 55). Despite the slight delineation, the essence of both motivational interviewing and health coaching is in the conversation. Miller and Rollnick (2013) clarify, "motivational interviewing is a collaborative conversation style for strengthening a person's own motivation and commitment to change" (p. 12). While strengthening motivation and commitment to change is important in all areas of a person's life, it especially enhances the health care field. As Rollnick, Miller, and Butler (2008) explain, "MI works by activating patients' own motivation for change and adherence to treatment" (p. 5). From this perspective of collaboration, a patient sees the health care provider as a partner, not an authority figure giving orders. Miller and Rollnick (2002) elaborate, "we define motivational interviewing as a client-centered, directive method for enhancing intrinsic motivation to change by exploring and resolving ambivalence" (p. 25). Or as Tindle (2013) addresses patients, "You know what you want to do. The big question is, how do you get there? MI helps answer that question. It's a tool that helps the road open up before you. MI shows you how to see the path and gives you a starting push in the right direction" (pp. 117-118). As they begin a treatment plan, this question is on the minds of numerous patients. They want to feel better, but how do they get there? Sometimes the road ahead can seem long and overwhelming. The key is following the road in small, manageable, yet productive steps.

Motivation is frequently connected to the sense of purpose a person has in life. Pink (2009) asks the question, "as you contemplate your purpose, begin with the big question: What's your sentence?" (p. 155). In other words, at the end of your life, if you could only have one sentence on your memorial stating what you accomplished in life, what would that sentence be? It may seem morbid to contemplate your mortality, but we don't always have as much time as we think, and looking backwards from a future point in time can help us figure out how we want to live in the present. My sentence would be: Helped others find their voices and use writing to heal both physically and emotionally while simultaneously living a strong life filled with family and faith.

Pink (2009) explores the concept of motivation by saying people can be divided into two personalities; Type I, motivated by intrinsic motivation, and Type X motivated by extrinsic motivation. He elaborates, "Type I behavior depends on three nutrients: autonomy, mastery, and purpose. Type I behavior is self-directed. It is devoted to becoming better and better at something that matters. And it connects that quest for excellence to a larger purpose" (pp. 78-79). Exploring this concept further, Pink continues, "Type X behavior is fueled more by extrinsic desires than intrinsic ones. It concerns itself less with the inherent satisfaction of an activity and more with the external rewards to which that activity leads" (p. 75). In contrast, "Type I behavior is fueled more by intrinsic desires than extrinsic ones. It concerns itself less with the external rewards to which an activity leads and more with the inherent satisfaction of the activity itself" (p. 75). I hope I would be doing this same writing if it remained on my computer screen and no one ever read these words except me, and that is intrinsic motivation. But I am also motivated by extrinsic motivation, and the knowledge that I have the chance for these same words to reach a larger audience and help people.

Other researchers argue that moving beyond extrinsic motivation to intrinsic motivation can make people happier. Enayati (2015) believes, "this reason to be happy – this essential "why" – is why we must be resolute in our quest to move beyond extrinsic motivations" (p. 135). Since extrinsic motivation involves doing something to either please someone else (getting a compliment from a doctor when complying with a medical treatment plan) or avoiding pain from someone else (getting a lecture from that same doctor when not complying with that medical treatment plan) we can experience stress. Enayati explains, "we volley emotions back and forth all the time, as part of every interaction – however brief or extended – that we have with one another. We can "catch" other people's stress, all with amazing speed" (p. 154). Visit a college campus around the time of midterms or finals, and witness students collectively getting stressed because while they are sharing the same community experience, that community experience is one of stress. Carter (2015) believes, "we also need intrinsic motivation, or passion – and the space to pursue our passions" (p. 183). This intrinsic motivation means finding the things that bring joy in life and provide both passion and purpose, such as signing up for a dance class for the pure joy of it or following a medical treatment plan for the desire to lead a healthier life regardless of what the doctor thinks. And pursuing passions can lead to improved health. As Carter explains, "when we are happy, we are more creative and motivated, more productive and skilled socially because blood flows freely to our pre-frontal cortex, allowing us to make better decisions than we would if we relied on the more primitive, instinctive regions of our brain that are activated when we are under stress" (p. 20). So while there are times in life where we may need extrinsic motivation from others to help us get through a situation, it also becomes essential to find the internal motivation that drives us to succeed and makes us happy.

Finding purpose and self-motivation can lead to growth. Dweck (2006) describes students with the growth mindset as "even if they thought the textbook was boring or the instructor was a stiff, they didn't let their motivation evaporate. That just made it all the more important to motivate themselves" (p. 61). The goal of learning eclipsed the potential barriers of a boring textbook or a passionless instructor. Of course, in an ideal education world, students would not have to deal with such obstacles. Every classroom would be like the one Johnson (1998) describes for teachers as, "you can harness the power of words to motivate and inspire your students by displaying inspirational quotations in your classroom where students will see them every day. Some teachers ask their students to discuss the quotations or write responses to them in their journals. Others let them speak for themselves. Whether you discuss them or not, your students will read them and think about them – although they may never admit that they do" (p. 141). The power of words is not limited to classrooms with desks. The power of words can be used with patients, clients, students, friends, family, colleagues, and anyone else we encounter in the classroom of life. By sharing words and stories, we support each other. We rely on our own intrinsic motivation but know where to find positive extrinsic motivation when needed. Sandberg (2013) states, "sharing emotions builds deeper relationships. Motivation comes from working on things we care about. It also comes from working with people we care about" (p. 88). There is a place for both extrinsic motivation and intrinsic motivation to coexist beautifully in supportive environments where people care about each other and encourage each other to achieve positive change.

Part II: Importance

Are we willing to change? The answer to that question is how important change is to a person. Miller and Rollnick (2002) explain, "one factor is the extent to which the person wants, desires, or wills change. We tend to talk about this dimension as the perceived importance of a particular change" (p. 10). We all know there are things we probably should do. But the importance of each thing to us determines if we make a change.

Connected to importance is another word that starts with I, intuition. People often have an intuitive sense of what is truly important to them. Individuals who have a strong sense of intuition can appear to others as having a psychic sixth sense of what to do and when to do it. While intuition is unique to each person and highly individualized, a significant amount of theory exists to explain the practice of intuition. Dimitrius (1998) provides the description, "what we call intuition is nearly always the surfacing of a submerged memory, a barely noticed event, or some combination of the two" (p. 216). Perhaps we have experienced something similar in the past, so we have a feeling of how we want to act in the present, even if we can't explain the feeling. Or maybe we notice something out of the corner of the eye that we know is significant information before the brain has the opportunity to process it. Dimitrius advises, "since your intuition depends on the quality and quantity of your information, your first step is clear: Improve the database" (p. 218). The more experiences people have, the more they are able to synthesize the experiences and file the information away in the database to help in the future. Starratt (1993) states, "professionals develop intuitions of what works over years of experience" (p. 39). What seems like magic or everything falling into a place is a result of a person collecting experiences and calling up those experiences when they are most needed to appear in a moment of intuitive insight.

As an FBI security expert, DeBecker (1997) tells people that intuition helps keep them safe and always provides helpful information. He explains, "intuition is always learning, and though it may occasionally send a signal that turns out to be less than urgent, everything it communicates to you is meaningful" (p. 70). So if something catches our attention, it is important to pay attention to it, because our intuition is trying to communicate something to us. DeBecker provides the valuable advice, "listen to your intuition" (p. 74).

Deep inside, we know the answers for what we truly feel is important in our lives. The key is to stop and listen. Baty (2003) concurs, "you hear it time and time again: Listen to your gut instinct, or intuition. Fact is, it works" (p. 3). Why does it work? Baty answers, "intuition just means acknowledging what you already know inside" (p. 4). If we ask ourselves the questions and trust our intuitive insights, we frequently get the answers right. But since what is important to one person may not be important to another, we can find our intuitive voices drowned out by the opinions of others or find ourselves not trusting someone else's intuition. DeBecker (1997) emphasizes the importance of listening without judgement because, "when free of judgment, we inherently respect the intuition of others" (p. 25). For example, as a clinician, if your patient has an intuitive sense that something is wrong even without specific evidence to prove it, you are more likely to ask follow up questions and find the source of the intuitive insight than if you have already judged your patient as a hypochondriac who can't provide facts for the feeling that there is a problem. DeBecker clarifies, "intuition is a gift we all have, whereas retention of knowledge is a skill" (p. 28). In fact, sometimes too much knowledge can cause people to question their intuition and ask for as many opinions as possible instead of trusting their own feelings. DeBecker describes this as, "even when intuition speaks in the clearest terms, even when the message gets through, we may still seek an outside opinion before we'll listen to ourselves" (p. 31). In medicine, it's always best to consult a medical professional if you have an intuitive sense something is wrong with your health. But if in your personal life, if you sense someone sinister behind you, listen to your intuition and keep yourself safe.

While security experts focus on the value of intuition to keep you safe, intuition can also help you assess what is important to achieve your goals in life. Beck (2001) believes, "your intuition has a more refined understanding of your right life than any other part of your consciousness" (p. 221). By listening to our intuition, we become aware of what we find important and what we value. If we are asked to do something we don't find important, intuition helps delineate whether we need to do that thing anyway to reach a goal or achieve a dream, or whether we think that thing is unimportant because it has no benefit. Beck describes this feeling as, "the more you listen to your intuition, the more it will change your life; and the more bravely you set forth into the territory of change, the more you'll come to rely on it" (p. 239). For example, maybe there is no logical reason for you to change careers, but your intuition tells you that a career change is part of your life's purpose. Being in a career that feels part of your highest purpose in life is something you value and find important, so you are more likely to achieve success if you listen to your intuition and follow the path that makes you happy instead of listening to anyone who doubts your insight. You know yourself better than anyone else.

How does intuition relate to the field of medicine? Groopman (2007) explains, "clinical intuition is a complex sense that becomes refined over years and years of practice, of listening to literally thousands of patients' stories, examining thousands of people, and most important, remembering when you were wrong" (p. 20). So for medical professionals, their clinical intuition becomes refined by learning from experiences and listening to patients. Groopman cautions against relying too heavily on intuition, because in the medical world, feelings about a diagnosis must often be supported with factual data. However, medical professionals place value on both their own and patients' intuition. Rankin (2015a) explains that people often feel fear in life and "although false fear can illuminate areas in your life that need your attention, healthy decisions that guide appropriate behavior never arise from false fear; they arise from intuition and integrity" (p. 51). Inherently, people know what they need to do to make healthy decisions and take care of themselves. And that sense of purpose helps them feel the importance of their actions. Rankin discovered, "the people I interviewed who had cultivated and learned to trust their intuition felt like they were always being guided, and they were supported by this guidance more than they were controlled by their fears" (pp. 142-143). Rankin admits that the busy pace of a doctor's schedule doesn't allow as much time with patients as doctors would like. But she learned that if she partnered with her patients and took the time to listen to their stories, it helped her make a diagnosis and adjust her treatment plan. Rankin (2015b) learned, "my new patient intake form was 12 pages long, and what these questions revealed about my patients' lives shocked me. When combined with the intuitive information I sometimes received from patients, I started to get a sense of the link between their physical health and their emotional health" (p. 120). Her story illustrates how a medical professional trusting her own clinical intuition and the intuition of her patients in the stories they shared with her helped patients heal.

Part III: Confidence

Do we feel we have the ability to change? The answer to that question is how confident a person feels about making a change. Miller and Rollnick (2002) explain, "sometimes a person feels willing but not able to change" (p. 11). We may feel that making a change is important, but we don't have the confidence we can make the change.

Connected to confidence is another word that starts with C, compassion. Connected to confidence is compassion, specifically the self-compassion we must have with ourselves when things don't go as planned. Life happens to all of us, and even the best organized plans can encounter unexpected barriers and obstacles. Often people can be their own worst critics, and when something doesn't happen the way we want it to happen, it becomes easy to give up and focus on self-blame instead of searching for methods to overcome the obstacles and other pathways to achieve the goal. Germer (2009) defines, "self-compassion is simply giving the same kindness to ourselves that we would give to others" (pp. 33-34). Since we cannot change the past, all we can do is move forward and show ourselves the same kindness that we demonstrate for others. Neff (2011) believes something meaningful can happen from a less than perfect experience and states, "by giving ourselves unconditional kindness and comfort while embracing the human experience, difficult as it is, we avoid destructive patterns of fear, negativity, and isolation. At the same time, self-compassion fosters positive mind-states such as happiness and optimism" (pp. 12-13). No one is immune from negative events, both the minor annoyances of daily life as well as the major life changing catastrophes, but keeping a positive attitude and demonstrating the kindness to ourselves that we would demonstrate to others can diminish the severity of an event's impact.

Germer (2009) explains the value of practicing self-compassion because, "research on self-compassion is demonstrating that it softens the impact of negative events in our lives. Self-compassionate people are more likely to recognize when their efforts turn out badly and to take responsibility for their part" (p. 98). Neff (2011) adds, "by giving ourselves unconditional kindness and comfort while embracing the human experience, difficult as it is, we avoid destructive patterns of fear, negativity, and isolation. At the same time, self-compassion fosters positive mind-states such as happiness and optimism. The nurturing quality of self-compassion allows us to flourish, to appreciate the beauty and richness of life, even in hard times. When we soothe our agitated minds with self-compassion, we're better able to notice what's right as well as what's wrong, so that we can orient ourselves toward that which gives us joy" (pp. 12-13). Self-compassion is not the same thing as self-confidence, but self-compassion can contribute to self-confidence. If a person practices self-compassion and sees that the hard times in life can be obstacles to overcome rather than insurmountable barriers, he or she can get creative in problem solving and build confidence in the process as each problem is solved. Once someone achieves or overcomes something, it becomes possible to draw on that memory of confidence to know something similar that was achieved in the past can be achieved in the future.

It can be easy to be faced with fear and lack of confidence when encountering a new situation. Cameron (2002) calls these moments creative U-turns; just like a car may need to make a U-turn when going the wrong direction on the road, people may have to make U-turns when going the wrong direction in life. Cameron encourages, "have compassion. Creative U-turns are always born from fear – fear of success or fear of failure. It doesn't really matter which. The net result is the same" (p. 157). The net result is that whatever caused the U-turn, it led to the discovery of a new way to overcome an obstacle along with the confidence of finding a solution to a problem.

Practicing compassion shows us we are not alone. When we demonstrate compassion for others and ourselves, we find a support system of people to walk with us on our journey. Brown (2012) believes, "self-compassion is key because when we're able to be gentle with ourselves in the midst of shame, we're more likely to reach out, connect, and experience empathy" (p. 75). When people accept us and our stories, we experience the confidence that we are okay as we are and that we do not need to be anyone other than ourselves. Our confidence decreases when we feel shame at what we have done or how we have acted. By finding the courage to share our stories and be compassionate with ourselves, we own our story and while we cannot rewrite what has already happened, we can find the confidence to pick up a pen and write a new ending. Brown (2012) describes this story sharing process as, "whether we're on the purging end or the receiving end of this experience, self-compassion is critical. We have to give ourselves a break when we share too much too soon, and we have to practice self-kindness when we feel like we weren't able to hold space for someone who hit us with the floodlight" (p. 161). When we find the right person with whom to share our story, we have the confidence that we will not be judged and that our words will be heard. By demonstrating compassion, people earn the right to hear our stories. Goldberg (2013) advises writers, "always have tremendous kindness for yourself. You'll get a lot more writing done" (p. 21). The same advice applies to all parts of life; demonstrating self-compassion means a lot less time thinking about regrets and a lot more time getting things accomplished.

How does compassion relate to the field of medicine? Tindle (2013) reports that self-compassion "has been linked to better self-care and healthier behaviors" (p. 77). How does this happen? Carter (2015) argues, "self-compassion – being warm and supportive toward ourselves, and actively soothing ourselves – has many benefits over self-criticism. It leads to less anxiety and depression, and greater piece of mind" (p. 219). And since emotional health is linked to physical health, if emotionally we are more compassionate to ourselves, physically we feel less tense from anxiety and stress. Self-compassion can provide the insight that a one day divergence need not derail an entire nutrition or exercise plan. Tindle (2013) reminds us, "self-compassion and the deep sense of self-worth that it fosters are at the very foundation of our physical and mental health" (p. 182). Because when people believe they have value, that confidence is reflected in their health.

Part IV: Expression

Are we ready to change? The answer to that question is the expression of where change falls on a person's priority list. Miller and Rollnick (2002) explain, "One can be willing and able to change, but not ready to do so" (p. 11). We may feel making a change is important and we may have the confidence to make the change, but we are not ready to take action.

Expression is articulating a plan for what is needed to be done in order to enact change. It means stating one's goals and making a commitment to the accountability of achieving them. This is often difficult for people, because it is one thing to say you will do something, but another thing to actually do it. Expression, however, can be fun because it allows for the exploration of possibilities. It puts experiences into words. This is often best done in writing. Goldberg (2016) believes, "you don't have to change a thing. Writing doesn't ask you to be any different from who you are right now" (p. 161). When writing, you are who you are. Looking at a piece of paper and seeing a plan for achieving goals in writing is a method of making the plan seem like a series of concrete steps to focus on and be accountable for instead of a series of ideas swirling around in one's head. Like a camera lens focusing on a subject, everything suddenly zooms into possibility. Seeing the words on the page allows an issue to become present and eliminate the maybe someday attitude people have when thinking of specific steps needed to put a dream into reality.

People can certainly experience success when speaking their goals or drawing pictures of them; however, expressive writing possesses power. Romano (2000) provides a description of expressive writing as, "we use expressive writing when we are trying to explain or render something for the first time, when we're seeking to recover information, make connections, generate ideas. Expressive writing is exploratory and new and focused on meaning" (p. 137). As all writers know, rarely is a first draft perfect. Elaborating on ideas is when the process of revision happens. Nevertheless, by capturing our words on paper, we not only share our story of what happened to us, but also explore what we want to happen next. Pennebaker and Evans (2014) explain, "expressive writing (EW) – can positively affect people's sleeping habits, work efficiency, and their connection to others. Indeed, when we put traumatic experiences into words, we tend to be less concerned with the emotional events that have been weighing us down" (pp. 3-4). Brown (2015) concurs that Pennebaker's work with writing as healing is "some of the most important and fascinating research I've seen on the power of expressive writing in the healing process" (p. 87). While Pennebaker and Evans have studied the positive effects of people writing about traumatic experiences, writing does not always have to be negative and people always have the power to rewrite their narratives. Gruwell (1999) named the students in her English class The Freedom Writers and helped them use writing to "create a sense of community and an outlet for expression" (p. 275). That outlet for expression enabled them to share their past experiences as well as future dreams and built a strong class community where they shared their stories with both themselves and each other to enact change in their lives and the lives of their community.

Indeed, while certain practitioners have always used the sharing of stories in the medical field, it is only recently becoming more of a mainstream practice. Therefore, the most interesting discussion of the value of expression comes from the field of writing. With healing, just as in writing, it becomes essential to trust the process. According to Goldberg (1986) "we must continue to open and trust in our own voice and process" (p. 12). She provides the encouragement, "understanding this process cultivates patience and produces less anxiety" (p. 15). Writers know that revision is always possible; the first few pages of a draft might not end up being used, but may provide an idea that can later be implemented. The same can apply when designing a plan for achieving a goal. The initial plan may not end up being used, but may provide an idea that can later be implemented. Sharp (2000) describes this writing process when telling the story of an author who "one day after rereading the first four hundred pages, she decided that the novel really began on page 401. She threw out the first four hundred pages, and the novel hit its stride. The author realized that she had to have written those first four hundred pages in order to have reached page 401" (p. 19). Similarly, a physical therapy patient may develop an initial plan of completing exercises at home in the evening before falling asleep. However, the competing priority of the need for sleep at the end of the day wins and that plan doesn't work. The patient uses the idea that it makes sense to complete exercises during an uninterrupted time instead of trying to fit exercises in during the day and adjusts the plan to complete exercises first thing in the morning. The initial draft didn't work, but in the revision, the essence of the idea remains to enable the enactment of change. Lamott (1994) agrees, "there may be something in the very last line of the very last paragraph on page six that you just love, that is so beautiful or wild that you now know what you're supposed to be writing about, more or less, or in what direction you might go – but there was no way to get to this without getting through the first five and a half pages" (p. 23). Capturing what Lamott refers to as the (expletive deleted) first draft of a piece leads to the beginning of idea exploration. The exploration of the initial draft may lead the writer to discover that he or she is believes a version of the story that is not entirely true. A simple example of this are physical therapy patients who tell themselves the story that they have no time to complete their at home exercise plans. Using expressive writing and capturing this idea on paper may reveal that while the no time argument may be believed to be true, there may in reality be moments of time when the exercises can be completed. Brown (2015) advises that when writing, "don't hold back. There is no rising strong without a true accounting of the stories we're making up" (p. 92). And when we hold ourselves accountable for the stories we're making up that we may emotionally believe to be true but that factually may not be true, we do become emotionally strong so we can become physically strong in our health as well.

Writing also allows the writer to turn negative emotions into positive ones. As Cameron (1998) observes, "we are so skilled in the art of negative imagination, we are so adroit at the art of writing out of anxiety, what might our writing and our world look like if we allowed ourselves to inhabit our positive imagination?" (pp. 125-126). And what might our world look like if we realized there is more than one road that can lead to our destination? Reframing the negative answer of not wanting to do something into the positive question of how that same thing can be made a priority will lead to an increased commitment to change. Goals are complex and require a series of detailed steps to accomplish. But expressing what needs to be done to make a goal a priority and accomplish it now and not later can cause a person to enact change in his or her life. Menasche (2013) asked his students to write a list of their priorities and "they were revealing themselves to their peers and trusting their classmates not to judge them – but that simple assignment gave the students flashes of insight into themselves, and it helped them to identify and empathize with each other. What had begun as an exercise in literature had evolved into a life lesson" (p. 71). In writing priority lists, students not only expressed their goals and values, but also learned how their priorities influenced their actions.

I AM

Writing helps us discover who we are. Our stories constantly evolve. Harrison (2002) writes, "think of the narrative structure as a mighty river whose tributaries branch forth in a variety of presentations" (p. 84). Writing captures narratives which constitute the flowing river of our lives and freezes moments in time like a beautiful photograph. Writing provides clarity and brings order to the chaos of life. Hale (2015) offers the advice, "I urge you to save some room for the unexpected. Stay open to plot twists, to edits, to rewrites, to uncertainty" (p. 194). Writing helps students in a classroom, patients in a hospital, and readers of this narrative who want to pick up a pen and write a new chapter. I conclude with a poem which reflects who I am at the time I write these words. This is who I am at this moment in time. This is my story. I encourage you to write yours.

I am an English teacher who encourages students to write in journals and interpret texts
I am a health coach who helps patients connect their vision and values to their goals
I am a Stephen Minister, a lay Christian caregiver at my church
I am also a devoted member of my family who wants to live her life purpose
Whenever I have the opportunity to help someone, I live my purpose
The seemingly divergent roles in my life converge to help me use writing as healing
But this prose poem won't help anyone if it remains in my journal
Time to share my story with others and inspire them to write their own stories

ACKNOWLEDGMENT

The author wishes to thank Ryan Urenda, DPT, and Eric Wanner, DPT. During their previous research and writing, Dr. Wanner's ideas inspired the author to further investigate the value of using narratives with physical therapy patients and advocate that every patient has a story. Once she wrote the words, Dr. Urenda's editing and advice assisted the author, an English professor, on the correct usage and discussion of physical therapy terminology. Both Dr. Urenda and Dr. Wanner are outstanding physical therapists who make a difference in the lives of the patients treated at their clinics.

REFERENCES

Adams, K. (1990). *Journal to the Self.* New York, NY: Warner Books.

Alexander, E. (2012). *Proof of Heaven.* New York, NY: Simon and Schuster.

Alexander, E. (2014). *The map of Heaven.* New York, NY: Simon and Schuster.

Anderson, C. M., & MacCurdy, M. M. (2000). Introduction. In C. M. Anderson & M. M. MacCurdy (Eds.), *Writing and healing* (pp. 1–22). Urbana, IL: National Council of Teachers of English.

Arterburn, S. (2011). *Healing is a choice.* Nashville, TN: Thomas Nelson.

Austen, J. (2005). *Pride and prejudice*. New York, NY: Penguin. (Original work published 1813). doi:10.5117/9781904633013

Baty, K. (2003). *A girl's gotta do what a girl's gotta do*. New York, NY: Rodale.

Beck, M. (2001). *Finding your own North Star*. New York, NY: Three Rivers Press.

Beck, M. (2008). *Steering by starlight*. New York, NY: Rodale.

Beck, M. (2012). *Finding your way in a wild new world*. New York, NY: Free Press.

Bird, J. L. (Ed.). (2015). *Innovative collaborative practice and reflection in patient education*. Hershey, PA: Information Science Reference. doi:10.4018/978-1-4666-7524-7

Bird, J. L., Wanner, E. T., Urenda, R., & Perry, R. (2015). Multigenre medicine. In J. L. Bird (Ed.), *Innovative collaborative practice and reflection in patient education* (pp. 1–19). Hershey, PA: Information Science Reference.

Brown, B. (2010). *The gifts of imperfection*. Center City, MN: Hazelden.

Brown, B. (2012). *Daring greatly*. New York, NY: Gotham Books.

Brown, B. (2015). *Rising strong*. New York, NY: Spiegel & Grau.

Caldwell, K., Gray, J., & Wolever, R.Q. (2013). The process of patient empowerment in integrative health coaching: how does it happen? *Global advances in health and medicine, 2*(3), 48-57.

Cameron, J. (1998). *The right to write*. New York: Tarcher/Putnam.

Cameron, J. (2002). *The artist's way* (2nd ed.). New York, NY: Tarcher/Putnam.

Carter, C. (2015). *The sweet spot*. New York, NY: Ballantine.

Charon, R. (2006). *Narrative medicine: honoring the stories of illness*. New York, NY: Oxford University Press.

Chopin, K. (1981). *The awakening*. New York, NY: Bantam. (Original work published 1899).

Clandinin, D. J., & Connelly, F. M. (2000). *Narrative inquiry*. San Francisco, CA: Jossey-Bass.

Connelly, F. M., & Clandinin, D. J. (1988). *Teachers as curriculum planners*. New York, NY: Teachers College.

Conner, J. (2008). *Writing down your soul*. San Francisco, CA: Conari.

DeBecker, G. (1997). *The gift of fear*. Boston, MA: Little, Brown and Company.

Dimitrius, J. (1998). *Reading people*. New York, NY: Ballantine.

DuMaurier, D. (1938). Rebecca. New York, NY: Avon.

Dweck, C. (2006). *Mindset*. New York, NY: Ballantine.

Enayati, A. (2015). *Seeking serenity*. New York, NY: New American Library.

Fitzgerald, F. S. (1925). *The great Gatsby*. New York, NY: Scribner.

Germer, C. K. (2009). *The Mindful path to self-compassion*. New York, NY: Guilford.

Gilbert, E. (2015). *Big magic: creative living beyond fear*. New York, NY: Riverhead Books.

Goldberg, N. (1986). *Writing down the bones*. Boston, MA: Shambhala.

Goldberg, N. (1990). *Wild mind*. New York, NY: Bantam.

Goldberg, N. (2000). *Thunder and lightning*. New York, NY: Bantam.

Goldberg, N. (2007). *Old friend from far away*. New York, NY: Free Press.

Goldberg, N. (2013). *The true secret of writing*. New York, NY: Atria.

Goldberg, N. (2016). *The great spring*. Boulder, CO: Shambhala.

Groopman, J. (2007). *How doctors think*. New York, NY: Mariner Books.

Gruwell, E. (2007). Teach with your heart. New York, NY: Broadway.

Gruwell, E., & the The Freedom Writers. (1999). The Freedom Writers diary. New York, NY: Broadway.

Hale, M. (2013). *The single woman*. Nashville, TN: Thomas Nelson.

Hale, M. (2015). *Beautiful uncertainty*. Nashville, TN: Thomas Nelson.

Handler, J. (2013). *Braving the fire*. New York, NY: St. Martin's Griffin.

Harrison, M. D. (2002). *Narrative based evaluation*. New York, NY: Peter Lang Publishing.

Haugk, K. C. (2000). *When and how to use mental health resources*. St. Louis, MO: Stephen Ministries.

Heard, G. (1995). *Writing toward home*. Portsmouth, NH: Heinemann.

Heard, G. (1999). *Awakening the heart*. Portsmouth, NH: Heinemann.

Helldorfer, M., & Moss, T. (2007). *Healing with heart*. Orinda, CA: Moss Communications.

Ibsen, H. (1958). A doll's house. In *Four great plays*. New York, NY: Bantam. (Original work published 1879)

Johnson, L. (1998). *Two parts textbook, one part love*. New York, NY: Hyperion.

Lamott, A. (1994). *Bird by bird*. New York: Anchor Books.

Madigan, S. (2011). *Narrative therapy*. Washington, DC: American Psychological Association.

Menasche, D. (2013). *The priority list*. New York, NY: Touchstone.

Michele, L. (2015). *You first: journal your way to your best life*. New York, NY: Crown Archetype.

Miller, W. R., & Rollnick, S. (2002). *Motivational interviewing* (2nd ed.). New York, NY: The Guilford Press.

Miller, W. R., & Rollnick, S. (2013). *Motivational interviewing* (3rd ed.). New York, NY: The Guilford Press.

Neff, K. (2011). *Self compassion: the proven power of being kind to yourself.* New York, NY: Harper-Collins.

O'Brien, T. (1990). *The things they carried.* New York, NY: Broadway Books.

Pennebaker, J. W. (1997). *Opening up: the healing power of expressing emotions.* New York, NY: The Guilford Press.

Pennebaker, J. W., & Evans, J. F. (2014). *Expressive writing: words that heal.* Enumclaw, WA: Idyll Arbor.

Pink, D. (2009). *Drive.* New York, NY: Riverhead Books.

Quindlen, A. (2004). *Loud and clear.* New York, NY: Ballentine Books.

Rankin, L. (2013). *Mind over medicine.* Carlsbad, CA: Hay House.

Rankin, L. (2015a). *The fear cure.* Carlsbad, CA: Hay House.

Rankin, L. (2015b). *The anatomy of a calling.* New York, NY: Rodale.

Rollnick, S., Miller, W. R., & Butler, C. C. (2008). *Motivational interviewing in health care: helping patients change behavior.* New York, NY: The Guilford Press.

Romano, T. (1987). *Clearing the way.* Portsmouth, NH: Heinemann.

Romano, T. (1995). *Writing with passion.* Portsmouth, NH: Heinemann.

Romano, T. (2000). *Blending genre, altering style.* Portsmouth, NH: Heinemann.

Romano, T. (2004). *Crafting authentic voice.* Portsmouth, NH: Heinemann.

Romano, T. (2008). *Zigzag.* Portsmouth, NH: Heinemann.

Romano, T. (2013). *Fearless writing.* Portsmouth, NH: Heinemann.

Rostand, E. (1950). *Cyrano de Bergerac.* New York, NY: Bantam. (Original work published 1898).

Rzeznik, J. (1998). Iris [Recorded by Goo Goo Dolls]. On City of angels soundtrack [CD]. Burbank, CA: Warner Brothers.

Sandberg, S. (2013). *Lean in.* New York, NY: Alfred A. Knopf.

Sharp, C. (2000). *A writer's workshop.* New York: St. Martin's Press.

Smith, L.L., Lake, N.H., Simmons, L.A., Perlman, A., Wroth, S., & Wolever, R.Q. (2013). Integrative health coach training: a model for shifting the paradigm toward patient-centricity and meeting new national prevention goals. *Global advances in health and medicine, 2*(3), 66-74.

Starratt, R. J. (1993). *The drama of leadership.* London, England: The Falmer Press.

Tindle, H. (2013). *Up: How positive outlook can transform our health and aging.* New York, NY: Hudson Street Press.

Weiner-Davis, M. (1995). *Fire your shrink.* New York, NY: Simon & Schuster.

Wharton, E. (1920). *The age of innocence.* New York, NY: Collier.

Wheelan, C. (2013). *Naked statistics.* New York, NY: W.W. Norton.

White, C. (2011). Epilogue: continuing conversations. In M. White (Ed.), *Narrative practice* (pp. 157–179). New York, NY: W.W. Norton & Company.

White, M., & Epston, D. (1990). *Narrative means to therapeutic ends.* New York, NY: W.W. Norton & Company.

Zimmermann, S. (2002). *Writing to heal the soul.* New York, NY: Three Rivers Press.

KEY TERMS AND DEFINITIONS

Confidence: The degree to which a person believes he or she is able to make a change in behavior.

Expression of Priorities: Whether or not a person feels ready to make a change in behavior by making it a priority.

Expressive Writing: Writing that is exploratory and focuses on meaning. It is the act of putting words to experiences.

Importance: The degree to which a person feels willing to make a change in behavior.

MICE: An acronym for motivation, importance, confidence, and expression.

Motivation: Motivation can be extrinsic or intrinsic. Extrinsic motivation relies on external factors, such as rewards or punishment, to motivate others to accomplish goals. Intrinsic motivation relies on internal drive when a person is self-motivated to accomplish goals.

Motivational Interviewing: A client-centered method of using reflective statements and open ended questions to enhance intrinsic motivation for change.

Self-Compassion: The act of demonstrating the same kindness toward oneself that one would demonstrate for others.

Chapter 2
Synergism through Therapeutic Visual Arts

Ashley Hartman
Florida State University, USA

Susannah Brown
Florida Atlantic University, USA

ABSTRACT

Oncology patients experience significant psychological distress in addition to physical symptoms associated with illness. Overwhelming emotions, negative moods, and other forms of psychological stressors are present due to uncertain future. Shock experienced after receiving diagnosis, distress associated with medical decision-making, lack of control over one's environment, and fears related to changes in lifestyle within the course of the illness are a few examples of the challenges faced by patients. Art therapy is a therapeutic treatment modality that accommodates the opportunity for patients to make autonomous decisions, organize and structure these choices, and obtain a sense of control over personal artwork as well as the therapeutic experience. In this paper, the authors explore the literature surrounding the impact of perceived control on psychological distress in oncology patients, the connection between decision-making and perceived control, and the potential for art therapy to increase perceived control through decision-making opportunities for oncology patients.

SYNERGISM THROUGH THERAPEUTIC VISUAL ARTS

Art therapists and art educators are aware of the relationship between art and development, particularly through creativity, self-expression, self-awareness, and personal discovery. The mind/body connection is intimately recognized through a holistic perspective in many fields. Gestalt theoretical orientations within art therapy stress how individuals innately seek health and possess the ability to self-regulate (Mann, 2010). Visual art can become a vehicle to proceed along a patient's healthcare journey. *Art serves a personal development and a path to well-being* (Brown, 2013, p.1). Creative expression in a variety of arts forms often leads to a discovery of new ideas. Art as a part of life integrates the whole self (affective, cognitive and physical). Self-expression and communication of ideas motivates a person's innate

DOI: 10.4018/978-1-5225-0640-9.ch002

desire to make something *special* (Dissanayake, 1992, p. 42). In this chapter, the authors explore the literature surrounding the impact of perceived control on psychological distress in oncology patients, the connection between decision-making and perceived control, and the potential for art therapy to increase perceived control through decision-making opportunities for oncology patients.

DISCUSSION

Perceived Control and Psychological Distress

Perceived control affects patients' healthcare attitudes that include personal decision-making concerning treatment and patient/physician experiences. Kirkland (1996) claimed that cancer diagnoses disrupted patient perceptions of control and autonomy. Malchoidi (1999) stated that patients with illness frequently experienced loss of control, which resulted in anxiety, depression, and altered body image. Health locus of control (HLOC) attributions are associated with an individual's perceived control over physical illnesses; accounts for the perception of which individuals consistently attribute their own health as a result of the environment or individual control (Hillen et al., 2014).

Health locus of control influenced cancer patients' trust in oncologists, attitude toward illness, expectations toward the future, and coping mechanisms (Hodges & Winstanley, 2012; Hillen et al., 2014). Individuals who perceived events as outside of their own control experienced greater psychological distress in the face of stressful events versus individuals who felt in control of their lives (Andrykowski & Brady, 1994).

Medical Decision-Making and Psychological Distress

Cancer patients are faced with various decisions that result in revisiting their challenges and making additional decisions: choice of medical practitioners, treatment choices, with whom to share information, reaction to diagnosis, potential changes in lifestyle, and from whom to receive support (Halkett et al., 2007). These overwhelming emotions interfere with medical decision-making process (Czmanski-Cohen, 2012). A patient often feels rushed when making decisions regarding treatment and needs time to accept the diagnosis. Fear of unpredictable and undesirable results, wavering and doubting individual values, and anxiety due to preoccupation with making decisions contributed to this psychological distress (Czmanski-Cohen, 2012). Moreover, coping with family members' reactions about illness was overwhelming for patients (Halkett et al., 2007) in addition to coping with their own emotional responses.

Decision-Making and Perceived Control

Recently legislation has been enacted that requires written consent by the patient before a treatment protocol begins (Krumholz, 2010). This ensures that the patient is an important part of the decision-making and thus, creating a process of joint decision-making between the patient and the medical practitioner (Czmanski-Cohen, 2012). The study by Pieterse, Baas-Thijssen, Marijnen, and Stiggelbout (2008) indicated that clinicians and patients preferred making shared decisions regarding oncology care; researchers (Sepucha, Belkora, Mutchnick, & Esserman, 2002; Step, Rose, Albert, Cheruvu, & Siminoff, 2009) confirmed that participation in shared decision-making produced less feelings of regret post-treatment (as cited in Czmanski-Cohen, 2012).

Ernst et al. (2013) confirmed the trend for cancer patients to demonstrate satisfaction with shared decision-making (SDM) regarding their illness. The SDM model was investigated in medical decision-making regarding the satisfaction with patient decisions in response to working with medical providers. The aim of the SDM model was to collaboratively and interactively engage patients and health care professionals in a joint decision-making process fostering trust and honesty in a positive and constructive working relationship. Components of the SDM model included acknowledging and respecting patient values and preferences, providing multiple choices for patients to choose from, outlining the process of decision-making in relationship to the illness and treatment plan, and respecting patient decisions. This process was created so that patients were able to feel a sense of control over the treatment options that they receive (Glass et al., 2012).

Ernst et al. (2013) claimed patients cope with loss of control over decision-making by allowing medical professionals to make decisions and valuing the patient-physician relationship beyond the traditional medical pact. Working together in an honest, open relationship was determined to be the best method because it combined the medical professional's expertise and the patient's values and beliefs. Patients frequently regained a sense of control and feelings of safety in an emotionally supportive patient-physician relationship (Ernst et al., 2013).

Art Therapy and Perceived Control

Art therapy provides a supported environment fostering a sense of regained control for individuals experiencing loss of control during the process of diagnosis, treatment, and hospitalization (Malchiodi, 2013). A prominent goal in art therapy within a medical setting included providing psychosocial care and emotional support for patients. Kern-Pilch (1980) and David and Ilusorio (1995) established that choice and control are intrinsic components of the art making process; these essential human needs can be provided for through art therapy interventions (as cited in Hilterbrand, 1999). Creative expression allows for personal realization and communication of ideas in unique ways. Various case studies (Hilterbrand, 1999) documented the benefits of visual art making and art therapy on enhancing perception of control, increasing feelings of safety and restoring order, and decreasing overwhelm and perceived helplessness for breast cancer patients.

Art therapy can assist in shifting patient perceptions of illness. Puig et al.'s (2006) pilot study included a series of four, 60-minute individual creative arts therapy sessions over four weeks. Patients reported an increase in well-being as well as the ability to perceive their experience with cancer more positively; they focused more focused on transformation. Art therapy improved physical and psychological health of the subjects as well as their perspectives of the future (Svensk et al., 2009).

Art Therapy and Decision Making

Hilterbrand (1999) posited that freedom of choice and control are human needs that are frequently diminished through physical illness. Sometimes, medical treatment and procedures do not leave patients with many choices and options. Art making provides various opportunities to experience control over one's environment through decision-making. Visual art making allows for the realization of artistic goals and meaning is derived from the process, thus empowering creative decision-making. Oncology patients sometimes experience limited opportunities to make choices and decisions. Providing patients with the ability to make decisions through choices of art media and thematic content enhances feelings of control. Nanis (2008) described the intentionality behind using art materials; providing broad choices facilitated empowerment through choice and control. Facilitating a safe space for patients to feel empowered throughout the day may enhance their decision-making ability as well as mood and overall well-being (Nanis, 2008).

Mindfulness Based Art Therapy

A study by Monti et al. (2006) was conducted to find the effect on quality of life in 111 cancer patients through an 8-week intervention of Mindfulness Based Art Therapy (MBAT). The MBAT was focused on health promotion and engaged in understanding personal awareness differentiating between the cognitive (objective) experience of the health program and the emotional (subjective) experience. Art therapy assisted patients by addressing self-regulation, focusing attention, gaining awareness, and obtaining acceptance. Results included the decreased in distress through a notable reduction in anxiety and depression scales (Monti et al., 2006). Thus, using mindfulness strategies to gain personal awareness and control over negative emotional states likely will enhance a patient's sense of control over their reactions and outlook regarding the experience of illness.

Mindfulness is an essential concept within visual art leading to aesthetic awareness, engagement, and heightened experience. Greene (1995) expands the concept of engagement and awareness as encircled by imagination to provide an impetus for action and make the world a better place for all. According to Greene (1995), the aesthetic experience (heightened and mindful appreciation of an art form) is affected by personal life events and influences. Each experience is aesthetically unique to each person and causes a sense of *wide-awakeness* (Greene, 2001, p.6). Aesthetic awareness alone is not enough unless combined with good intention and positive action for the betterment of all involved (Greene, 1995).

Meditation and Mindfulness Based Art Therapy

Meditative experiences have been provided as a successful strategy in treating anxiety, depression, and chronic pain (Malchiodi, 1999). The benefits of meditation centered on mindfulness include increased awareness and concentration, focused and regulated breathing, and heightened positive emotions while a patient concentrated on positive and empowering statements. The emotional benefits of meditation are many; mindfulness training assists with reducing anxiety and symptoms associated with chronic pain. The roles of meditation in medical clinics are various. For example, it can be used by patients and family members to help them work through anxiety and frustration. Guided meditations frequently assist individuals when they begin mindfulness practices. The immediate results are defined in increasing concentration and awareness. Mindfulness assists with healing, quieting the mind, and distracting from pain. Emotions directly influence physical symptoms, and by using mindfulness to moderate negative emotions and increase positive emotions, the healing process is drastically improved (Gardner-Nix, 2009).

Monti et al. (2006) confirmed the positive results of a mindfulness based art therapy (MBAT) treatment plan on 111 cancer patents and found that MBAT reduced symptoms of distress and improved the health and quality of life in patients. McCown and Reibel (2010) summarized MBAT interventions that were effective in stress-reduction and decreasing symptoms associated with medical conditions. This is in addition to the observed benefits of meditation on stress reduction.

Phenomenological Art Therapy

Goodman et al. (1998) inquired into the use of art making as a means of personal exploration and investigated how the art museum could facilitate meaningful experiences for visitors by engaging them with art objects and building individualized connections. Phenomenological art therapy in the art gallery facilitates intentional looking, a mindfulness based approach that emphasized the exploring of senses, thoughts, and memories while fully experiencing art works. Individuals could make personal connections with the art works, resulting in meaningful and lasting responses. Phenomenology is a theoretical orientation within the field of art therapy concerned with the perception of objects such as, works of art (Betensky, 1995, 1999). Clients are encouraged to project their own interpretations and comprehensions of art objects and imagery; this enhances a client's ability to gain insight into their own thoughts and feelings. Guttmann and Regev (2004) cited various authors' descriptions of phenomenological perspectives as focusing on the perception of individuals and how they view the world. Components derived from this approach include distancing or focusing on a point reference beyond actual physical experience, intentional motivated looking/viewing, and exploring concepts in the present moment. Figure 1 represents the style of artwork that can be used to promote this intentional motivated looking/viewing. Visual art practices may be used for reducing stress, increasing reflective ability and self-efficacy, distracting from pain, and improving the quality of life of patients.

Figure 1. Gabrielle Wu Lee, Subliming, 1984, enamel on three canvas panels (relief) 72 x 72 inches
Courtesy of Paul Z. Lee, PhD, all copyrights reserved.

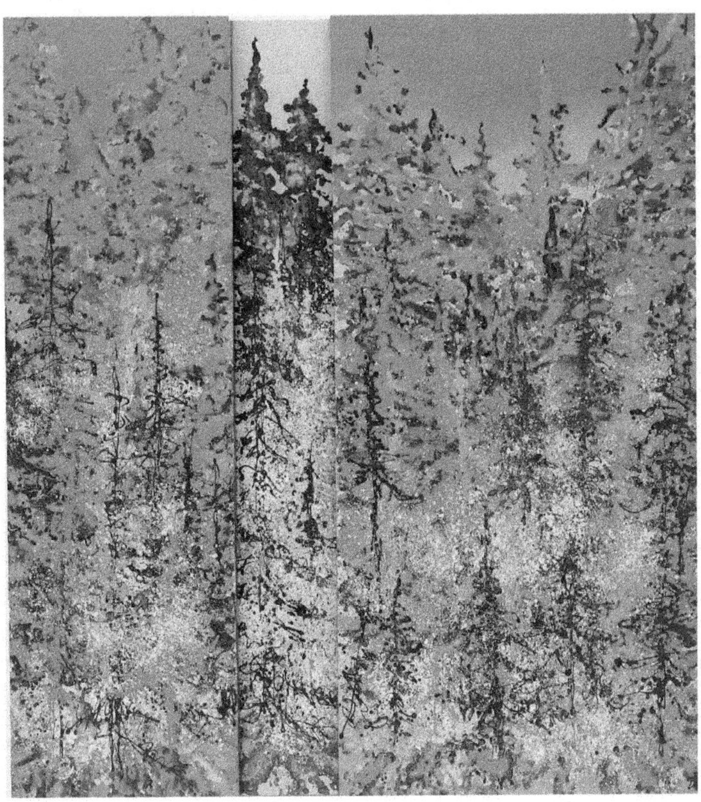

Visual Arts Based Synergistic Partnerships

Since the emergence of Arts in Medicine programs, collaborative efforts between art museums and hospitals have begun to facilitate art therapy services, either directly or indirectly. In this section, the authors describe several different programs to provide support for visual art therapy partnerships with healthcare facilities and museums. The benefits of collaborative partnerships between art therapy and art museum education have been recognized, particularly by organizations facilitating funding that promotes these endeavors. Although there are many types of collaborative programs, the authors focus on collaborative efforts between hospitals, museums, and art therapy programs seeking to improve the well-being and quality of life for patients and their families.

Benefits of Art Museum Education and Art Therapy Partnerships

Numerous benefits exist in developing collaborative interdisciplinary partnerships with arts, healthcare, education, and community organizations such as museums. For instance, art gallery viewing provided psychological benefits for caregivers of family members with complex mental health issues (Roberts, Camic, & Springham, 2011). According to Chatterjee, Vreeland, and Noble (2009), engaging with objects in the museum contributed to perceived life satisfaction and health status inside inpatient medical settings. Another art therapy and museum education collaborative effort aimed to increase self-actualization and socialization skills for youth living with HIV/ AIDS through the McMichael Canadian Art Collection Gallery, in which a therapeutic arts program was developed. Due to the benefits of this program, in 1995, an art therapy program for hospitalized cancer patients was established (Treadon, Rosal, & Wylder, 2006).

Another program is the *Art That Heals*, a model program developed at the University of California Los Angeles (UCLA) that promoted five services: art-as-therapy, an art cart, exhibitions by patients with cancer, strolling musicians program, and the exhibit *Confronting Cancer Through Art*. The program's art-as-therapy model promoted verbal and artistic exploration of the journey through cancer (Deane, Fitch & Carman, 2000a).

Rosenblatt (2014) acknowledged that art museums make significant contributions to healthcare by integrating museum education, art education, and art therapy. *The Creative Aging* program at The Phillips Collection in Washington, D.C. is a sample collaborative program that provides viewing and reflective art experiences followed by art making as a way for social support, creative self-expression, a sense of pride through accomplishment, and empowerment.

Deane, Fitch and Carman (2000b) described another art therapy and art museum education program developed in 1996 at the McMichael Canadian Art Collection and Toronto-Sunnybrook Regional Caner Center-Bayview Support Network. The program included three rounds of 16 sessions led by an art therapist. An existential/ phenomenological approach was provided, assisting patients in accepting and confronting death in order to lead more meaningful lives. The program emphasized the healing aspect of art as well as the holistic experience of creative expression. Individuals processed painful, distressing experiences of cancer through visual art. The program used the *Art That Heals* model described earlier in this section and adapted it to align with the McMichael Canadian Art Collection's museum education program mission. This program incorporated the mission of the museum education department and art therapy values: self-expression, creative play for adults, positive self-esteem, a sense of accomplishment through creation of aesthetically pleasing work, the ability to reflect on artwork, and confronting pain and psychological distress through imagery. The process of reflecting on the artwork prompted patients to express concerns related to illness through creating artwork focusing on body image and physical pain. The museum education department provided an educative component in the museum gallery experience featuring artwork about landscapes, body image related to illness, spirituality, loss, and sociopolitical issues. These themes were further explored using reflective studio art-making experiences (Deane, Fitch & Carman, 2000b).

Another example of the integration of visual arts therapy and healthcare was designed by The National Gallery of Australia, which developed *The Arts of Health* project that integrated social work, and assisted people with chronic illness by raising awareness regarding the link between lifestyle and health. This program laid the groundwork to develop strengths as a resource for creativity, expression, and learning. The project's mission advocated that Maslow's (1954) hierarchy of needs should be addressed in art museums: ego, self-esteem, belongingness, and self-actualization (Treadon, Rosal, & Wylder, 2006).

A trend in hospital, art museum, and art therapy programs exists with children's hospitals and children's museums in larger cities. For instance, the St. Louis Children's Museum and St. Louis Children's Hospital developed a program including an interactive exhibit where children could engage and use play to experiment with roles of health professionals and caretakers of infants. Children dress up in doctor and nurse outfits, and use pretend play to rock, dress, weigh, and take care of infants. These activities display St. Louis Children's Hospital's model of Family-Centered Care (St. Louis Children's Hospital, 2015).

Also, Children's Hospital through the University Hospitals of Cleveland and The Children's Museum of Cleveland promoted the museum's educational mission by enhancing creativity and learning for children through hands-on play and connection with parents and caregivers. The museum's educational program valued an interdisciplinary educative experience with math, history, science, and arts integrated curricula. Creative play inside the exhibit included interacting with house chores like cooking, making beds, getting dressed, role-playing about the future days, and running errands (Children's Museum Cleveland, 2015).

Another example of museum and healthcare collaboration began in 2012 when the Denver Art Museum (DAM) and Children's Hospital Colorado partnered to build confidence and engage family connection through art and creativity. The program valued self-care, holistic wellbeing, and the overall therapeutic value of arts. The Ponzio Creative Arts Therapy Program at Children's Hospital Colorado worked with the DAM to create art making sessions. Target audiences included families of patients undergoing treatment, and utilized DAM collection artwork, lectures, visits, and art making for children and families at the hospital (Denver Art Museum, 2012).

In further support of art therapy, museum and healthcare partnerships, The Museum of Fine Arts in Boston's Artful Healing at Boston's Children Hospital, Massachusetts General Hospital, and Dana-Farber Cancer Institute hosted a collaborative effort to enhance the experiences for patients and families at the medical center (Museum of Fine Arts Boston, 2015). The Boston MFA's mission seeks to accommodate and provide access for visitors with disabilities. The MFA collection determines themes related to art making and exploratory experiences. Patients can watch a slide show of the collection and participate in bedside studio art making session with various materials such as Chinese brush painting, printmaking, wire sculpture, paint, and clay. Off-site workshops are located in the various healthcare centers for patients undergoing treatments and their family members.

A larger collaboration involved The Ann & Robert H. Lurie Children's Hospital of Chicago in partnership with 21 museums and arts facilities in the Chicago area to enhance the environment for patients and their families through design, educational programs and interactive exhibits (Lalley, 2012). The program used various images, photographs, illustrations, 3D dioramas, murals, and installations. Some partners were the Art Institute of Chicago and the Museum of Contemporary Art Chicago (MCA). The

MCA provides family programs that focus on viewing and interpreting contemporary artwork followed by response art making. Additionally, the DuSable Museum of African American History funded and assisted with mural creation in the hospital. One of the mural themes titled *Little Black Pearl,* was designed symbolically to exemplify the patients' transformation through the experience of surgery. Butterflies symbolically represent endurance, change, hope, and life in the mural. The hospital's design resembles a children's museum with each of the 23 floors including art installations (Lalley, 2012).

Focusing on long term care partnerships, Moss Rehab's Einstein Healthcare Art Therapy Program and the Philadelphia Museum of Art (PMA) was established to accommodate individuals with physical and cognitive disabilities (Einstein Healthcare, 2015). Each of the organizations promoted self-expression, and an opportunity to experience a high quality art institution. The Moss Rehab Art Therapy Program includes a tour at the PMA and participation in art making. The patients are also provided the opportunity to submit artwork to the *Bridges* exhibition at PMA along with professional artists with disabilities (Moss Rehab, 2012).

Finally, Magee's Art Therapy and the PMA collaborated to provide museum tours and art therapy sessions with art making regarding what individuals experienced at the PMA (Magee Rehabilitation, 2013). Magee Rehabilitation Hospitals Art Therapy Program and the PMA share the mission of promoting the healing benefits of the arts, specifically for individuals with physical disabilities. Magee's Art Therapy Program uses the art making process to help patients express themselves and cope with their new limitations.

COLLABORATIVE PARTNERSHIP: SYNERGY IN ACTION

In an effort to bridge the gap between the fields of medicine, education, and community engagement through the museum and arts, a collaborative pilot program was established through partnerships between the graduate level art therapy program at Florida State University (FSU), the Birmingham Museum of Art (BMA), and the University of Alabama (UAB) radiology lab. Aligning with the mission values of each organization involved, this collaboration was developed to advance the hospital and cancer center while providing a healing space for patients and their families.

Goals of the project included the facilitation of stress and anxiety-reduction strategies, providing distraction from distressing psychological symptoms associated with invasive medical procedures, and the improvement in the overall quality of life of the patients and their family members. This program serves a diverse audience within the Birmingham community, as well as patients from the southeastern United States, seeking quality medical treatment for various illnesses. Patients, family members, and caregivers of patients undergoing medical procedures in the UAB facility have access to the curated artworks, the audio tour, guided viewing prompts, and meditation experiences through an internet-based mobile application.

Missions of the Birmingham Museum of Art, University of Alabama PET Testing Lab and the Florida State University's Art Therapy Graduate Program

Due to the collaborative nature of the program, it is important to understand the missions of each organization and program to better connect the potential impact on patient healthcare. The mission of the BMA is to *provide an unparalleled cultural and educational experience to a diverse community by collecting, presenting, interpreting, and preserving works of art of the highest quality* (Birmingham Museum of Art, 2014). The Museum Education Department provides services to the community by bringing art to Birmingham's community. The department engages with community-based service projects within local schools in surrounding neighborhoods (Birmingham Museum of Art, 2014).

UAB's PET Testing Lab provides outstanding clinical care, excellence in teaching and mentoring, and serves as a premier academic radiology program emphasizing patient well-being, respect, and high ethical principles (University of Alabama Department of Radiology, 2014).

FSU's Graduate Art Therapy program provides superior education to graduate students and offers exemplary services to the community and university through the enhancement of theory, research, and clinical practices (Treadon, Rosal, & Wylder, 2006).

Overview of the Pilot Program

Integrating collaborative partnerships among art therapy, medical settings, and museums provides positive outcomes for patients and the community. Treadon, Rosal, and Wylder (2006) outlined various populations who directly benefitted from these partnerships: cancer patients, individuals with various chronic illnesses, and individuals with HIV/ AIDS. A pilot program developed by one of the authors through the University of Alabama PET Testing Radiology Lab, Birmingham Museum of Art, and Florida State University demonstrates a collaborative effort to benefit the patients, families, and caregivers served in the community. It directly complements medical services through its aim to bridge the gap between education, medicine, and community engagement with the use of the arts.

The BMA, UAB, and FSU Collaborative Project

A FSU graduate level art therapy intern and one of the authors for this chapter worked with the Birmingham Museum of Art (BMA) to curate eight works of art from the museum aligning with the theme: *The Art of Meditation*. In addition to the use of these artworks inside the waiting room of the Radiology Lab at the University of Alabama PET Testing Lab, a series of guided imagery scripts, mobile tour guided prompts, transcripts for audio tours, and content for the Smart Guide Mobile App through BMA's website was developed.

In alignment with the theme *The Art of Meditation*, a series of guided prompts were transcribed in order to provide auditory and visual experiences of the curated artworks. In addition, mindfulness and relaxation meditation scripts were developed and recorded for family members to experience while waiting in the clinic. The development of these mindfulness and relaxation scripts included questions that were inspired by the idea of linking audio guides to guided imagery prompts that lead the listener while viewing each painting. Patients could experience the paintings and engage with colors and nature imagery by visually and mentally transporting themselves into the paintings. Questions directed the viewer towards exploration of the painting while engaging in a meditative, stress reducing experience. The scripts were designed to guide the individual through the exploration of the sensory and personal meanings associated with each image. The goal was not to inform or to explore the technical aspects of artwork, but to assist the visitors and clients in engaging with mindfulness, guided imagery, and meditative processes.

Artist Gabrielle Wu Lee's work (see Figure 2) represents how the use of specific artworks can assist patients in alleviating stress during treatment in a hospital or clinic setting. Figure 2 represents a sample

Figure 2. Gabrielle Wu Lee, Emerald Beach, Florida, No. 35, 2004, 48 x 60 inches

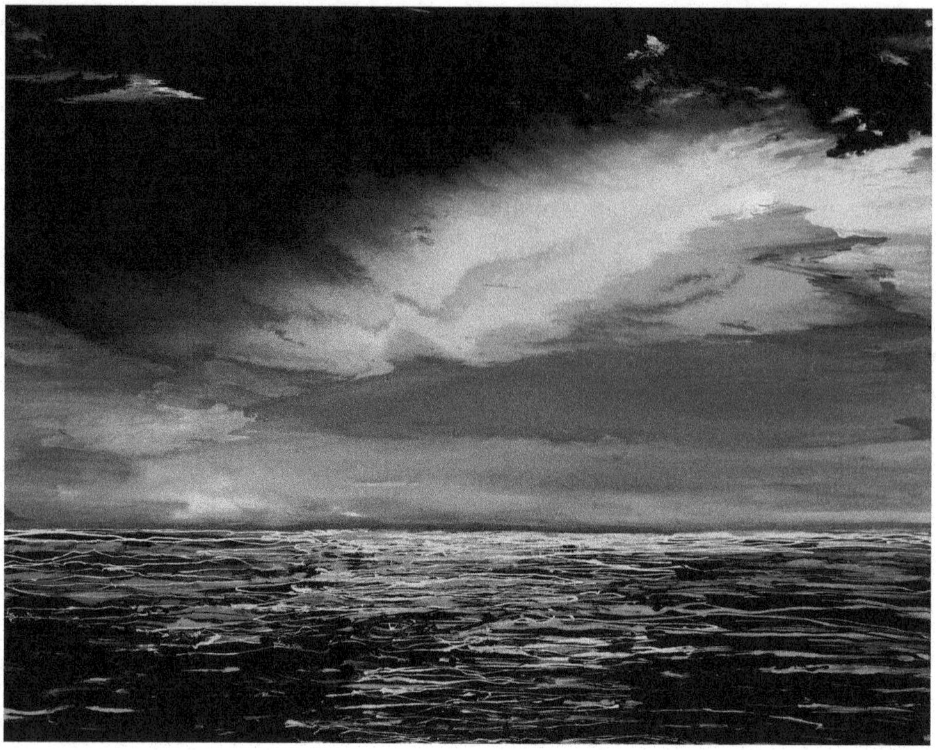

of how meditation, mindfulness and visualization strategies can aid in increasing patient well-being during invasive medical procedures.

Creative approaches involving mindfulness, meditation and visualization are described to help transcend beyond the illness and treatment program and inspire relaxation and awareness of aesthetic beauty within visual art. Included in this section is a sample excerpt that is used while the patient is attentive to an artwork similar to the image of Gabrielle Wu Lee's *Emerald Beach, Florida,* No. 35, (2004).

Start by relaxing. Notice anywhere your body is holding tension. Focus on this area. Slowly, inhale deeply and exhale any stress you're holding in this area. Become aware of your breath as you inhale and exhale. During each exhale, release any stress you're holding onto. As you inhale and exhale, visualize tension and stress leaving your body. Take time to relax and quiet your mind. Pause the recording, and repeat this process as many times as you need before you begin to explore the artwork.

Now that you're relaxed, look closely at the artwork. Take in the colors, and notice where your eyes focus. Are you drawn to the yellows? The blues? In which direction do your eyes naturally move? As you view the colors, notice where in your body these colors bring sensations. Which words would you use to describe how the yellows make you feel? Take a few deep breaths. Has your breath shifted while viewing the artwork? Pause the recording until you're ready to move on.

What does this artwork remind you of? We often associate specific colors with experiences, sensations, and feelings. Meditate on color, and imagine those experiences, sensations, and feelings, or objects in nature that come to mind (Hartman, personal communication, February 9, 2016).

Gabrielle Wu Lee's artwork is appropriate for mindful meditation strategies because of the abstract style which allows viewers to interpret their own thoughts and emotions. Lee is an artist and medical doctor who suffered from rheumatic myocarditis which confined her to bed for years. She understands the important connection between art and medicine. Lee confides that her proactive attitude, deep understanding of medicine and her love of beauty, nature and humanity created her optimistic hope for the future against all odds. "Art is an expression of love, beauty, faith, hope, understanding, and analysis. This is the ultimate reason it can be used as therapy" (Lee, personal communication, January 20, 2016).

Allowing individuals the opportunity to engage and make personal connections to suit their comfort levels allows patients to focus on the guided imagery through the artworks to inspire anxiety reduction and inspiration. The process of intentional looking aligns well the BMA's Slow Art events (Birmingham Museum of Art, 2014). Intentional looking is a process in art therapy that enhances the client's ability to use phenomenological examination for meaningful experiences and articulate those meanings through engagement with the imagery.

CONCLUSION

Art Therapy as Adjunct Complementary Therapy in Healthcare

Art therapy has been established as an increasingly significant treatment modality in adjunct with traditional medical treatment in oncology settings. A large percentage of cancer patients use complementary therapies in addition to standard medical treatments (Nanis et al., 2006). Benefits of creative therapies include increasing sense of control, distracting attention from distressing emotions, developing coping skills, reducing negative emotions, strengthening patient cooperation with medical interventions (Kreitler, Oppenheim, & Segev-Shoham, 2012), enhancing self-care, heightening feelings of empowerment, and increasing quality of life (Wood & Molassiotis, 2011).

According to Drake and Winner (2012), drawing was used as a therapeutic component to redirect thoughts from rumination while increasing positive mood states. Patients reported improvements in pain, fatigue, depression, and anxiety when comparing one-hour prior to post art therapy sessions (Rhondali, Rhondali, & Lasserre, 2013). For patients with extended hospital stays, art therapy provided relaxation and distraction from pain (Malchiodi, 1999). Specifically, a Cognitive Behavioral (CBT) expressive therapy intervention provided distraction from chronic pain and decreased pain perception (Camic, 1999), which are frequent symptoms experienced by cancer patients.

Wood et al. (2013) summarized findings of art therapy interventions in psycho-oncology care. Art therapy influenced significant improvements in quality of life, body image, physical symptoms (Svensk et al., 2009), coping resources (Oster et al., 2009), improvement in eight of nine health and psychological symptoms (Nanis et al., 2006), immune functioning (Virago & Dunkley, 2008), and self-expression (as cited in Wood et al., 2013). Visual art therapy was also helpful in decreasing distressing emotions (Gabriel et al., 2001), reducing anxiety, depression, and anger (Puig et al., 2006), and diminishing psychological distress (Monti et al., 2006). Art therapy induced personal empowerment, self-expression, and openness. The process of art making was a healing process involving the body, mind, and spirit. The non-verbal, unconscious experience of art therapy allowed patients to contain feelings associated with psychological distress: anxiety, apprehension, fear, and confusion (Malchiodi, 1999).

Benefits of Visual Arts in Healthcare

According to Malchiodi (1999), art experiences allow patients to confront illness and enjoy life by, overcoming the pain, fear, and anxiety associated with illness. This transformation in thinking influences the immune system. Overall, this transformation has a positive impact on the health of the body, and psychological well-being. Art therapy helps patients and their families increase awareness of self, cope with symptoms, and adapt to stressful and traumatic experiences (Nanis et al., 2006).

Emotions influence the dynamics of the immune system. For instance, stress has a negative impact on the immune system, which causes a downstream change in bodily functions (Rubert, Long, & Hutchinson, 2007). Stress also compounds with this immune dysfunction by negatively altering a patient's ability to heal. Processing sensory information can reduce stress and positively impact emotional responses either positively or negatively.

Exposure to visual arts in healthcare settings influenced patient perception of control and power (Daykin, Byrne, Souteriou, & O'Conner, 2008). Artistic expression induced a relaxation response in patients, mitigated negative health symptoms, and increased patient immune system functionalities (Malchiodi, 1999).

Psychological distress accompanying the diagnosis of a serious illness is problematic to patient health, self-identity, and future expectations of survival. The shock of receiving a cancer diagnosis is often traumatic and unexpected. Halkett, Arbon, Scutter, and Borg (2007) described various contributors influencing psychological distress: confusing and overwhelming emotions, anxiety regarding treatment options, attitude toward survival, preparation for future obstacles, acceptance of diagnosis, and receiving adequate information regarding medical treatment options.

FUTURE IMPLICATIONS FOR VISUAL ARTS IN HEALTHCARE

According to Poggi, (2006), viewing nature scenes improved patient outcomes and enhanced a healing environment by reducing stress and anxiety, lowering blood pressure, reducing the need for pain medication, increasing patient trust and hope, and by providing a distraction. Also using calming colors such as blue, green, and violet in healthcare settings and artwork displayed in these settings can possess healing benefits such as stress-reduction and a calming effect (Rubert, Long, & Hutchinson, 2007).

Both color and landscape contributed towards patient healing by having an impact on the perception of healing within the healthcare design. *The Lancet* (Lejsted & Johannes, 2006) published a document confirming that patients viewing nature images experienced less anxiety and received fewer strong pain medication doses. Visual imagery depicting nature was perceived as healing and improved health outcomes (Urist, 2014).

Imagery exercises have been implemented in interventions in medicine and health psychology (Long, 2004). The use of imagery within art promotes healing by the concretizing of art processes through the imagination. Halm (2009) noted that relaxation and imagery were highly prioritized components of anxiety reduction strategies for cardiac patients.

Besides viewing and engaging with artworks, patients benefit from creating their own works of art. Malchiodi (1999) claimed that reflection in art making assisted in balancing internal and external locus of control, which affected the tendency to actively participate in health care and self-care strategies (as cited in McNutt, 2013).

The art making processes of creating collages, mandalas and visual journals provide a benefit for patients. Engaging in the collage process through art therapy provided a safe experience for a cancer patient's emotions through expression of colors, shapes, and images. The process of collage alleviates the need to draw realistically and includes sorting, choosing, organizing, and collecting printed images from a variety of sources (brochures, magazines, newspapers, and photographs). Allowing patients to browse through magazine images offers structure, freedom, and choice (Elkis-Abuhoff et al., 2009; Foster, 1992) without interfering with perceived expectations clients may have regarding artistic abilities in drawing tasks (Malchiodi, 2013; Rubin, 2001). Individuals engaged in collage experienced "control through decision-making" (as cited in Stallings, in press, p. 29).

Forzoni et al (2010) reported of 157 chemotherapy patients engaged in art therapy sessions, the majority of patients (94.5%) reported that participating in free collage was helpful. Approximately 37% of patients perceived art therapy collage as relaxing, 33% reported the benefit of the client-therapist relationship, and approximately 30% of patients reported the benefits of art serving as a structure through which to express emotions and reflect on meanings visually represented in the narrative (Forzoni et al., 2010).

Creating mandalas was also helpful in obtaining a sense of order and balance during emotional conflicts (Elkis-Abuhoff et. al., 2009). Mandalas or circular designs are a prime reflection of gestalt art therapy (Jung, 1972). Mandalas reflect the healthy individual, one who is able to integrate all the body systems into one dynamic act of creativity. These circular designs exemplify core identities within the whole self, integrated together. Constructing mandalas can lead to insight, help to process unfinished business, and move patients towards self-exploration (Fincher, 2007). Interpretations of individual mandalas are guided by the artist/patient as this process is a personal journey of image and color association through language (Fincher, 2010).

Visual journaling is another creative expression that provides benefits for patients. Visual journals or artistic design journals are a combination the characteristics of a written entries and the visual elements of the artistic expression. Hand-bound journals are especially meaningful for the artist/patient since the process of binding the book is rewarding and personal (Brown, 2015). According to Brazelton (2004) and Chilton (2007), altered books, scrapbooking, and journaling offered the opportunity for free expression, creativity, and structure (as cited in Stallings, in press). The containment or structure provided by the borders of the page allowed patients to control their environments through a defined space (the blank page). Art therapy provided empowerment through creative expression, discounting the loss of control experienced by patients. The non-verbal and relaxation benefits of art therapy allowed the patient to express painful themes such as loss, change, depression, and fear, thus increasing perceived control over the experience (Malchiodi, 1999).

The integration of color design, artwork selection, art making for creative expression, and mindful meditation provides a unique combination of benefits for patients in art therapy and healthcare collaborations. The flexibility in thinking that is promoted through creative expression may be appropriate in maintaining a more stable HLOC throughout the course of diagnosis, treatment, and survivorship periods of illness. Future research connecting art therapy with healthcare facilities and museums is encouraged to further the support medical treatment that heals the body, mind and spirit through creativity and innovation.

REFERENCES

Andrykowski, M. A., & Brady, M. J. (1994). Health locus of control and psychological distress in cancer patients: Interactive effects of context. *Journal of Behavioral Medicine*, *17*(5), 439–458. doi:10.1007/BF01857919 PMID:7877155

Betensky, M. G. (1995). What do you see? Phenomenology of therapeutic art expression. London: Jessica Kingsley Publishers. Retrieved from http://search.proquest.com/docview/618763898?accountid=4840

Betensky, M. G. (1999). Phenomenological art therapy. In J. A. Rubin (Ed.), *Approaches to art therapy* (2nd ed.). Philadelphia: Brunner-Routledge.

Birmingham Museum of Art. (2014). *Accessibility*. Retrieved from http://www.artsbma.org/access/

Brazelton, B. (2004). *Altered Books Workshop*. New York, NY: F+ W Media, Inc.

Brown, S. (2013). *Teaching art integration in the schools*. Mason, Ohio: Cengage Learning.

Brown, S. (2015). Healing through Self-discovery and Artistic Design Journals. In J.L. Bird (Ed.), Innovative collaborative practice and reflection in patient education (pp. 103-119). Hershey, PA, USA: IGI Global.

Camic, P. M. (1999). Expanding treatment possibilities for chronic pain through the expressive arts. In C. A. Malchiodi (Ed.), *Medical art therapy with adults* (pp. 43–61). London: Jessica Kingsley.

Camic, P. M., Tischler, V., & Pearman, C. H. (2013). Viewing and making art together: A multi-session art-gallery-based intervention for people with dementia and their carers. *Aging & Mental Health*, *18*(2), 161–168. doi:10.1080/13607863.2013.818101 PMID:23869748

Chatterjee, H., Vreeland, S., & Noble, G. (2009). Museopathy: Exploring the healing potential of handling museum objects. *Museum & Society*, *7*(3), 164–177.

Children's Museum of Cleveland. (2015). House and hospital. Retrieved from http://www.clevelandchildrensmuseum.org/exhibit/house-and-hospital/

Chilton, G. (2007). Altered books in art therapy with adolescents. *Art Therapy: Journal of the American Art Therapy Association*, *24*(2), 59–63. doi:10.1080/07421656.2007.10129588

Czamanski-Cohen, J. (2012). The use of art in the medical decision-making process of oncology patients. *Art Therapy: Journal of the American Art Therapy Association*, *29*(2), 60–67. doi:10.1080/07421656.2012.680049

David, I. R., & Ilusorio, S. (1995). Tuberculosis: Art therapy with patients in isolation. *Art Therapy: Journal of the American Art Therapy Association*, *12*(1), 24–31. doi:10.1080/07421656.1995.10759120

Daykin, N., Byrne, E., Souteriou, T., & O'Connor, S. (2008). Review: The impact of art, design and environment in mental healthcare: a systematic review of the literature. *Perspectives in Public Health*, *128*(2), 85–94. PMID:18402179

Deane, K., Fitch, M., & Carman, M. (2000a). An innovative art therapy program for cancer patients. *Canadian Oncology Nursing Journal, 10*(4), 147–151, 152–157. doi:10.5737/1181912x104147151 PMID:11894321

Deane, K., Fitch, M., & Carman, M. (2000b). The cancer journey: Bridging art therapy and museum education. *Canadian Oncology Nursing Journal, 10*(4), 140–142, 143–146. doi:10.5737/1181912x104140142 PMID:11894320

Denver Art Museum. (2012). *Denver Art Museum and Children's Hospital Colorado team up to focus on the restorative and transformational powers of art.* Retrieved from http://denverartmuseum.org/article/press-release/denver-art-museum-and-children-s-hospital-colorado-team-focus-restorative-and

Dissanayake, E. (1992). *Homoaesthetics: Where art comes from and why.* New York: Macmillan Inc.

Drake, J. E., & Winner, E. (2012). Confronting sadness through art-making: Distraction is more beneficial than venting. *Psychology of Aesthetics, Creativity, and the Arts, 6*(3), 255–261. doi:10.1037/a0026909

Einstein Healthcare. (2013, July 11). Moss Rehab's art therapy program with Philadelphia museum of art receives award. Retrieved from http://www.einstein.edu/news/mossrehab%E2%80%99s-art-therapy-program-with-philadelphia-museum-of-art-receives-award/

Elkis-Abuhoff, D., Gaydos, M., Goldblatt, R., Chen, M., & Rose, S. (2009). Mandala drawings as an assessment tool for women with breast cancer. *The Arts in Psychotherapy, 36*(4), 231–238. doi:10.1016/j.aip.2009.04.004

Ernst, J., Berger, S., Weißflog, G., Schröder, C., Körner, A., Niederwieser, D., & Singer, S. (2013). Patient participation in the medical decision-making process in haemato-oncology—A qualitative study. *European Journal of Cancer Care, 22*(5), 684–690. doi:10.1111/ecc.12077 PMID:23731258

Fincher, S. (2010). *Creating mandalas for insight, healing and self-expression.* Boston, MA: Shambhala Publications, Inc.

Fincher, S. F. (2007). Mandalas and the gestalt of self. *International Gestalt Journal, 30*(2), 65–78.

Forzoni, S., Perez, M., Martignetti, A., & Crispino, S. (2010). Art therapy with cancer patients during chemotherapy sessions: An analysis of the patients' perception of helpfulness. *Palliative & Supportive Care, 8*(1), 41–48. doi:10.1017/S1478951509990691 PMID:20163759

Foster, M. T. (1992). Experiencing a "creative high.". *The Journal of Creative Behavior, 26*(1), 29–39. doi:10.1002/j.2162-6057.1992.tb01154.x

Gabriel, B., Bromberg, E., Vandenbovenkamp, J., Walka, P., Kornblith, A. B., & Luzzatto, P. (2001). Art therapy with adult bone marrow transplant patients in isolation: A pilot study. *Psycho-Oncology, 10*(2), 114–123. doi:10.1002/pon.498 PMID:11268138

Gardner-Nix, J. (2009). The mindfulness solution to pain: Step-by-step techniques for chronic pain management. Oakland, CA: New Harbinger Publications; Retrieved from http://search.proquest.com/docview/622056475?accountid=4840

Glass, K. E., Wills, C. E., Holloman, C., Olson, J., Hechmer, C., Miller, C. K., & Duchemin, A. M. (2012). Shared decision making and other variables as correlates of satisfaction with health care decisions in a United States national survey. *Patient Education and Counseling*, *88*(1), 100–105. doi:10.1016/j.pec.2012.02.010 PMID:22410642

Goodman, R., Williams, K., Agell, G., & Gantt, L. (1998). Talk, talk, talk, when do we draw? *American Journal of Art Therapy*, *37*(2), 39.

Greene, M. (1995). *Releasing the imagination: Essays on education, the arts, and social change*. New York: Wiley.

Greene, M. (2001). *Variations on a blue guitar: The Lincoln Center Institute lectures on aesthetic education*. New York: Teachers College Press.

Guttmann, J., & Regev, D. (2004). The phenomenological approach to art therapy. *Journal of Contemporary Psychotherapy*, *34*(2), 153–162. doi:10.1023/B:JOCP.0000022314.69354.41

Halkett, G. K. B., Arbon, P., Scutter, S. D., & Borg, M. (2007). The phenomenon of making decisions during the experience of early breast cancer. *European Journal of Cancer Care*, *16*(4), 322–330. doi:10.1111/j.1365-2354.2007.00778.x PMID:17587355

Halm, M. A. (2009). Relaxation: A self-care healing modality reduces harmful effects of anxiety. *American Journal of Critical Care*, *18*(2), 169–172. doi:10.4037/ajcc2009867 PMID:19255107

Hillen, M. A., de Haes, H. C. J. M., Stalpers, L. J. A., Klinkenbijl, J. H. G., Eddes, E., Verdam, M. G. E., & Smets, E. M. A. (2014). How attachment style and locus of control influence patients' trust in their oncologist. *Journal of Psychosomatic Research*, *76*(3), 221–226. doi:10.1016/j.jpsychores.2013.11.014 PMID:24529041

Hilterbrand, E. U. (1999). Coping with Cancer through image manipulation. In C. A. Malchiodi (Ed.), *Medical art therapy with adults* (pp. 113–135). London: Jessica Kingsley.

Hodges, K., & Winstanley, S. (2012). Effects of optimism, social support, fighting spirit, cancer worry and internal health locus of control on positive affect in cancer survivors: A path analysis. *Stress and Health: Journal of the International Society for the Investigation of Stress*, *28*(5), 408–415. doi:10.1002/smi.2471 PMID:23129560

Jung, C. (1972). *Mandala symbolism*. Princeton, NJ: Princeton University Press.

Kern-Pilch, K. (1980). Art therapy with a terminally ill patient. *American Journal of Art Therapy*, *20*(1), 3–11. PMID:10251680

Kirkland, B. J. (1996, May). Psychological adjustment to breast cancer: Congruence of locus of control and information and decision making participation. *Dissertation Abstracts International: Section B: The Sciences and Engineering*.

Kreitler, S., Oppenheim, D., & Segev-Shoham, E. (2012). *Fantasy, art therapies, and other expressive and creative psychosocial interventions*. Somerset, NJ: Wiley-Blackwell. doi:10.1002/9781119941033.ch13

Krumholz, H. M. (2010). Informed consent to promote patient- centered care. *Journal of the American Medical Association, 303*(12), 1190–1191. doi:10.1001/jama.2010.309 PMID:20332406

Lalley, H. (2012, May 13). Chicago civic groups contribute art to Ann and Robert H. Lurie Children's Hospital. Retrieved from https://www.luriechildrens.org/en-us/our-home/Pages/community-partner-spaces.aspx

Lejsted, M., & Johannes, N. (2006, December). Art created by psychiatric patients. *Lancet, 368*, S10–S11. doi:10.1016/S0140-6736(06)69906-6

Long, J. K. (2004). Medical art therapy: Using imagery and visual expression in healing. In P. M. Camic & S. J. Knight (Eds.), *Clinical handbook of health psychology; a practical guide to effective interventions* (2nd ed., pp. 315–342). Portland, OR: Ringgold Inc.

Magee Rehabilitation. (2013). Maggee rehabilitation art therapy program becomes a community partner of Philadelphia museum of art. Retrieved from: http://www.mageerehab.org/page.php?id=1420

Malchiodi, C. (1999). Art therapy, arts medicine, and arts in healthcare: A vision for collaboration in the next millennium. *International Journal of Arts Medicine, 6*(2), 13–16.

Malchiodi, C. A. (Ed.), (2013). *Art therapy and health care*. New York: Guilford Press.

Mann, D. (2010). *Gestalt therapy: 100 key points & techniques* (1st ed.). New York: Routledge.

Maslow, A. (1954). *Motivation and personality*. New York, NY: Harper.

McCown, D., & Reibel, D. (2010). Mindfulness and mindfulness-based stress reduction. Integrative psychiatry (pp. 289–338). New York, NY: Oxford University Press. Retrieved from http://search.proquest.com/docview/622134155?accountid=4840

McNutt, J. V. (2013). Art therapy as a form of visual narrative in oncology care. In C. A. Malchiodi (Ed.), *Art therapy and health care* (pp. 127–135). New York: Guilford Press.

Monti, D. A., Peterson, C., Kunkel, E. J. S., Hauck, W. W., Pequignot, E., Rhodes, L., & Brainard, G. C. (2006). A randomized, controlled trial of mindfulness-based art therapy (MBAT) for women with cancer. *Psycho-Oncology, 15*(5), 363–373. doi:10.1002/pon.988 PMID:16288447

Moss Rehab. (2012). Art therapy program. Retrieved from http://www.mossrehab.com/special-services/mossrehab-outpatient-art-therapy-program.html

Museum of Fine Arts Boston. (2015). Artful healing. Retrieved from http://www.mfa.org/programs/community-programs/artful-healing

Nainis, N., Paice, J. A., Ratner, J., Wirth, J. H., Lai, J., & Shott, S. (2006). Relieving symptoms in cancer: Innovative use of art therapy. *Journal of Pain and Symptom Management, 31*(2), 162–169. doi:10.1016/j.jpainsymman.2005.07.006 PMID:16488349

Nainis, N. A. (2008). Approaches to art therapy for cancer inpatients: Research and practice Considerations. *Journal of the American Art Therapy Association, 25*(3), 115–121. doi:10.1080/07421656.2008.10129597

Öster, I., Egberg Thyme, K., Sundin, E. C., & Lindh, J. (2009). Individual brief art therapy can be helpful for women with breast cancer. *Palliative & Supportive Care*, *7*(1), 87–95. doi:10.1017/S147895150900011X PMID:19619378

Pieterse, A. H., Baas-Thijssen, M. C. M., Marijnen, C. A. M., & Stiggelbout, A. M. (2008). Clinician and cancer patient views on patient participation in treatment decision-making: A quantitative and qualitative exploration. *British Journal of Cancer*, *99*(6), 875–882. doi:10.1038/sj.bjc.6604611 PMID:18781148

Poggi, E. (2006). Beyond traditional treatment: Establishing art as therapy. *Healthcare Design*, *6*(7), 23–25.

Puig, A., Lee, S. M., Goodwin, L., & Sherrard, P. A. D. (2006). The efficacy of creative arts therapies to enhance emotional expression, spirituality, and psychological well-being of newly diagnosed stage I and stage II breast cancer patients: A preliminary study. *The Arts in Psychotherapy*, *33*(3), 218–228. doi:10.1016/j.aip.2006.02.004

Rhondali, W., Rhondali, W., & Lasserre. (2013). Art therapy among palliative care inpatients with advanced cancer. *Palliative Medicine, 27*(6), 571; 571-572; 572.

Roberts, S., Camic, P. M., & Springham, N. (2011). New roles for art galleries: Art-viewing as a community intervention for family carers of people with mental health problems. *Arts & Health: An International Journal for Research. Policy & Practice*, *3*(2), 146–159.

Rosenblatt, B. (2014). Museum education and art therapy: Promoting wellness in older adults. *Journal of Museum Education*, *39*(3), 293–301. doi:10.1080/10598650.2014.11510821

Rubert, R., Long, D. L., & Hutchinson, M. L. (2007). Creating a healing environment in the ICU. In R. Kaplow & S. R. Hardin (Eds.), *Critical care nursing; synergy for optimal outcomes (2007)* (pp. 27–39). Portland, OR: Ringold, Inc.

Rubin, J. (2001). *Approaches to art therapy: Theory and technique* (2nd ed.). New York: Brunner-Routledge.

Sepucha, K. R., Belkora, J. K., Mutchnick, S., & Esserman, L. J. (2002). Consultation planning to help breast cancer patients prepare for medical consultations: Effect on communication and satisfaction for patients and physicians. *Journal of Clinical Oncology*, *20*(11), 2695–2700. doi:10.1200/JCO.2002.10.068 PMID:12039932

St. Louis Children's Hospital. (2015). The magic house, St. Louis children's museum. Retrieved from http://www.stlouischildrens.org/health-resources/community-education/community-partnerships/the-magic-house-st-louis-childrens-museum

Stallings, J. (in press). Collage as expressive medium in art therapy. In D. Gussak and M. Rosal's (Eds). The Wiley-Blackwell Handbook of Art Therapy. Oxford England: Wiley Blackwell Publishing. doi:10.1002/9781118306543.ch16

Step, M. M., Rose, J. H., Albert, J. M., Cheruvu, V. K., & Siminoff, L. A. (2009). Modeling patient-centered communication: Oncologist relational communication and patient communication involvement in breast cancer adjuvant therapy decision-making. *Patient Education and Counseling*, *77*(3), 369–378. doi:10.1016/j.pec.2009.09.010 PMID:19811883

Svensk, A. C., Oster, I., Thyme, K. E., Magnusson, E., Sjodin, M., Eisemann, M., & Lindh, J. et al. (2009). Art therapy improves experienced quality of life among women undergoing treatment for breast cancer: A randomized controlled study. *European Journal of Cancer Care, 18*(1), 69–77. doi:10.1111/j.1365-2354.2008.00952.x PMID:19473224

Treadon, C. B., Rosal, M., & Wylder, V. D. T. (2006). Opening the doors of art museums for therapeutic processes. *The Arts in Psychotherapy, 33*(4), 288–301. doi:10.1016/j.aip.2006.03.003

University of Alabama Department of Radiology. (2014). *Department of Radiology Mission, Vision & Values Statement.* Retrieved from https://www.uab.edu/medicine/radiology/about/mission-vision-values

Urist, J. (2014, September 23). The healing power of art: Can hospital collections help? Retrieved from http://www.nbcnews.com/health/health-news/healing-power-art-can-hospital-collections-help-n208966

Virago, M., & Dunkley, M. (2008, March). A journey past the sun and back: Using art psychotherapy to investigate the connection between immunological and psychosocial function following a diagnosis of melanoma. *Psycho-Oncology, 17*(3), S27–S28.

Wood, M. J. M., Low, J., Molassiotis, A., & Tookman, A. (2013). Art therapy's contribution to the psychological care of adults with cancer: A survey of therapists and service users in the UK. *International Journal of Art Therapy, 18*(2), 42–53. doi:10.1080/17454832.2013.781657

Wood, M. J. M., & Molassiotis, A. (2011). What research evidence is there for the use of art therapy in the management of symptoms in adults with cancer? A systematic review. *Psycho-Oncology, 20*(2), 135-145.

KEY TERMS AND DEFINITIONS

Art Therapy: A therapeutic treatment modality that accommodates the opportunity for patients to make autonomous decisions, organize and structure these choices, and obtain a sense of control over personal artwork as well as therapeutic experiences.

Arts in Healing: The use of creative expression (arts forms) to gain understanding of emotions, thoughts and physical conditions in order to promote positive changes in a person's attitudes and health.

Collaborative Healthcare: Engaging patients and physicians by networking in a jointly defined community (i.e.; family, friends, medical caretakers, other patients, researchers) to increase the benefits of healthcare.

Creative Expression: Designing and creating artwork using a variety of media (forms) to communicate one's emotions, experiences, inspirations, and thoughts.

Health Locus of Control (HLOC): Attributions associated with an individual's perceived control over physical illnesses; accounts for the perception of which individuals consistently attribute their own health as a result of the environment or individual control (Hillen et al., 2014).

Mindfulness: A therapeutic strategy that calmly focuses a person's cognitive capacities on the present experiences, while recognizing emotions, thoughts and physical senses.

Perceived Control: Patients' healthcare attitudes that include personal decision making concerning treatment and patient/physician experiences.

Phenomenology: A theoretical orientation within the field of art therapy concerned with the perception of objects such as, works of art (Betensky, 1999).

Shared-Decision Making (SDM): Collaboratively and interactively engage patients and healthcare professionals in a joint decision-making process fostering trust and honesty in a positive working relationship.

Visual Journaling: Using visual art media (i.e.; collage, drawing, painting, photography, sketching) and writing to creatively record emotions and thoughts in a sketchbook or journal.

Chapter 3
HeartMath®: A University Initiative

Beth M. King
Florida Atlantic University, USA

Jo Ann M. Bamdas
Florida Atlantic University, USA

Charlotte D. Barry
Florida Atlantic University, USA

Kimberly Bronner
Florida Atlantic University, USA

Karethy A. Edwards
Florida Atlantic University, USA

ABSTRACT

HeartMath® is a program designed to build resilience and enhance coping skills in response to stress, challenges and adversity (Institute of HeartMath®, 2014) through self-regulation and the use of biofeedback technology. Many faculty from the Florida Atlantic University's Christine E. Lynn College of Nursing have become certified HeartMath® trainers and have committed to bring this program to their college community: Students, staff and faculty. This chapter describes HeartMath® and its implementation at the college. Exemplars are offered that explicate the value of the program and inspire the development of future initiatives within the University and broader community.

As I sat in the meeting listening to the requirements of a new faculty member, I could feel my anxiety building – my headache was pounding, and I was having difficulty swallowing. Would I ever be able to meet all these expectations, publish all those articles, find research money, and be a great teacher? Then I remembered, HeartMath®, and to BREATHE, change my emotional response, and recall the feel of my daughter's arms reaching around me and telling me how much she loved me. I continued to breathe and felt myself relax, bathed in the feeling of love that thinking about her gave me. I am a good teacher, I can write an article, I can get funding – my colleagues will help me.

Okay, I can do this – one step at a time. - Anonymous

DOI: 10.4018/978-1-5225-0640-9.ch003

INTRODUCTION

University educators, students, and healthcare professionals experience stress and anxiety on a daily basis and are challenged to develop strategies to enhance self-care and well-being for those they serve. The Christine E. Lynn College of Nursing (CON) at Florida Atlantic University (FAU) initiated a strategy to bring HeartMath® to the college. HeartMath® is a program designed to build resilience and enhance coping skills in response to stress, challenges, and adversity (Institute of HeartMath®, 2014) through the use of technology and self-regulation. The HeartMath® program originated from the HeartMath® Institute, a nonprofit organization based in California whose mission is to "help people bring their physical, mental, and emotional systems into balanced alignment with their heart's intuitive guidance" (HeartMath Institute, 2016, para 1). The program, based on self-regulation and self-management theory and biofeedback techniques, can be used in educational settings to better prepare healthcare professionals and all students to cope with stress and anxiety.

Two faculty members from the CON had attended the HeartMath® Institute in California and returned to the college with the intent to share their knowledge with students and to improve their own self-care. In the fall, 2014 a new FAU administration team arrived. They had utilized HeartMath® at their previous university and were aware of the outcomes HeartMath® interventions could provide: increased test scores and graduation rates and a strategy to cope with stress and anxiety. In the fall of 2014, the HeartMath® program was presented to the CON faculty and by spring 2015 a strategy to bring the certified trainer program to the CON and university was implemented. Twenty-three nursing faculty and key administrators and faculty from other departments and colleges were trained as Certified HeartMath® trainers in May of 2015. Since that time a strategic plan has been developed to fully implement the program at the CON and to extend the program to the broader university and community.

THEORETICAL FRAMEWORK

The theoretical framework guiding the introduction of HeartMath® into the CON's approach to caring for self and others is guided by three distinct yet unifying approaches to caring: The FAU CON philosophic framework, Bandura's (1991) social cognitive theory, and Grey, Schulman-Green, Knafl, and Reynolds (2015) self-management model. The usefulness of the three approaches provides a solid grounding and variable guidance for self-management interactions.

FAU CON Philosophic Framework

Nurturing the wholeness and well-being of others in caring is the focus of nursing at FAU (FAU, 2012). This definition guides the practice of nursing in which the nurse responds uniquely to the call for caring from the one nursed. This approach is patient/client focused, grounded in compassion, and draws on the broad knowledge base of the nurse, who provides care for the whole patient/client: mind, body, and soul. The nurse asks the patient/client "What matters most to you at this moment and how can I be helpful to you?" The verbal and/or written responses to the questions then form the essence of a plan of care directed toward nurturing the wholeness and wellbeing of the patient/client. In the authors' experience everyone has hopes and dreams of caring for themselves and of living a balanced life. Tenets of social cognition and self-regulation are helpful in supporting an individual's desire for living a coherent life in harmony with self, others, and the environment.

Self-Regulation Theory

Self-regulation, a conceptual domain within Bandura's (1990) social cognitive theory supports the tenets of the HeartMath® program. Self-regulation focuses on three principles to impact change in behavior: self-monitoring of one's own behavior, its determinants, and its effects, and judgment of one's behavior and affective response to the event. The success of self-regulation is based on the "fidelity, consistency and temporal proximity of self-monitoring" (Bandura, 1991, p. 250) along with a person's "beliefs that they can exert control over their motivation and behavior and over their social environment" (Bandura, 1990, p. 9).

Self-regulation theory supports the fundamental tenet of HeartMath®, which is that by learning to control one's emotions lies greater potential for positive health behavior change. HeartMath® includes a process of personal self-reflection of emotional energy draining and building events and the actions of heart-focused breathing techniques with positive affirmation and using self-monitoring equipment (emWave), which displays heart rate variability and coherence functioning.

Self-Management Model

Grey et al.'s (2015) self-management revised framework focuses on identification of facilitators and barriers to self-management, processes impacting self-management, and outcomes of self-management. The HeartMath® program promotes self-management by promoting the understanding of the psychological and physiological effects of stress and anxiety. The outcome is to empower the patient/client to manage stress and anxiety by utilizing the self-management techniques of HeartMath®.

HEARTMATH® PROGRAM

The HeartMath® program is multi-faceted: understanding the body's physiological and emotional response to stress and learning stress reduction techniques and emotional self-regulation. The program consists of (a) learning modules that describe the theory, research, and techniques related to the program; (b) learning activities that encourage self-reflection of energy draining and energy enhancing situations; (c) practice of paced heart-focused breathing techniques with emotional affirmations; and (d) demonstration and practice of the biofeedback/self-monitoring equipment (emWave), which displays HRV and coherence.

The outcomes of the program are focused on HRV and coherence and the ability to increase emotional self-regulation for the participants. HRV is a measure of cardiac autonomic innervation by the brain (Gorman & Sloan, 2000) and is an indicator of physiological resiliency and a person's ability to adapt to stress (Institute of HeartMath®, 2014). Heart rate coherence leads to an "optimal state for healing, learning, emotional transformation and peak performance" (Childre & Rozman, 2007, p. 45). Coherence also is described as "the degree of order, harmony, and stability among the various rhythmic activities in the body" (Bedell & Kaszkin-Bettag, 2010, p. 27) and is accompanied by "feelings of calmness, mental clarity and ease" (Thurber, Bodenhamer-Davis, Johnson, Chesky, & Chandler, 2010, p. 30).

According to Good and Zauszniewski (2014), HRV biofeedback was first studied by scientists in the Soviet Union in the 80s and represents the "interaction between the sympathetic and parasympathetic systems" (p. 154). Heart rate variability is the beat-to-beat changes within the heart based on the body's response to emotions and physiological changes. "It is the patterning of the rhythm (the ordering of changes in rate over time), rather than the rate (at any point in time), that is most directly related to emotional dynamics and physiological synchronization" (McCraty & Childre, 2010, p. 12).

Emotions have been identified as major contributors to physiological and psychological illness. This program utilizes positive emotions to increase HRV and coherence. Experiencing anew the positive feelings of being loved, appreciated, or affirmed, along with intentional paced breathing, are used to shift the body into a state of coherence in a stressful, emotional situation.

The first step of the program is to learn about the body's response to anxiety and stress: chaotic heart rate patterns, increased cortisol levels, and emotional turmoil. The stress response involves the neuroendocrine hypothalamic pituitary adrenal axis (HPA) and the autonomic nervous system (parasympathetic and sympathetic system). Understanding the physiological response to anxiety assists one to learn how to self-regulate responses to stress and anxiety.

The second step of the program is to ask the participant to reflect upon situations that are energy draining and energy renewing. Reflection allows for time to review what in life is depleting the energy level (physical and emotional) and/or energizing, such as work situations, relationships, school, and/or personal responsibilities. The other component of this step is to think about what steps might be taken to alter the energy depleting situations and to increase the energy renewing situations.

The third step is to have the participant learn heart-focused breathing and shifting of emotions to a positive/affirming affect. The participant focuses on the area of the heart and is asked to breath in and out through the heart, establishing a pace and depth comfortable for them. "Conscious regulation of one's respiration at a 10 seconds rhythm (0.1 HZ) increases cardiac coherence and starts the process of shifting into a more coherent state" (McCraty & Zayas, 2014, p. 10). At the same time, the individual needs to shift toward a positive emotion, which has been shown to increase cardiac coherence (McCraty & Zayas, 2014). This a very individual matter as the person must think of a situation in which he/she has experienced a positive/affirming emotion such as feelings of love, happiness. As the individual focuses on heart-focused paced breathing and feels the positive/affirming emotion, HRV increases and becomes more synchronized and coherent. This shift to positive/affirming emotion "induces enhancements in perception and cognition that enable more effective memory, reasoning, decision making, and action when confronted with stressful or challenging situations" (Bradley, Galvin, Atkinson, & Tomasino, 2012, p. 40).

Learning how to utilize the biofeedback equipment that aids in learning the breathing technique and HRV/coherence completes the final fourth step in the process. The emWave biofeedback equipment consists of a sensor placed on the ear, which transmits the heart rhythm to a computer and presents a visual picture of the level of coherence.

Through continued practice of the techniques, an individual can re-pattern the brain to a new set point in which the system strives to achieve (Bradley et al., 2012). By learning to regulate one's emotions in response to stress, the body's physiological response can be altered, which can lead to the potential for positive health behavior change and outcomes.

LITERATURE REVIEW

A growing body of literature describes the effectiveness of the HeartMath® program in a variety of settings and among diverse populations. This section focuses on HeartMath® studies in educational settings, in the broader community, and with healthcare professionals.

Educational Settings and HeartMath®

Studies using HeartMath® as an intervention have been conducted across the educational spectrum, from preschools to universities, by researchers seeking to improve student learning. This section describes the findings of several studies conducted with students, highlighting the effect of this program on stress reduction and student learning.

An adaptation of the HeartMath® program, called Early HeartSmarts (Institute of HeartMath®, 2014) has been implemented in pre-school and elementary school settings. Bradley et al. (2012) conducted a quasi-experimental longitudinal field study to examine the effectiveness of the program for pre-school children 3-6 years old. This program for children uses positive affirmation techniques called "Shift and Shine and Heart Warmer" to help children understand and regulate basic emotions. The intervention group was drawn from students in three classes (n=66). The children were identified as being from ethnic minorities and a lower socioeconomic class. The control group was drawn from 16 pre-school classes (n=309). Teachers with the intervention group were taught the program and implemented the techniques for one school year. The Creative Curriculum Assessment (TCCA) test (Bradley et al., 2012), which measures the four dimensions of social and emotional development, physical development, cognitive development, and language development, measured the efficacy of the program at baseline, pre-intervention, and post intervention. The researchers reported data analysis indicated significant differences between the intervention and control group on the TCCA, thus supporting the efficacy of the Early HeartSmarts program.

Another randomized control study by Lloyd, Brett, and Wesnes (2010) arrived at similar results, this time with children with a diagnosis of attention deficit hyperactivity disorder (n=38) in Grades 6 to 8. The student participants were taught HeartMath® techniques to increase their HRV and coherence. The researchers reported findings that indicated a significant improvement in behavior and cognitive functioning.

The HeartMath® techniques have had positive outcomes among college/university students. A major goal of the study by Edwards et al. (2009) was to increase the BSN graduation rates of undergraduate nursing students with the aim of improving the healthcare for minority and vulnerable underserved populations. Student participants received an intensive orientation that incorporated HeartMath® techniques and Buzan's mind mapping (as cited in Edwards et al., 2009); both techniques were utilized to enhance student cognitive performance. Following the second year of the program, the number of minority graduates increased from 45 to 70, of which 96% passed the NCLEX the first time (Edwards et al., 2012, p. 66).

Another study by Ratanasiripong, Sverduk, Prince, and Hayashino (2012) focused on 30 diverse students, ranging in age from 18-42, who were experiencing stress and anxiety and sought assistance from the university's counseling center. The students were randomly assigned to either the placebo group, which received four sessions of individual counseling, or to the treatment group, which received both individual counseling (four sessions) and four sessions of biofeedback. The biofeedback sessions involved learning breathing techniques to increase heart rate variability and coherence. The Beck Anxiety Inventory (as cited in Ratanasiripong, Sverduk et al., 2012) was administered both pre and post treatment. The researchers indicated that both the control group and treatment group had a significant reduction in anxiety symptoms, but the participants receiving the biofeedback training in addition to the counseling had a significantly higher mean improvement score, illustrating the power of biofeedback to increase heart rate variability and coherence.

The Thurber et al. (2010) study was similar in that the researchers used HRV, coherence, biofeedback training, and emotional self-regulation techniques with 14 college student musicians to see if music performance anxiety (MPA) would be improved. After a baseline performance, students were randomly assigned to either the control or treatment group. Assessment measurements included portions of the State-Trait Inventory, Flow State Scale, and Performance Anxiety Inventory in addition to HRV. The treatment group received four to five 1-hour training sessions, which included HRV coherence training and emotional regulation techniques. The researchers reported that data analysis indicated a significant statistical difference between the treatment and control group, and that biofeedback and emotional regulation techniques accounted for a large portion of the difference (Thurber et al., 2010, p. 33). In addition, the treatment group's average subjective MPA decreased 71% and their average subjective performance improved by 62% (Thurber et al., 2010, p. 1).

A similar study by Paul, Elam, and Vehulst (2007) investigated the use of deep breathing and focused mediation in decreasing the stress levels of minority students enrolled in a post baccalaureate program preparing students for the Medical College Admission Test (MCAT). As part of the curriculum, students were encouraged to use deep breathing, measured by the Heart Math Stress Management System and deep breathing mediation (DBM) as a stress management technique (as cited in Paul et al., 2007). The results of pre and posttests and the follow-up survey indicated that students experienced a decrease in test anxiety, decrease in self-doubt, and an increase in ability to concentrate. The researchers reported a major study limitation was the lack of direct measurement and observation data and the use of self-reported perceptions. Despite the limitations, the students report is rich with meaning. They reported "they believed DBM would be helpful in medical school and as a physician; they also anticipated using it in the future" (Paul et al., 2007, p. 290).

Finally, a randomized control study by Ratanasiripong, Ratanasiripong, and Kathalae (2012) investigated the use of biofeedback as an intervention to reduce the stress and anxiety levels of 60 second-year nursing students in a college in Thailand. The intervention group received two training programs on the use of biofeedback equipment and regulation of HRV and was instructed to utilize the equipment three times each day over a 5-week period. Pre and post surveys were conducted using the Perceived Stress Scale and the State Anxiety Scale (as cited in Ratanasiripong, Ratanasiripong, et al., 2012). The investigators reported findings indicating that students utilizing the biofeedback equipment had a significant reduction in anxiety.

Each of the empirical studies described previously shows positive correlations to HeartMath® tools and technique that increase coherence among various populations in several types of educational settings. Biofeedback, regulation of HRV, deep breathing, and emotional self-regulation provide successful tools to aid in lowering anxiety and stress levels.

Broader Community and HeartMath®

In addition to educational settings, HeartMath® techniques have been successful with adults in the workplace. McCraty, Atkinson, and Tomasino (2003) examined the impact of a workplace stress management program with 32 employees with high blood pressure. Randomly assigned, the treatment group received a 16-hour program on emotional regulation and the use of biofeedback equipment to learn to regulate HRV and coherence. Data measurements included blood pressure measurements and a psychological survey, the Personal and Organizational Quality Assessment (POQA) tool. Both the treatment and control group experienced a reduction in blood pressure, but the systolic blood pressure reduction in the treatment group was significantly larger ($p<.05$) than the control group. The data were obtained every week for four weeks and post three months after the program. The researchers measured both blood pressure and emotional health, finding that both systolic and diastolic blood pressure decreased by an average of 10 points. The POAQ results showed a significant improvement in the indicators of well being and organizational effectiveness.

Lastly, in 2007, a whole community located in Grinnell, Iowa, initiated a program titled, The Heart of Grinnell: A Community – Wide Rural Health Wellness Initiative. The objectives were to increase community coherence, improve morale, and increase wellness behaviors within the community. Local colleges, schools, churches, businesses, social service agencies, government, and hospital were part of this initiative. Community-wide training in stress reduction technique and coherence using HeartMath® techniques were initiated (Linden, Jackson, Rutledge, Nath, & Lof, 2010).

Healthcare Professionals and HeartMath®

Healthcare professionals experience stress routinely in practice. The random controlled study by Lemaire, Wallace, Lewin, de Grood, and Schaefer (2011) demonstrated the value of the HeartMath® program. They examined the use of a biofeedback stress management intervention and reduction in the stress levels of 40 physicians at a tertiary care center. The intervention group received an introduction to the biofeedback device and a training session on the use of quick coherence methodology. They were instructed to use the devise for 28 days at least three times each day for five minutes. In addition, the participants completed 15 items from the Perceived Stress Scale and 25 items from the POQA-revised questionnaire. Other measures included heart rate, blood pressure, and cortisol levels. The findings reported revealed that the intervention group experienced a significant reduction in stress ($p=0.013$).

The HeartMath® program research indicates measurable differences in quality of life, stress levels, and increased emotional self-regulation within a variety of settings and among diverse populations. The ability to teach these techniques to adults and children alike, combined with the relative ease of practice, creates an exciting field to develop for the world of health, wellness, and disease prevention.

COLLEGE OF NURSING: IMPLEMENTATION OF THE HEARTMATH® PROGRAM

Healthcare professionals practice within an environment that can be stressful and filled with day-to-day challenges such as unpredictable health crises, time constraints, and institutional pressures. By implementing the techniques of HeartMath®, faculty and nursing students in the CON have examined their response to stress and anxiety, communication with each other, and their HRV and coherence.

The journey began with two faculty members who became certified as HeartMath® trainers. This, in turn, led to an invitation to the entire nursing faculty to participate in a week-long training program to become Certified HeartMath® trainers. Many of the faculty responded to the invitation, along with key leaders throughout the university. The HeartMath® Institute trainers and two CON certified HeartMath® trainers presented the week-long program and pre-preparation prior to the sessions. The trainers met with all participants at least three times prior to the week-long training to review the materials. All participants were encouraged to practice the stress reduction and resilience building techniques prior to the week-long class. Since that time, faculty continue to practice the techniques at the beginning of meetings and during stressful situations.

Today, students receive an overview of the HeartMath® program at their respective orientation programs, and then each are encouraged to utilize the technique to assist with stress and anxiety and to build their resilience capacity. Courses throughout the undergraduate and graduate program utilize HeartMath® prior to exams, during clinical practice, and stressful activities. However, no formative or summative assessments have been developed at this time. In addition, specific courses review the components of the HeartMath® program. For example, the undergraduate students review the HeartMath® program during the *Psychiatric Mental Health Nursing* course and then are encouraged to utilize the techniques with clients in clinical practice. In addition, the *Creative Healing Environment* course encourages the practice of the HeartMath® techniques as students are completing their studies and are preparing to enter the nursing profession.

The following exemplar provides one nursing student's perception of the usefulness of HeartMath® in her life:

As a BSN student at the Christine E. Lynn College of Nursing, I became familiar with HeartMath® as part of my education and practice. As a class, we are introduced to HeartMath at the beginning of the nursing program, and we are encouraged by faculty to use it whenever we feel it could be beneficial for ourselves, or our patients, in the clinical setting.

My introduction to HeartMath was a welcome change of pace from the usual rigor of nursing school. As a class, students were asked to visualize a time when we were honestly at peace and felt total contentment. We were encouraged to creatively express these peaceful settings and share them with one another. My peaceful place is in my parent's home where I grew up, at the dinner table with my extended family looking at everyone's faces and all of the wonderful food my mom makes. With these pictures in our minds, we were guided to find a comfortable position focus on our heart and breathe deeper and slower The energy in the room changed quickly. After a few deep breaths, we were led to maintain that feeling of contentment in our minds and, in addition, visualize breathing into our heart with warm, deep breaths. I had never felt so relaxed at school. This practice is a gift.

We then, as a group, were able to take turns using the HeartMath® monitor with our results on the screen above for the class to share. This was an excellent way to demonstrate how the relaxed feelings we experienced translated into tangible and favorable changes within our vital signs. Even as new nursing students, we were able to appreciate the impact within ourselves on a personal level and, in addition, see the beneficial effects this simple practice could bring to others.

Since having this gratifying introduction to HeartMath®, we are continuously invited to take some time for ourselves before stressful situations within [the] nursing school and utilize those same techniques. Our professors will encourage a few moments of HeartMath® before an exam or presentation. During stressful clinicals we are able to call on this skill to really prohibit stress from taking over our bodies and our minds. We are also able to encourage our patients who may need peace to take a moment, visualize a place of contentment, close their eyes, and breathe into their hearts.

In addition, faculty has embraced the technique and utilizes HeartMath® for self-care and faculty coherence. The faculty begin their meetings utilizing the quick coherence technique of heart focused breathing and activation of a positive or renewing feeling which can lead to more coherence and receptivity at the meetings.

Building upon the success of the HeartMath® program within the CON, the program continues to grow in the university and in the broader community. The following exemplars demonstrate the value of the HeartMath® program.

UNIVERSITY: IMPLEMENTATION OF THE HEARTMATH® PROGRAM

Owls Care Health Promotion Program

The Director of the Owls Care Health Promotion program was familiar with the HeartMath® program and attended the HeartMath® Certified Trainer program. The Healthy Owls program (FAU, 2014) is located on campus, easily accessible to students, and offers many programs related to health promotion including a variety of stress management programs. While the Owls Care Health Promotion program already had the biofeedback equipment for HeartMath®, utilization of the program with students increased following the program. The director reported students find that the program helps with feelings of anxiety and stress.

Florida Atlantic University Police Department

The deputy chief of the Florida Atlantic University Police Department participated in the HeartMath® program and planned to implement the program with fellow officers. He expressed the following about the program, "I'm more cognizant of who I am, what's going on internally, and how I can translate that to the outside . . . HeartMath® resets your internal battery, making you more aware of your emotions, and helps you learn what's depleting you and what's energizing you" (Weeks, 2015).

COMMUNITY: IMPLEMENTATION OF HEARTMATH®

This section of the chapter describes the use of HeartMath® with community partners at a local school, orientation programs for school nurses, and with other departments within the university.

School Nurses

HeartMath® was an integral component of a School Nurse Orientation and Back to School continuing education program in the summer of 2015. Approximately 160 Florida school nurses participated in an introduction to HeartMath® techniques for stress reduction and finding balance within the context of a busy school-based health center and other life commitments.

The session began with instructions and demonstration of heart-focused paced breathing. After demonstrating the technique, the nurses were invited to try it as the instructor led in a slow rhythmic timed pattern. After three rounds of this intentional paced breathing, the nurses were invited to recall a time and feeling when each felt loved, cared for, or generally at peace. Once again the instructor led heart-focused paced breathing, but this time the school nurses were invited to simultaneously experience anew the recollection of feeling acknowledged, affirmed, loved, or at peace. This emotional shift and paced breathing leads to increased HRV and coherence. The school nurses said they felt relaxed, felt the power of HeartMath®, and said they would use it.

Local Elementary Schools

A faculty member was invited to help 3rd graders prepare for the Florida Comprehensive Assessment Test (FCAT). The principal explained that it was the 3rd graders' first experience with taking the test and the first time students could be retained in a grade depending on their test scores.

HeartMath® was introduced as a onetime presentation with an interactive lecture and slide presentation by FAU CON faculty. The idea of how feeling anxious could block one's memory was explained and how the instructor had a great technique to help them with their memory while taking the test. Paced heart-focused breathing was demonstrated and the students all practiced it. Then the students were asked to recall a time that each felt really happy or to think of something that made them feel very happy, like having ice cream or getting a kiss from Mommy. The students each shared a happy time and were instructed to remember it when they felt stumped on a test question. They were told that feeling the happy time would open up their memory and they would know the answer to the test question. The session concluded with playing the song *Happy* (Williams, 2013) and everyone got up and danced to it. The session ended on a very uplifting note and the principal reported that the 3rd graders had the highest scores on the FCAT that the school had ever seen.

Community Nurse Partners

Quarterly, community nurse leaders meet with the administrators of the CON. Knowing the value of the HeartMath® program, we were anxious to share the value of the program with the leaders of local community hospitals and agencies. A PowerPoint presentation with a demonstration of the techniques was presented in fall, 2015. Following the program, several leaders indicated an interest in the program and thought it would be beneficial for their employees and agencies.

FUTURE PLANS: INTERPROFESSIONAL EDUCATION AND COLLABORATIVE PRACTICE PROGRAM

At FAU, the Christine E. Lynn College of Nursing, the Charles E. Schmidt College of Medicine, and the School of Social Work in the College of Design and Social Inquiry implemented an Interprofessional Education (IPE) and Collaborative Practice (IPECP) program five years ago. Jacomino, Bamdas, Keller, Hamlin, Hawkins, Gordon, and Ouslander (2015) describes the FAU Office of Interprofessional Education's IPE program and outcome of meeting this accreditation standard for the American Association of Colleges of Nursing, Association of American Medical Colleges, and American Association of Colleges of Pharmacy. These interprofessional education programs offer a fertile context for student growth as a professional. The HeartMath® program teaches techniques to achieve coherence in one's professional and personal life.

Suggestions for Creating Space for HeartMath®

Creating space for HeartMath® is a valuable initiative for the IPE and IPECP program. The benefits of this program for both faculty and student include improved academic performance and enhanced emotional and physiological coherence.

One possibility for including HeartMath® is expanding and enhancing existing relationships between the CON, College of Medicine, and the School of Social Work within the Office of Interprofessional Education, hosted in the Provost's Office and supported by each college's dean and administrative levels. Students as well as faculty suffer stress-related situations needing coping strategies every day, from having to juggle classes and the IPE program, clinical rotations, and field internship experiences. Having faculty certified as HeartMath® trainers to work with the IPE program will secure the space for the implementation of this program. This initial training then transfers throughout the university and its broad community base as the IPE program and other IPE-inspired and expanded programming moves forward. The plan for the next five years is to expand IPECP initiatives further, and HeartMath® would be an exemplary initiative for faculty and students.

Another way to expand the reach of HeartMath® is to invite nursing students who have been trained and use HeartMath® to become leaders for the other students and faculty in the other professions. The literature review also describes the successful implementation of Heart Math® in other venues and offers practical approaches to extend the HeartMath® program.

The interprofessional education program has a captive audience each academic year when approximately 250 students enter a program that is designed to take place over six face-to-face visits either at the university with team members or with older members of the community and their teams in the older adult's home environment. Faculty attends facilitator training and students learn about the competencies of IPECP. While we have the students and faculty in sessions, we could schedule time to introduce HeartMath® techniques which initiate self-reflection of energy draining and energy enhancing personal and professional situations. For example, students who are focused on gaining professional competence, share that they prefer to be out in the "real world" rather than studying or working together in classroom practice situations. Trained faculty could listen to their concerns and help them understand the fullness of "helping professions' competency" includes caring for the whole person both self and patient/client. During brief pauses in the IEP sessions, one or two activities could be used to encourage self-reflection and facilitate direction inward.

Students and faculty also can be guided into practicing breathing techniques and emotional shifts, components of the HeartMath® program. Incorporating HeartMath® for students and faculty in classes and in outside programs can provide a space for building self-awareness where there can be found times and places to cope with stress and to circumvent the chaotic emotions in which students and faculty sometimes find themselves embroiled.

HeartMath® promotes better learning and performance. At the beginning of sessions or even within a blended learning environment, students could be prompted with breathing exercises and remembrances to be reflective practitioners. With multi-media today, creative solutions such as apps, software, tools, and techniques recommended by HeartMath® and other digital health companies can be placed on Blackboard sites. No synchronous or asynchronous environment is too small a space for faculty, staff, and students to locate stress and anxiety-reducing techniques. These environments provide spaces where program directors and trainers can show how better learning and performance can be attained with the tools and techniques of HeartMath®. Learning and performance promotion do not have to happen in face-to-face settings but can be incorporated into online courses too.

In addition, although at times stressful, the IPE sessions afford chances for sustained well-being and positive feelings of care over time while students collaborate either with their team members in face-to-face groups or with their volunteer mentors. When students are in-step and in-tune with one another, then health and wellness is felt both individually and by the group members.

Since students learn how to work together as a team and to communicate with each other on interpersonal and intrapersonal levels, programs such as team-based learning in IPECP programs build many opportunities for self-regulation and self-management. Once found and developed over the course of a university education and in clinical practice, the positive feelings that emerge and the excitement that something like this works can be transferred over time into the community when students move to healthcare professions.

Part of the HeartMath® training includes a section on "authentic communication." In this case, communication means how to enhance relationships and reduce stress after conflict negotiation and outcomes of miscommunication. University students begin learning communication problems in their fields. The nursing students are steeped in *Team Strategies and Tools to Enhance Performance and Patient Safety (TeamSTEPPS™)* from the Agency for Healthcare Research Quality (AHRQ, 2016). The mission of the AHRQ is to produce evidence to make healthcare safer, higher quality, more accessible, equitable, and affordable. A component of AHRQ's initiatives is the TeamSTEPPS training, tools, and techniques. TeamSTEPPS (AHRQ, 2016) is a teamwork system designed for healthcare professionals to improve communication and teamwork skills.

Areas of authentic communication are needed and would be well served by HeartMath® when undertaking discussions of diversity, bias, and stereotyping. These are highly sensitive topics often inducing conflict, anxiety, and stress. A recent example of polypharmacy situations that endanger patient safety illustrates diversity in communication that is somewhat unthinkingly disregarded as unnecessary discussion. A nursing professor was at a seminar with students in medicine, nursing, social work, and pharmacy and told the following situation: Dr. Susan said that she had sat in on discussions between an interprofessional healthcare team and a woman who could only speak Spanish and her son who was trilingual and listened and spoke for his mother. The team told Mrs. Hernandez and her son William that she had to take one medicine *doce* times a day. At the end of the week Mrs. Hernandez fell ill and was rushed to the hospital. When the team saw her again in the hospital, they discovered that the patient had taken a dose of *12* pills. By not clarifying and accounting for the discussion about dose/*doce,* a lack of comprehending instructions and mixed linguistic messages and meaning ended up negatively affecting patient safety. Fortunately, Mrs. Hernandez received proper care in time. Many patient safety issues can be connected to avoidance – avoiding uncomfortable areas of communication with diverse populations and lack of language awareness. This area of concern or risk assessment for patient safety remains a largely untapped area of education and research that would be well served by interprofessional education and collaborative practices with tools and techniques of HeartMath® led by experienced certified trainers and willing partners. Along with TeamSTEPPS® and other types of programs that focus on interpersonal communication with non-verbal clues and enhanced listening techniques, situations like the one described can be eliminated early. Also, when these types of programs are placed in interprofessional educative programs, a more in-depth understanding of interpersonal communication arises. By adding authentic communication to an IPECP program for nursing, medicine, and social work students, the IPECP program with training using HeartMath® can provide payback to students, faculty, staff, facilitators, and trainers, which will broaden effective educational programs.

HeartMath® at our university with certified HeartMath® faculty, students, and staff creates partnerships with the community to reach out to different settings and different populations to go beyond the university's promotion of health, wellness, and fitness. An example of community outreach with HeartMath® program within our immediate university's campuses is health and wellness organizations that can offer space and participants with whom our certified HeartMath® trainers can promote a healthy attitude. One center close by seeks to help older adults within an adult day care program. This same center could be a significant placement for a HeartMath® trainer to train others who, in turn, also will become HeartMath® providers. Numerous facilities are open to partnership with our university to incorporate HeartMath®, including adults in independent living facilities and community centers where our university students can meet aging populations. These older adults may have numerous mental and physical challenges that may induce anxiety and invoke the need for authentic communication, along with the other HeartMath® tools and techniques. The possibilities of university-community partnerships for implementation of the HeartMath ® program are limited only by imagination.

SUMMARY

The HeartMath® program was embraced by the FAU administration and the CON and has branched out into the university at large and into our broader community. A great opportunity exists for partnering with other faculty, students, organizations, and community partners to study and research the impact of HeartMath® on the health and well being of each one. As we have shown in this chapter, HeartMath® offers numerous positive benefits. Educational settings and educators trained in the tools and techniques of HeartMath® open vast spaces and opportunities to affect positive change in reducing anxiety and stress, increasing coping skills, and increasing resilience for students, faculty, healthcare professionals and individuals within our communities.

REFERENCES

Agency for Healthcare Research Quality. (2016). *Team STEPPS 2.0.* Retrieved from http://www.ahrq.gov/professionals/education/curriculum-tools/teamstepps/instructor/index.html

Bandura, A. (1990). Perceived self-efficacy in the exercise of control over AIDS infection. *Evaluation and Program Planning*, *13*(1), 9–17. doi:10.1016/0149-7189(90)90004-G

Bandura, A. (1991). Social cognitive theory of self-regulation. *Organizational Behavior and Human Decision Processes*, *50*(2), 248–287. doi:10.1016/0749-5978(91)90022-L

Bedell, W., & Kaszkin-Bettag, M. (2010). Coherence and health care cost-RCA actuarial study: A cost effectiveness cohort study. *The Journal of Alternative Therapies*, *16*(4), 26–31. PMID:20653293

Bradley, R. T., Galvin, P., Atkinson, M., & Tomasino, D. (2012). Efficacy of an emotional self-regulation program for promoting development in preschool children. *Global Advances in Health and Medicine*, *1*(1), 36–50. doi:10.7453/gahmj.2012.1.1.010 PMID:24278801

Center for Advancement of Interprofessional Education. (2016). *The definition and principles of interprofessional education.* Retrieved from http://caipe.org.uk/about-us/the-definition-and-principles-of-interprofessional-education/

Childre, D., & Rozman, D. (2007). *Transforming depression. The HeartMath® solution to feeling overwhelmed, sad, and stressed.* Oakland, CA: New Harbinger.

Edwards, K., Radcliffe, S., Patchell, B., Broussard, K., Wood, E., & Ogans, J. (2009). Outcomes: The recruitment enhancement cultural affirmation project. *Journal of Cultural Diversity*, *16*(2), 64–67.

Florida Atlantic University. (2012). *Christine E. Lynn College of Nursing philosophy.* Retrieved http://nursing.fau.edu/index.php?main=1&nav=635

Florida Atlantic University. (2014). *Owls care health promotion.* Retrieved from http://www.fau.edu/owlscare/

Florida Atlantic University. (2016). *Office of Interprofessional Education.* Retrieved http://fau.edu/provost/academic-affairs/interprofessional-education.php

Good, M., & Zauszniewski, J. A. (2014). Biofeedback. In R. Lindquist, M. Snyder, & M. F. Tracy (Eds.), *Complementary & alternative therapies in nursing* (pp. 153–166). New York, NY: Springer Publishing Company.

Gorman, J. M., & Sloan, R. P. (2000). Heart rate variability in depressive and anxiety disorders. *American Heart Journal*, *140*(4Suppl.), 77–83. doi:10.1067/mhj.2000.109981 PMID:11011352

Grey, M., Schulman-Green, D., Knafl, K., & Reynolds, N. R. (2015). A revised self-and family management framework. *Nursing Outlook*, *63*(2), 162–170. doi:10.1016/j.outlook.2014.10.003 PMID:25771190

HeartMath® Institute. (2016). *HeartMath Institute's mission and vision.* Retrieved from https://www.heartmath.org/about-us/hmi-mission/

Institute of HeartMath®. (2014). *The resilience advantage: Skills for personal and professional effectiveness.* Boulder Creek, CA: Institute of HeartMath®.

Interprofessional Education Collaborative. (2011). *Core competencies for interprofessional collaborative practice: Report of an expert panel.* Retrieved from http://www.aacn.nche.edu/education-resources/ipecreport.pdf

Jacomino, M., Bamdas, J. M., Keller, K., Hamlin, E., Hawkins, M., Gordon, S., & Ouslander, J. (2015). An innovative interprofessional education program for university medical, nursing, and social work students learning in teams during sessions and visits with geriatric mentors. *Journal of Interprofessional Education & Practice*, *1*(3-4), 100–103. doi:10.1016/j.xjep.2015.10.003

Lemaire, J. B., Wallace, J. E., Lewin, A. M., de Grood, J., & Schaefer, J. P. (2011). The effect of a biofeedback-based stress management tool on physician stress: A randomized controlled clinical trial. *Open Medicine*, *5*(4), E154–E163. PMID:22567069

Linden, T. C., Jackson, C., Rutledge, S., Nath, C., & Lof, L. N. (2010). The heart of Grinnell: A community–wide rural health wellness initiative: A pilot observational study and a prospective study design. *The Journal of Alternative Therapies*, *16*(4), 46–49. PMID:20653295

Lloyd, A., Brett, D., & Wesnes, K. (2010). Coherence training in children with attention-deficit hyperactivity disorder: Cognitive functions and behavioral changes. *Alternatives Therapies*, *16*(4), 34–42. PMID:20653294

McCraty, R., Atkinson, M., & Tomasino, D. (2003). Impact of a workplace stress reduction program on blood pressure and emotional health in hypertensive employees. *Journal of Alternative and Complementary Medicine*, *9*(3), 355–369. doi:10.1089/107555303765551589 PMID:12816624

McCraty, R., & Childre, D. (2010). Coherence: Bridging personal, social and global health. *The Journal of Alternative Therapies*, *16*(4), 10–22. PMID:20653292

McCraty, R., & Zayas, M. A. (2014). Cardiac coherence, self-regulation, autonomic stability, and psychosocial well-being. *Frontiers in Psychology*, *5*, 1–12. doi:10.3389/fpsyg.2014.01090 PMID:25324802

Paul, G., Elam, B., & Vehulst, S. (2007). A longitudinal study of student's perceptions of using deep breathing meditation to reduce testing stress. *Teaching and Learning in Medicine: An International Journal*, *19*(3), 287–292. doi:10.1080/10401330701366754 PMID:17594225

Ratanasiripong, P., Ratanasiripong, N., & Kathalae, D. (2012). Biofeedback intervention for stress and anxiety among nursing students: A randomized controlled study. *International Scholarly Research Network*. Retrieved from http://www.heartmath.com/wp-content/uploads/2014/04/biofeedback_intervention_stress_nursing_students.pdf

Ratanasiripong, P., Sverduk, K., Prince, J., & Hayashino, D. (2012). Biofeedback and counseling for stress and anxiety among college students. *Journal of College Student Development*, *53*(5), 742–749. doi:10.1353/csd.2012.0070

Thurber, M. R., Bodenhamer-Davis, E., Johnson, M., Chesky, K., & Chandler, C. (2010). Effects of heart rate variability coherence biofeedback training and emotional management techniques to decrease music performance anxiety. *Biofeedback*, *38*(1), 28–39. doi:10.5298/1081-5937-38.1.28

Weeks, K. (2015). *University initiatives: FAU implements university-wide HeartMath training*. Retrieved from http://www.fau.edu/newsdesk/articles/university-wide-heartmath-training.php

Williams, P. (2013). *Happy. On Despicable Me 2 (Movie soundtrack)*. New York, NY: Columbia Record.

KEY TERMS AND DEFINITIONS

Coherence: The degree of order, harmony, and stability among the various rhythmic activities in the body (Bedell & Kaszkin-Bettag, 2010, p. 27).

HeartMath®: A program designed to build resilience and enhance coping skills in response to stress, challenges, and adversity (Institute of HeartMath®, 2014).

Heart Rate Variability (HRV): HRV is the heart beat-to-beat changes based on the body's response to emotions and physiological changes (Institute of HeartMath®, 2014).

Interprofessional Education (IPE/IPECP): Interprofessional Education and Interprofessional Collaborative Practice go hand and hand and terms that are used often interchangeably. IPE/IPECP is defined as a process that occurs when two or more professions learn with, from, and about each other to improve collaboration and the quality of patient care (Centre for the Advancement of Interprofessional Education, 2002).

Resilience: The capacity to prepare for, recover from, and adapt in the face of stress, challenge, and adversity (Institute of HeartMath®, 2014).

Self-Regulation: Self-monitoring of one's own behavior, its determinants and its effects; and judgment of one's behavior and affective response to the event (Institute of HeartMath®, 2014).

Chapter 4
A Need for Greater Collaboration:
Initiatives to Improve Transitions of Care

Mariette Sourial
Palm Beach Atlantic University, USA

Angelica Constanzo
University of Kansas Hospital, USA

Jo Ann M. Bamdas
Florida Atlantic University, USA

Marina E. Ishak
Palm Beach Atlantic University, USA

ABSTRACT

Patient safety concerns have risen to such levels that multiple organizations and initiatives have been created to reduce hospital readmissions and medication errors in the United States healthcare system. Interprofessional education and collaborative practice (IPECP) has become a center of focus in health-care education and the competency-based programs help health providers function more effectively as a team, train new university and college healthcare students to become ready for collaborative practice, and assist in making new policies and practices to improve today's healthcare system. This chapter provides a comprehensive overview of healthcare initiatives created to help lower hospital readmission rates and polypharmacy errors. These projects, programs, and initiatives optimize patient care while minimizing costs. With pharmacists, physicians, nurses, social workers, and other professionals and caregivers build better teams with improved communication and understanding each other's roles and responsibilities, the global healthcare system will overcome the numerous challenges.

INTRODUCTION

A Patient's Story

TP is a 78-year old African American female who presented to the hospital complaining of shortness of breath. Her shortness of breath in addition to throbbing headaches began a few days ago and worsened today, for which she was admitted. Her past medical history is significant for hypertension, reduced ejection fraction heart failure, non-valvular atrial fibrillation, and hypothyroidism. Patient denies smoking

DOI: 10.4018/978-1-5225-0640-9.ch004

or using illicit drug. She reported compliant with her medications and was taking the following, which were written on a piece of a paper: lisinopril 10 mg by mouth daily, carvedilol 6.25 mg by mouth twice daily, furosemide 80 mg by mouth twice daily, diltiazem hydrochloride 120 mg by mouth once daily, rivaroxaban 15 mg by mouth daily, and levothyroxine 75 mcg by mouth every morning. Her pulse upon admission varied from 151 to 92 and her blood pressure between 144/76 mmHg to 160/91 mmHg. Her serum creatinine was 1.9 and her blood urea nitrogen was 35 (her baseline was a serum creatinine of 1.7). Other pertinent labs were within normal limits. ECG showed atrial fibrillation with rapid ventricular response. Upon hospitalization, some of her medication regimens were changed – carvedilol was increased to 12.5 mg by mouth twice daily, lisinopril was decreased to 5 mg by mouth once daily, and furosemide 80 mg by mouth once daily was switched to bumetanide 1 mg by mouth once daily. The discharge instructions were provided by the healthcare team, yet the patient could not recall the discussion. She was confused with regard to the complexity of her medical conditions and the changes in her medication regimen, which were necessary for her post-discharge home care.

Two days later, the patient was readmitted to the hospital with similar symptoms. Upon further discussion, it appears that the patient was confused in her medication regimens and was taking her medications inappropriately. Luckily, she had brought with her the medication bottles, and was referred to the clinical pharmacist for medication reconciliation. The patient was taking carvedilol 12.5 mg by mouth twice daily along with her original regimen of 6.25 mg by mouth twice daily, for a total of 18.75 mg by mouth twice daily. We also discovered that the rivaroxaban 15 mg required prior authorization, but she was going off a physician sample that had a few pills left. Her diltiazem bottle was found to be emptied and dated since last month. When asked, the patient claimed it did not have refills and she had not had been able to visit her cardiologist yet.

Problem

TP's story powerfully reminds the importance of safe and effective transitions of care. She left the healthcare setting without being fully able to care for her conditions due to the lack of appropriate education based on her level of understanding and to gaps in communication between the healthcare providers. In order to be proactive in her own care, TP could have used a notebook to write down important information for discussion with her healthcare providers.

Predominantly, communication gaps are one of the major causes of ineffective transitions of care. Healthcare providers may not communicate information completely between the members of the team, to the patient, or their caregivers. Various risk factors that may contribute to such communication breakdowns include different expectations between senders and receivers, a culture that lacks teamwork and respect, a culture that does not promote a successful hand-off, inadequate time, and lack of standardized procedures (The Joint Commission, Joint Commission Center for Transforming Healthcare, & Joint Commission Resources, n.d.).

Secondly, a patient's level of understanding of the provided education is another major challenge in transitions of care. The patient's understanding can affect the way their health is managed. Sometimes, patients and caregivers receive conflicting information about their health, are excluded from the decision making, and are confused in their medication regimens, as seen in this patient. TP had multiple comorbid conditions and was taking multiple medications with various dosing regimens, placing her at risk for medication errors. Patients and caregivers sometimes are also excluded from the decisions making. Furthermore, unclear instructions related to timely follow-up may pose an obstacle to the patient's health (The Joint Commission et al., n.d.).

Solution

This story provides several examples of many real world polypharmacy problems occurring daily. This unfortunate readmission could have been prevented with a proper and accurate medication history as well as improved communication among health professionals. A healthcare team including a physician, nurse, pharmacist, and others as appropriate also should include the patient in their decision making. Furthermore, the team should collaborate with effective communication techniques from the moment the patient enters into their care. Each member of a healthcare team needs to be held accountable for ensuring that the patient's healthcare needs are coordinated and met across the different settings. While the healthcare team is accountable for the care of the patient, the patient also has the responsibility of taking care of their own health. Each of the various professionals are entrusted with a unique body of knowledge that they use in practice. For example, pharmacists in TP's case should have looked at her medication therapy and should have ensured that the prescribed medications indicated for her medical conditions were safe, effective, affordable, and that TP could adhere to the regimen.

Other topics of concern needing solutions for this patient center on patient education, on the patient's voice in decision making, and on discharge planning. Appropriate patient education given at the level of TP's understanding should have been done for her medications and medical conditions. A great need exists for the healthcare team to empower and hear the patient's voice and place them at the core of any health decision making. Moreover, proper discharge planning is needed with steps taken to ensure that the patient has sufficient knowledge and understanding of their medical condition and care plan as well as access to contact information and follow up. These areas of concern addressed are just a few that can lead to many preventable readmissions; this stresses the need for better coordination of care with all team members participating across settings to save costs as well as improve the quality and safety of patient care.

Implications

It is important to understand the term care transition or transitions of care. According to the American Society of Health System Pharmacists (ASHP, 2016), a resource for pharmacists, student pharmacists, and others, the term care transitions:

… is the movement of a patient from one setting of care to another. In concert with physicians, nurses, and others who contribute to the overall medical care of patients, pharmacists optimize medication therapy that translates into improved outcomes, reduced readmissions, and the overall goal of improved quality of life for patients.

According to Coleman and Boult (2003), the American Geriatrics Society published a position statement defining transitional care as a "set of actions designed to ensure the coordination and continuity of healthcare as patients transfer between different locations or different levels of care within the same location" (p. 556).

In a study by Jencks, Williams, and Coleman (2009), almost one fifth of the Medicare patients who had been discharged from a hospital were rehospitalized within 30 days. During transitions of care patients become vulnerable, especially to medication-related errors. In a study conducted by Foster, Murff, Peterson, Gandhi, and Bates (2003), nearly one out of five patients experienced an adverse drug event post discharge, ranging from abnormal laboratory findings to permanent disabilities (pp. 164-165). During hospitalization, drugs may be added or discontinued from a patient's medication regimen or dosing may be altered. A systematic review by Tam et al. (2005) revealed that 10-67% of patients had at least one error in their prescription medication histories (p. 511). Patients with complex medical conditions often find themselves cared for in many different healthcare settings and/or see different practitioners. Despite collaborative care teams, communication can be less than ideal. In an acute care setting, hospitalists often focus on the critical diagnosis while deferring chronic disease management to the patient's primary care provider. Several studies discussed later explore the use a transitional care pharmacist and demonstrate the benefit of pharmacist involvement in the continuum of care process. Incorporating accurate medication reconciliation into hospital practice improves transitions of care, yet chart reviews reveal that over half of all hospital medication errors occur at the interfaces of care (Rozich & Resar, 2001). To address deficiencies, cooperative systems should be put in place between different settings and professionals.

PATIENT PROTECTION AND AFFORDABLE CARE ACT

Under the Patient Protection and Affordable Care Act (2010), new financial incentives and penalties have been implemented to optimize the healthcare system and improve patient outcomes. One important initiative through the Centers for Medicare & Medicaid Services (CMS, 2016b) has been Medicare's Hospital Readmissions Reduction Program (HRRP), which began in October 2012. This program penalizes hospitals with excess unplanned 30-day readmissions for *initial* hospitalization. The penalties apply due to specific health conditions such as pneumonia, heart attacks, heart failure, chronic obstructive pulmonary disease, and hip/knee replacement regardless of whether the patient was readmitted to the same or another hospital as well as regardless of the reason for the readmission. The reduction in Medicare payments for Inpatient Prospective Payment System (IPPS) hospitals has been increasing each year, with a 1% reduction in 2013, 2% in 2014, and 3% in 2015 (CMS, 2016b). Thus, the main focus of several hospitals has been to lower those readmission rates. In turn, new opportunities have been created for collaboration among healthcare providers and even at the education level among students of various healthcare disciplines. Hospitals work at improving their discharge processes such as creating patient-friendly educational health videos, printing patient-tailored brochures, and incorporating transitional care initiatives to follow-up post-discharge either through phone calls or with a visit.

INNOVATIVE COMMUNITY TRANSITIONS OF CARE INITIATIVES

Several innovative initiatives designed by hospitals, as well as through colleges and universities, help increase patient safety and decrease readmission rates. Some include improving the medication reconciliation process, enhancing patient health education, improving patient discharge communication, coordinating care with the patient's providers, and reducing medical complications during the hospital stay. Many care coordination and transitions of care initiatives have emerged to address the challenges that have risen by the HRRP. These initiatives such as Project RED (Re-Engineered Discharge) (Project RED, 2014), and others such as Avoid Readmission through Collaboration (ARC, 2013b), Project BOOST (Better Outcomes for Older adults through Safe Transitions) (Society of Hospital Medicine, 2015), Script Your Future (Script Your Future, 2016), and Pharm2Pharm (University of Hawai'i at Hilo, 2012) have proven to be successful in overcoming some of those challenges and are discussed in this chapter. These are by no means a comprehensive list as there are other numerous successful initiatives currently available. With a continued push to collaborate, healthcare organizations should continue to seek collaborative partnerships and invest in sustaining them. Furthermore, to prepare health professional students for collaborative partnership in practice, many academic institutions are investing in interprofessional education as means to set the standard for such team-based practice and patient safety.

In the next few sections, collaborative opportunities are explored and discussed. In addition, proven transitional care initiatives designed specifically to address the challenges in the HRRP are highlighted in order to benefit the institutions, providers, and, ultimately, patients.

DISCUSSION

Interprofessional Collaboration

As the healthcare system has evolved, providers' integration has occurred through the formation of interdisciplinary teams. Institutions have been adopting new models in order to increase efficiency and improve patient outcomes (McDaniel & Robertson, 1995). These healthcare professionals share the same primary goal of serving patients. While each provider has their own set of duties and primary focus, their overall commitment to healthcare allows for collaborative work to ensure optimum patient care. An interprofessional team includes a physician, nurse, pharmacist, social worker, and others as appropriate. This interactive team communicates, collaborates, and coordinates a patient's care plan. The team begins this at admission and continues it throughout the entire inpatient stay, then focuses on a successful transition to outpatient (The Joint Commission et al., n.d.).

The health care team should be interprofessional and include a physician, a nurse, and a pharmacist, among other providers. An overview of the roles, responsibilities, education, and brief overview of these team members are discussed next.

Physician

The primary leader in an interprofessional team is the physician. The educational background of a physician is built on the foundation of medical school. Medical school consists of a total of four years: two being didactic, where students learn in the classroom setting, and two experiential, where they go on rotations in different focused medical settings. Post-graduation and upon licensure, physicians earn the title of Medical Doctor (MD) or Doctor of Osteopathic Medicine (DO). These physicians must undergo multiple post graduate years (PGY) of residency training where they practice, but also focus on sharpening their skills before completing final training. If a physician wants to specialize in a specific field of medicine, additional training is necessary. Physicians are considered a team leader as their primary role focuses on diagnosing. After determining a diagnosis, it is the responsibility of the physician to prescribe and coordinate the patient's overall healthcare plan with other providers on the team. Other duties a physician may have on a collaborative team includes providing referrals to other specialized practitioners who are specific to the patient's needs (The University of Texas at Austin, n.d.).

Over the past decade, there has been an increase in the amount of patients needing medical attention. This rise in the number of patients have outnumbered the amount of physicians available to attend to them.

Physician Assistants (PAs)

Physician assistants (PAs) can play a prominent role in healthcare when physicians are scarce. PAs undergo similar training as physicians; however, instead of a total of a 4-year program, it is a total of three years. The first two years are devoted to didactic coursework and the remaining year to clinical experience with participation in rotations in different settings. After completion of a PA program, PAs are not required to undertake a residency and can immediately start working (American Academy of Physician Assistants, 2006). While medical doctors can practice independently, PAs cannot. Each must share the responsibility of the patient with a supervising physician to provide optimum patient care. The responsibility of the PA includes diagnosing, interpreting and ordering labs, and prescribing. When a PA prescribes a medication, they are acting on behalf of the supervising physician. However, some variation of prescribing controlled substances may differ among states.

Physician's duties sometimes can become overwhelming due to an influx of patients or lack of time. One potential solution to this problem includes incorporating PAs on an interdisciplinary team where more patients can be seen and treated, thereby maximizing time and resources that are given to each patient. Although physicians and PAs provide the initial provider encounter for the patient, nurses have the most direct contact with the patient.

Nurse

In addition, nurses play a crucial role of a healthcare team as they ensure patient needs and communicate requests to other members of the healthcare team. Nurses are able to capture this component as their educational background allows for it. Nurses typically undergo a 3- to 4-year program that is divided into didactic and clinical experience (American Association of Colleges of Nursing [AACN], 2016). Upon completion of the program, nurses earn the title of being a registered nurse (RN). The roles and responsibilities of nurses depend on the designation of the nurse (Registered Nurse, Nurse Practitioner, and others). Some nurses may desire to expand their duties and go through more schooling to become an advanced registered nurse practitioner (ARNP) or doctor of nurse practitioner (DNP). ARNPs and DNPs have extended responsibilities because of being able to diagnose and prescribe medications; however, some differences exist between states regarding the ability to prescribe controlled substances. All types of nurses, however, are able to practice in different settings including, but not limited to hospitals, nursing homes, and clinics. Nurses monitor vitals, labs, and symptoms of the patient that may require immediate attention. Ever since Medicare started penalizing institutions for readmissions, hospitals have reset their focus on reducing readmissions rates. Nurses can play a pivotal role in avoiding this penalty by engaging in the patient's discharge process. Nurses collect discharge information, receive reconciled medications, and review the discharge plan with the patient; they also are commonly the ones leading the discharge when a patient is ready to leave the hospital. Because of how accessible nurses are, they are able to collaborate with the patient's family and the healthcare team to ensure the line of communication is clear to all.

Another study by Balaban, Weissman, Samuel, and Woolhandler (2008) examined nurses taking initiative for the patient's discharge care plan. A comprehensive discharge form was filled out by the physician and given to the nurse to review with the patient. This form included new medications to be taken and addressed communication issues that commonly occur during care transitions. After discharge, a follow up phone call was set up by the nurse to assess the patient's status, review the discharge form, and answer any concerns the patient may have had (Balaban et al., 2008)

Pharmacist

Another primary member of the healthcare team is the pharmacist. Pharmacists go to pharmacy school, which consists of a total of four years, similar to physicians. A traditional program typically consists of three years of didactic coursework and one year of experiential practice. Upon licensure pharmacists earn the title of Doctor of Pharmacy (PharmD). After completion of the PharmD degree, pharmacists have the option of doing a residency. The roles and responsibilities of the pharmacist vary by the setting of which they work. Overall, pharmacists serve as the medication experts on the healthcare team and their duties include ensuring that the patient's medications are appropriate for their indication, effective, and safe as well as cost-effective. Pharmacists ensure the correct medication is given with the appropriate dose for the right indication; also each can adjust doses as necessary. In addition, these doctors monitor for drug and disease interactions and potential allergic reactions. They also can order specific labs to ensure therapeutic levels of drugs are met. Pharmacists are trained heavily in the area of pharmacokinetics and understand factors that affect the medications in regards to absorption, distribution, and elimination, and how medications are affected throughout these parameters (General Pharmaceutical Council, 2016).

Pharmacists play an integral role in ensuring that patients receive therapeutic amounts of their medications and contribute in various transitions of care models due to their vast knowledge in pharmacotherapy and ability to manage medication regimens while optimizing patient care and reducing healthcare costs. Pharmacists have been reported to have reduced readmission rates by 86% through the integration of their services on a team (Zillich et al., 2014). A prospective pilot study by Sebaaly et al. (2015) viewed the number and severity of medication errors identified by a pharmacist prior to patient discharge. Medication errors encompassed omission of medications; extra medications; and inappropriate medications based on age, weight, antibiotic susceptibilities, wrong dose, frequency, or dosage form. A total of 84 errors were identified in a group of 67 patients, with the highest medication error being in chronic disease management. This was translated to a total of $42,300 in cost avoidance simply by allowing a pharmacist to perform a detailed comprehensive medication review (CMR). This detailed CMR allowed the pharmacist to be able to determine the reason for discrepancies in the admission and discharge medication orders (Sebaaly et al., 2015). Another study by Kilcup, Schultz, Carlson, and Wilson (2003) studied the rate of hospital readmission and financial savings with pharmacist intervention. By implementing post-discharge medication reconciliation, pharmacists could follow up with patients regarding medication management after transitioning out of the hospital. By utilizing a pharmacist, four readmissions were prevented per 100 patients. This equates to a financial saving of $35,478 per 100 patients after considering the cost of readmission and cost of labor of a clinical pharmacist (Kilcup et al., 2003). Integrating pharmacists on an interprofessional team has proven to reduce the cost of healthcare and readmission rates, while improving patient outcomes.

It is important to leverage the skills of each member of the interprofessional team and maximize their roles and responsibilities. This is one of the many reasons why the members of an interprofessional team need to know each other's roles and responsibilities. Many other healthcare professionals such as social workers, physical therapists, nutritionists, and certified diabetic educators contribute meaningfully to the care of patients. Through collaborative efforts between the healthcare professionals and the patients as well as their caretakers, the patient's care experience can be improved, the populations' health also can be improved, and healthcare expenditures can decrease, all of which are the critical objectives of what is known as the "Triple Aim" by the Institute for Healthcare Improvement (IHI, 2016).

Interprofessional Education (IPE) and Collaborative Practice (CP)

Interprofessional collaboration has been shown to be essential in optimizing patient care and patient safety while improving healthcare costs. Many academic institutions have incorporated interprofessional education as a foundational component of their curricula. The Interprofessional Education Collaborative (2016) has created four core competencies for interprofessional education, which includes shared ethics and values, roles and responsibilities, and communication as well as teams and teamwork. As healthcare continues to evolve, there are new opportunities constantly for health providers to work together with the same ultimate goal in mind – better patient care.

Patient safety and transitions of care have been significant aspects of IPECP competency concerns for many professional organizations and initiatives including the AACN (2016a), American Association of Colleges of Osteopathic Medicine (AACOM, 2016), American Association of Colleges of Pharmacy (AACP, 2016), American Dental Education Association (ADEA, 2016), Association of American Medical Colleges (AAMC, 2016), Association of Schools of Public Health (ASPH, 2016), and Agency for Healthcare Research and Quality (ARHQ, 2016). ARHQ has been proactive, particularly for many team-based learning opportunities at basic, master, and advanced levels of training educators and leaders to make patient safety a priority with the TeamSTEPPS® Strategies and Tools to Enhance Performance and Patient Safety (ARHQ, 2016). Interprofessional Education (IPE) also has become an area of focus for the AACP, with several groups, including these authors from the AACP Interprofessional Education Task Force, working on developing resources to promote and support IPE planning and development. In a review by Buring et al. (2009), there is fundamental information and background on the definition of IPE, evidence to support IPE and its need, student competencies and objectives for IPE, barriers to implementation of IPE, and elements critical for successfully implementing IPE.

The field of IPECP has been around for approximately 40 years (Brandt, 2015). Interprofessional education has been initiated, developed, and instituted around the world fueled by calls from the World Health Organization's (WHO, 2010) "Framework for Action on Interprofessional Education and Collaborative Practice." Like the United States and Canada, international efforts have been ongoing in Europe equally as long. Arguably, the largest influence in Europe is the professional organization, the Centre for the Advancement of Interprofessional Education (CAIPE, 2016) in the United Kingdom, which grows in advocacy and advancement every year. Also, the European Interprofessional Education Network (EIPEN, n.d.) was "one of the first interprofessional education networks to be formed." Furthermore, EIPEN (n.d.) has stated, "Initially . . . EIPEN . . . was led by the UK Higher Education Academy, a group of universities and CAIPE obtained European funding to set up a network in approximately 2007." Throughout the years, EIPEN has undergone change such as expansion and development of conferences around the world. CAIPE and EIPEN, along with major initiatives from professional organizations in Canada such as the Canadian Interprofessional Education Health Collaborative (CIHC, 2016), have propelled the movement forward. The growth of interprofessional education and collaborative practice is evidenced by both a National Center for Interprofessional Education and Practice (2015) that was founded in 2012 and funded by several agencies including the Josiah Macy Jr. Foundation, Robert Wood Johnson Foundation, and Gordon and Betty More Foundation. In addition, two new journals were created in 2015; namely, the *Journal of Interprofessional Education and Practice* and the *Journal of Research in Interprofessional Practice and Education.* In the last year or two only one major journal has focused on interprofessional education and/or collaborative practice; namely, the *Journal of Interprofessional Care*, which is available to a researcher when becoming an annual CAIPE member.

In the United States, several key milestones for IPE and IPECP stemmed from a major report, "Educating for the Health Team" by the Institute of Medicine (IOM, 1972). In 1999, the Institute of Medicine created another report "To Err is Human: Building a Safer Health System," and then in 2001 created the Crossing the Quality Chasm. Other organizations such as AHRQ created efforts on retraining to building interprofessional (IP) teamwork and team-based care through TeamSTEPPS training face-to-face and with masters and advanced training face-to-face and online. Finally, the American Recovery and Reinvestment Act (ARRA) of 2009 and the Patient Protection and Affordable Care Act (2010) have placed emphasis on medical home, population health, improved primary care outcomes, and more.

Universities throughout the United States have been creating and instituting IPE/IPCP programs for a number of years. Two of the most prominent and experienced initiatives developed over time are the University of Washington's (UW, 2016) Center for Health Science Interprofessional Education, Research, and Practice and the University of Minnesota (2015) where the National Center for Interprofessional Practice and Education is housed. The Center was founded by Dr. Pam Mitchell, who is the current director for the Center for Health Sciences Interprofessional Education. Dedicated individuals like Dr. Pam Mitchell and dedicated professional organizations fuel the IPECP movement forward, including those initiated and growing in Florida.

Several large Florida universities built IPECP programs, courses, and certificates while some smaller universities have instituted interprofessional education programs as well. One of the first universities in Florida to create an interprofessional education program across their university was University of Florida (Davidson & Waddell, 2005). These programs provide students in pre-professional programs and professional programs with the competencies needed to prepare future clinicians to move into various health professions. In 2011, FAU created an Interprofessional Education program for medical, nursing, and social work students and faculty to begin training and developing future practitioners for the healthcare system (Jacomino et al., 2015).

Palm Beach Atlantic University (PBAU), a private university, created an IPE program with faculty from the Colleges of Nursing and Pharmacy after shadowing FAU's program and leadership. After consulting with FAU's Office of Interprofessional Education director, PBAU's School of Pharmacy students and faculty were invited by FAU's director to participate in FAU's IPE development session on healthcare policy and quality, which focused on the readmission rate and care transition problems. The students were prepared for the problems of care transition and readmission and then instructed to create a care transition plan together. In the 2014-2015 academic year 16 pharmacy students attended the March IPE session, along with faculty who served as team facilitators. For the 2015-2016 academic year, PBAU was invited back to FAU's care transition and reducing hospital readmission discussions for the third Interprofessional Education Development Session (IPEDS) series in February. The first session had 12 students and three faculty members participating. PBAU's Dr. Mariette Sourial wrote to FAU's Dr.

Jo Ann Bamdas that she felt "we planted seeds in the session that would be fruitful by the time the students went into practice. We believe that students learned new ways of thinking that made them realize the value of each discipline present" (email communication, February 17, 2016). Having pharmacy students on the team added a layer of team building that benefited both private and public university students and faculty. Since FAU does not have a school of pharmacy and PBAU does not have a medical school or school of social work, new knowledge was shared and transferred into practice that would not have been accomplished without collaborating across institutional borders.

The intent of the public university's final workshop session in a series of three was to discuss the Patient Protection and Affordable Care Act (2010) and the challenge to hospitals for a patient's readmission within 30 days of release. Each academic year, FAU serves approximately 250 medicine, nursing, and social work students, who work in teams of 3-5. The program includes a welcome and introduction to a panel of the session's committee members from each of the colleges/schools. After an introduction into the problem of care transition and readmission, students are asked to create a care transition plan directed at a local hospital. Next the panel members listen to the students' recommendations. At the conclusion of volunteering the transition plans, panel members ask students to debrief.

Because students consistently ask to participate in real-world situations rather than simulated exercises or didactic lessons from PowerPoint presentations, Palm Beach Atlantic University and Florida Atlantic University have tried to create opportunities to learn from community partners. Also, in the past two years, FAU has partnered with a local hospital whose interprofessional staff, led by the nursing department, joined the university faculty members to listen to students' plans and give feedback in real-world terms. The hospital leadership team models for students the process for an interprofessional team collaborating. The pharmacist, physician, social worker/cases manager, and nurse from the hospital include an introduction of each other's education, roles and responsibilities, and communication as they work collaboratively in a team.

In the current year's 2015-2016 collaboration between the two universities, both PBAU and FAU have decided to continue partnering and IPECP expansion, which will benefit university, students, faculty, and staff. In that vein, the goal has been to cross the public versus private university system divide. One major change currently is underway: Mariette Sourial has been invited to join the committee that plans the third workshop for students and faculty on transitions of care. This change also adds the voice of pharmacy to the original IPE working group team when viewing real case studies from the local hospital volunteering to participate. After two years working with one local hospital, this year the universities will work with another hospital in the community to view how the leadership collaborates for transitions of care and counteracts readmission rates. The development of the universities' partnership no doubt will include several hospitals in the future since students, faculty, administrators, and hospital leaders want to prepare and be prepared for improving the healthcare system. Hospitals and universities can form initiatives for working together so that each can learn together as a team.

TRANSITIONS OF CARE INITIATIVES THROUGH INTERPROFESSIONAL COLLABORATION

Currently, many initiatives exist to increase the awareness of healthcare collaboration as the patient transitions from one care setting to another and to emphasize the Triple Aim (IHI, 2016). According to the IHI (2016), the Triple Aim approach strives to optimize health system performance, and consists of "three critical objectives: (a) improving the patient experience of care (including quality and satisfaction), (b) improving the health of populations, and (c) reducing the per capita cost of health care."

By implementing transition of care models, readmission rates can be greatly decreased as well. Integrating interprofessional collaborative practice in these initiatives ensures optimum patient care and patient safety. Many initiatives have emerged, which focus on improving transitions of care through collaborative efforts. The ARC (2013b) initiative, based in California, focuses on reducing readmission rates after discharge. In 2013, ARC helped reduce over 6,400 readmissions in a 3-year period. This initiative not only reduced readmission, but helped save healthcare over $62 million. ARC works by enlisting a number of hospitals that participate in the ARC Action Network. This network allows participating hospitals to submit their readmission information through the ARC website where five measures are entered. These five ARC measures include:

1. Percent of 30-day readmissions.
2. Percent of 90-day readmissions.
3. Responses to HCAHPS patient survey question #23: "During this hospital stay, staff took my preferences and those of my family or caregiver into account in deciding what my healthcare needs would be when I left."
4. Responses to HCAHPS patient survey question #24: "When I left the hospital, I had a good understanding of the things I was responsible for in managing my health."
5. Responses to HCAHPS patient survey question # 25: "When I left the hospital, I clearly understood the purpose for taking each of my medications." (ARC, 2013a)

Additionally, other hospitals may add other unique measures that their hospital uses to oversee readmissions. In this database, hospitals can view their own readmission information and collaborative care over a period of time and compare their information to others to see others performing in comparison.

Another transitions of care initiative is Project RED (2104), developed by a research group at Boston University Medical Center. This initiative focuses on revamping the workflow in a transition of care setting in order to improve patient safety, while reducing readmission rates. At the time of discharge, the nurse discharging the patient is the main caregiver responsible for their transition out of the hospital. The charge nurse must oversee 11 components that are to be reviewed with the patient. These include:

1. Educating the patient about his/her diagnosis.
2. Making follow up appointments and any post-discharge testing for follow-up and post-discharge testing.
3. Discussing any tests or studies that have been completed in the hospital.
4. Organizing post-discharge services.
5. Confirming their medication plan.
6. Reconciling the discharge plan with standard of care guidelines.
7. Reviewing what to do should a problem arise.
8. Expediting discharge summary to physicians.
9. Assessing the degree of understanding of patient through the "teach-back" method.
10. Giving the patient a written discharge plan at the time of discharge.
11. Providing reinforcement via telephone two to three days after discharge. (Project RED, 2014).

This initiative aims for optimum care and strives to reduce healthcare costs. It has been reported through a study that Project RED has saved up to $412 per patient, equivalent to a 33.9% reduction in overall costs (Brian et al., 2009, p. 184).

Another initiative, Project BOOST (Better Outcomes for Older adults through Safe Transitions) is led by the Society of Hospital Medicine (SHM, 2015). Their mission seeks to improve the care of patients when transitioning from inpatient to outpatient. The primary focus of this initiative includes identifying high risk patients prone to re-hospitalization, reducing potential adverse events, reducing 30-day readmission rates, improving HCAHPS measures associated with discharge, and improving communication and work flow among healthcare providers.

The board members on Project BOOST's consist of medical doctors along with representatives from AHRQ, Blue Cross and Blue Shield Association, CMS, Centers for Disease Control and Prevention (CDC), IHI, The Joint Commission, Kaiser Permanente, and many more. These mentors assist in providing evidence-based clinical interventions for hospitals to integrate into their systems.

Project BOOST encompasses a comprehensive intervention tool that was developed by experts practicing evidence-based medicine. It also provides a variety of management tools including the teach-back training method for interdisciplinary teams to implement with patients and other providers. To ensure continuity in care while minimizing gaps in miscommunication, BOOST allows sites to communicate with and learn from each other via the BOOST Listserv and BOOST Community site. Hospitals may choose to use any or all of these resources. Much of this information can be accessed on the BOOST Data Center, which is an online resource that allows different sites to store and benchmark data and to generate reports. In 2012 almost 4,000 sites had adapted the project BOOST toolkit, with reports of a 21% reduction in 30-day all cause readmission rates after implementation of BOOST. BOOST not only improves readmission rates, but also specifically caters to patients to have an increased level of medical service through collaboration (Society of Hospital Medicine, 2015).

Collaboration among Pharmacists

The ASHP (2010) 2015 initiative empowers pharmacists to be the medication experts during transitions of care (Goal 1, objective 1.6). Pharmacists are well suited to identify and resolve medication-related problems related to transitional care, activities that are core fundamentals to pharmaceutical care. Their roles ultimately can lead to identifying and resolving medication-related errors, decreasing adverse drug events upon discharge, and reducing unnecessary emergency room visits. Pharmacists are trained to evaluate a patient's drug therapy to ensure it is indicated, safe, and effective, and that the patient can adhere to it. Through patient interactions, pharmacists also can see whether the patient is able to use the medications as intended. For example, upon interviewing a patient, the pharmacist may discover that a particular patient was on an insulin regimen at home, which was not included in the medication list at the hospital. If, upon discharge, a different insulin regimen was prescribed, it could lead to the patient taking both regimens and being place at risk of having a hypoglycemic event, which could lead to a readmission. Therefore, if a pharmacist is involved in discharge counseling, this could be addressed and an adverse drug event could have been prevented. Furthermore, The Joint Commission's (2016) National Patient Safety Goals in Ambulatory Healthcare stresses the importance of medication reconciliation and the role of communicating effectively the medications to the next provider. Pharmacy organizations such as these have strived to put together in place a system to help with safer practices and to engage the patients in healthcare decisions (The Joint Commission, 2016).

As an integral function, medication management needs to be seen at all interfaces of change as patients' transition from one care setting to another. Adverse drug events are a major cause of avoidable hospital readmissions and lack of medication adherence has been a lead cause of post-discharge adverse events.

The University of Hawaii at Hilo (2012) created an innovative project focused on pharmacist-to-pharmacist collaboration, known as "Pharm2Pharm." The model is geared toward transitions of care and care coordination and aims at improving patient safety while reducing medication-related hospitalizations and emergency room visits, especially in rural communities. It involves the collaboration between hospital pharmacists and community pharmacists to close the medication-related gaps as patients transition from the hospital to the community setting. This establishment of hospital and community pharmacists' teamwork is a great exemplary model for other institutions to follow as well (University of Hawai'I at Hilo, 2012).

Another study conducted by Calvert et al. (2012), titled "PILOT-EBM: Patient Focused Intervention to Improve Long-term Adherence to Evidence Based Medications," evaluated the effectiveness of a program to help patients with heart disease stay on their medications. The lead coordinator was the inpatient pharmacist for medication management, who was involved in a collaborative effort with the community pharmacist identified by the patient. The inpatient pharmacist addressed patient and caregiver barriers to adherence identified by the care team. These adherence barriers then were discussed by the inpatient pharmacist with the community pharmacist and information was sent to the primary care. The community monitored refill records and communicated discrepancies to the patient's care team (Calvert et al., 2012).

Collaboration with Patients and Caregivers

A pharmacist integrated into a patient's healthcare team has the potential to improve patient's health and to increase their healthcare delivery. This integration also promotes collaboration between other healthcare providers, professionals, patients, and their caregivers (CDC, 2013). It is not every day that caregivers are considered to play an active role in the chain to achieving adequate healthcare. Yet, caregivers generally are the main ingredient to a patient's healthcare. They usually take over the transition of patient care, so why are they not engaged as partners of care during this vital transition for patients? Discharge processes vary between institutions; yet, how often do these processes involve patients and their caregivers? Practical ways to achieve patient and caregiver engagement include asking questions about their care, using the "teach-back" method (restating the information learned), and sharing beliefs and concerns with the healthcare team. Oftentimes, it is the goal to educate the patient on their health. While that is true, there have been discussions about the need to start looking at the big picture to see the entire line of transition (American Pharmacists Association [APhA], 2014).

Several major questions often asked within the health field include: Who is ultimately responsible for managing a patient's healthcare? Is the patient only responsible? Does the physician or pharmacist make sure any information is relayed to the patient? Is the family member of the patient the responsible caregiver? No one exact answer exists to these questions. It is a joint effort of all those involved in the care of patient to make sure the best care is provided (Interprofessional Education Collaborative, 2016). Patient self-management of their healthcare success requires collaboration to promote and achieve better transitions of care. Successful self-management can prevent costly readmissions, improve healthcare outcomes, and enhance patient satisfaction and experiences with their healthcare (Naylor & Keating, 2008).

Transitions of care remains a critical area of concern that healthcare providers and institutions continually focus their efforts to maximize results. During transitions of care, healthcare information, accountability, responsibility, and authority are transferred to the patient (Schulz et al., 1997). Unfortunately, sometimes the transitions of these three major components do not occur as smoothly as anticipated and follow up to care or confusion potentially can occur. The Joint Commission et al. (n.d.) implemented a 3-year initiative to define ways in which to achieve effective transition of patients between different healthcare settings in order to provide safe and quality care for patients regardless of the setting. Today, with a growing awareness of the importance of transition of care, several tools to facilitate seamless care continue to be developed. Various tools readily available to patients, providers, and caregivers can assist and smooth out the processes associated with the transition of care.

TOOLS AND PROGRAMS FOR HEALTH PROVIDERS

While several tools currently are under development, many resources and tools now assist and ensure effective transitions of care. One organization, AHRQ (2007), has developed a toolkit, which is focused on assessing a patient's health literacy in order to ease communication between patients and providers to improve health outcomes.

In addition to AHRQ's toolkit, several tests have been developed for healthcare providers to assist in assessing the health literacy of their patients and their caregivers. One test, the Rapid Estimate of Adult Literacy in Medicine Short Form (REALM-SF), is a 7-item recognition assessment that provides some indication of the person's health literacy. Another test, the Short Assessment of Health Literacy Spanish and English (SAHL-S&E) is longer and is comprised of an 18-item assessment of a patient's health literacy (AHRQ, 2007).

Also, other implemented programs help health professionals and patients during care transitions. In collaboration, two major pharmaceutical organizations, the ASHP and APhA developed a program called the Medication Management in Care Transitions (MMCT). This program assists in the transitions of care by pharmacists and in collaboration with patients and their caregivers (ASHP & APha, n.d.).

Another program that emerged through the Affordable Care Act by the Centers for Medicare & Medicaid Services is called the Community-based Care Transitions Program (CCTP). This program examines and identifies ways to improve patient care transitions in hopes of reducing readmissions for Medicare patients/beneficiaries (CMS, 2016a).

A national campaign, Script Your Future, led by the National Consumers League, helps patients take an active role in their healthcare by encouraging medication adherence to promote a healthier life (Script Your Future, 2016). This campaign aims to help people manage chronic and debilitating disease states such as diabetes, chronic obstructive pulmonary disease (COPD), asthma, and hypertension by supporting the importance of taking medications as prescribed and directed by their physician. Patients not taking their medications as prescribed or directed put their health and, more importantly, their future at risk. Healthcare costs rise daily in today's society. The United States spends more on healthcare than most other countries (Anderson, 2005). One way to contain healthcare costs includes adhering to the prescribed medication regimen, which, in turn, can prevent a readmission.

The Script Your Future (2016) campaign includes a website that allows patients and their caregivers to create a personal pledge to take medications as prescribed to help reinforce its importance. Some other tools available on their website include text reminders, Script Your Future wallet cards in languages such as Spanish and English, an adherence estimator, and a pocket size medication list have available at all times and to bring to doctor visits. Recently, the campaign has begun providing pharmacy students and faculty around the country with a unique opportunity to participate in a competition held nationally. The competition encourages teams to develop ideas and initiatives for raising awareness about the importance of medication adherence in the transitions of care of patients (Script Your Future, 2014).

The City of New York Health and Mental Hygiene in conjunction with the Fund for Public Health in New York (FPHNY) developed an initiative, the Medication Adherence Project (Starr & Sacks, 2010), for patients with several chronic and debilitating disease states, reinforcing effective communication by pharmacists and all healthcare providers. A major barrier to successful patient care identified by the MAP Initiative was lack of medication adherence. To overcome the barrier, MAP provides tools and resources to achieve optimal patient results in outcomes in this specific patient population. MAP created several objectives to facilitate the transition of care process and adherence barrier. The tools and resources available by the MAP initiative are targeted for everyone on the healthcare team. A 2-part guide assists in increasing effective communication. The first part is the guide, which contains medication adherence basics for providers, tools, and icebreakers to facilitate the training. The second part of the guide consists of the actual trainer curriculum, which serves as a guide to create MAP training sessions for anyone on the healthcare team (Starr & Sacks, 2010).

HEALTH LITERACY

One major influence of adherence to a prescribed regimen is the patient's health literacy. Limited literacy has been associated with poor health status, poor outcomes, and a barrier to successful transition of care. Individuals with limited literacy also tend to have higher incidences of illness and hospitalizations compared to individuals with higher literacy and reading skills. The National Adult Literacy Survey found that roughly 44 million Americans, or about one quarter of the adult population, are considered by definition to be illiterate (National Center for Education Statistics [NCES], n.d.). Many of the health brochures, health information, and education information printed for patients traditionally have been written at a 10th grade reading level or above (NCES, n.d.). Often, providers supply information to educate the patient and assist in understanding their disease states or next steps, but actually the patient may not comprehend what it means. AHRQ (2007) has developed resources including four tools to assist in measuring health literacy in our patient population.

Health literacy evaluation occurs in several ways including education level, reading level, barriers in language, and more. Oftentimes healthcare professionals may engage the patient they want to educate and assist; however, sometimes the person responsible for administering the patient's medication or daily activities does not understand what they are being told or are not informed at all; as a result, issues such as medication adherence and proper patient therapy are affected. Patients who may have difficulty in obtaining, processing, and understanding basic health information and services can have a health coach help them navigate through the health system or can designate a caregiver who can build relationships with the patient's healthcare providers. Health providers also should be cognizant of the patient's and caregiver's health literacy level and tailor the information they provide in a manner that they can understand and use. For example, the use of pictures to illustrate how to take a medication is a great way to help visualize the drug regimen. The American Medical Association has recognized that limited patient literacy is an actual barrier to effective treatment for patients (Parker, 2000).

PATIENT ENGAGEMENT

Patients need to play a more active role in their health. They are the central hub for all their health information and services. It not only is important for them to become involved in decision making, but also to be their own health advocate. One example of how to achieve this is through the use of the "teach-back" method, where patients and/or caregivers are asked to demonstrate their understanding of the instructions by explaining back in their own words what they have been informed. Patient's goals and preferences need to be accounted for during the decision making as they may directly influence the medication regimen. In an IOM report entitled "To Err is Human," patients with low level of involvement in their care become a major obstacle as well as the lack of awareness of the patient's voice during decision making (Kohn, Corrigan, & Donaldson, 2000). Achieving therapeutic goals are not necessarily the goals of the individual patient. Every patient should understand the information being received, which includes the diagnosis and the degree of uncertainty of their medical problems, the risks and benefits of the treatments options, the expected recovery time, and the healthcare providers and the costs involved. Patients should be empowered to share their beliefs and concerns with their healthcare providers. Whenever a new medication is prescribed, patients should ask their provider: "What am I taking?" "What am I taking this for?" "When should I take it?" "Are there any side effects?" "Are there any special instructions?" "What if I miss a dose?" The patients also should be aware of any past medications used and discontinued as well as any allergies and what happened to them when they had an allergic reaction. Through informed consent, each patient should become involved with their healthcare providers in making decisions about their healthcare and be the 'champions' in their own care, a movement led by the World Health Organization (WHO, 2016) called Patients for Patient Safety.

CONCLUSION

Everyone either may be a caregiver at some point in their lives or may need one during their lifetime. Sometimes caregiving can occur gradually, while other times it may happen rapidly. Studies have shown that most caregivers are not as prepared for their role as they would like to be. Caregiver participation has shown improvement in outcomes for patients, especially those with physical, mental, and cognitive disorders. Also, participation contributes to greater patient satisfaction and improves the patient's continuity of care. Caregivers are just as vital in the line of communication as patients when it comes to providing effective care. Caregiver education is needed to achieve goals, obtain desired results, and ensure effective patient transition when caregivers are involved. Proper education and incorporation of caregivers into the healthcare of an individual is not only convenient but necessary (Pinquart & Sorensen, 2003).

Many other great organization and initiatives are taking place now. As healthcare systems begin to adjust their practices to help reduce readmissions and overall healthcare costs as well as to improve patient care and safety, a much greater need exists for the healthcare professional to be accountable, collaborate as a team, and engage patients and their caregivers. Healthcare in the United States still is fragmented despite all these national efforts; however, there is progress being made in coming together and achieving the "Triple Aim" to improve the patient experience of care, including quality and satisfaction; to improve the health of populations; and to reduce the per capita cost of healthcare.

FUTURE TRENDS

Healthcare professional organizations have identified several topics of great concern for an interprofessional healthcare team's competencies. Some of the concerns discussed in this chapter are situations involving a growing aging population and chronic disease management, along with many patient safety issues such as polypharmacy and miscommunication. But healthcare reforms and focusing on better care, better health, and lower costs as well as transitions of care and the likelihood of 30-day readmission rates will be a continuing concern in the future. In addition to highlighting some gaps in healthcare, this chapter also has pointed to solutions to create a seamless healthcare system between provider, educator, patient, and caregiver. Experts in other disciplines have pointed to other trends in the healthcare system of which all interprofessional team members need to be cognizant. One profession investigated by Stanton and Lammon (2008) showed "predicted changes in [nurse] case management" (p. 161). Three of these trends included: "transitions of care, informatics in healthcare …, and the impact of an aging population …" (Stanton & Lammon, 2008, pp. 163-164).

As one gazes into the future, one may predict several opportunities and problems that will continue to be with us such as the growth of technology in healthcare. With the new informatics, telehealth, mobile health, and digital health market growing seemingly every day, knowledge, skill, and imagination will increase benefits to those who have access. But some tools may create challenges and barriers that conflict with each other. In fact, in some ways one may not think about the ramifications of some unforeseen medical dilemmas. As technology develops, particularly online courses, and training programs emerge, pharmacists, nurses, social workers, literally everyone, will need to be able to work together to benefit all stakeholders. With the advent of technology making healthcare systems seemingly easier to use, complications certainly will emerge. These conflicts and obstacles will continue affecting transitions of care and readmission rates for hospitals as well as for educators.

With the challenges at hand today, one also can gaze into the future to predict the effect of childhood chronic disease as well as physical and mental health problems. Arguably those most at risk are youth with a number of cognitive and physical disabilities. Other challenges will continue, such as access and equitable arrangements for those living in rural areas versus those in affluent areas, and will have a major impact on policy and politics. In addition, the population growth of aging Baby Boomers needing additional medical care professionals and those individuals ready to retire from the healthcare professions will invariably cause concern for transitions of care and the need for interprofessional teams to work together to solve problems.

Finally, the future of education and training will continue being affected deeply by the push for an interprofessional education and collaborative practice framework and its competencies in institutions and in the workforce. Simply put, healthcare professionals and educators cannot continue working in isolation, with silo mentalities, or within hierarchical structures and systems. As described in the *Business Dictionary*, silo mentalities are:

a mind-set present in some companies when certain departments or sectors do not wish to share information with others in the same company. This type of mentality will reduce the efficiency of the overall operation, reduce morale, and may contribute to the demise of a productive company culture. ("Silo mentality," 2016)

But many chances to improve group and team communication abound. Creating initiatives at the local and state level will bring healthcare professionals together. Workforce development state and educational initiatives such as the recent State University System of Florida's "Think Florida" (n.d.) will call on universities to reflect on the partnerships between student's knowledge, skill, and attitudes, along with workforce development. The process by which healthcare and education systems communicate and collaborate as a team will move the country forward.

This chapter has highlighted the need for patients to have a strong interprofessional team where everyone understands each other's role and responsibility and collaborates. This chapter also has captured the need for patients to take ownership of their health, the need to understand the comprehensive growth of communication and collaboration in the healthcare system today, and the need to move into the future.

REFERENCES

Agency for Healthcare Research and Quality. (2007). *Health literacy measurement tools (revised)*. Retrieved from http://www.ahrq.gov/professionals/quality-patient-safety/quality-resources/tools/literacy/index.html

Agency for Healthcare Research and Quality. (2016). *TeamSTEPPS® strategies and tools to enhance performance and patient safety*. Retrieved from http://www.ahrq.gov/professionals/education/curriculum-tools/teamstepps/index.html

American Academy of Physician Assistants. (2006). *Q&A about physician assistants: The most commonly asked questions about PAs*. Retrieved from http://www.gidoctor.net/client_files/file/Physician-Assistants.pdf

American Association of Colleges of Nursing. (2016). *Home page*. Retrieved from http://www.aacn.nche.edu/

American Association of Colleges of Osteopathic Medicine. (2016). *Home page*. Retrieved from https://www.aacom.org/

American Association of Colleges of Pharmacy. (2016). *Home page*. Retrieved from http://www.aacp.org/Pages/Default.aspx

American Dental Education Association. (2016). *Home page*. Retrieved from http://www.adea.org/

American Pharmacists Association. (2014). *Pharmacists' patient care processes*. Retrieved from http://www.pharmacist.com/sites/default/files/files/PatientCareProcess.pdf

American Recovery and Reinvestment Act (ARRA) of 2009, Pub. L. No. 111-5, 123 Stat. 115, 516 (2009).

American Society of Health-System Pharmacists. (2010). *2015 ASHP health-system pharmacy initiative*. Retrieved from http://www.ashp.org/doclibrary/policy/2015/2015goals.aspx

American Society of Health-System Pharmacists. (2016). *Transitions of care resource center*. Retrieved from http://www.ashp.org/menu/PracticePolicy/ResourceCenters/Transitions-of-Care

American Society of Health-System Pharmacists, & the American Pharmacists Association. (n.d.). *ASHP-APhA medication management in care transitions best practices*. Retrieved from http://media.pharmacist.com/practice/ASHP_APhA_MedicationManagementinCareTransitionsBestPracticesReport2_2013.pdf

Anderson, G. (2005). *U.S. still spends more on health care than any other country* [Press release]. Retrieved from http://www.jhsph.edu/news/news-releases/2005/anderson-health-spending.html

Association of American Medical Colleges. (2016). *Home page*. Retrieved from https://www.aamc.org/

Association of Schools of Public Health. (2016). *Home page*. Retrieved from http://www.aspph.org/

Avoid Readmission through Collaboration. (2013a). How ARC measures improvement. Retrieved from http://www.avoidreadmissions.com/arc-action-network.html

Avoid Readmission through Collaboration. (2013b). *Initiatives*. Retrieved from http://www.avoidreadmissions.com/improving-transitions-of-care/initiatives.html

Balaban, R. B., Weissman, J. S., Samuel, P. A., & Woolhandler, S. (2008). Redefining and redesigning hospital discharge to enhance patient care: A randomized controlled study. *Journal of General Internal Medicine*, *23*(8), 1228–1233. doi:10.1007/s11606-008-0618-9 PMID:18452048

Brandt, B. F. (2015). Interprofessional education and collaborative practice: Welcome to the 'new' forty-year old field. *The Advisor*. Retrieved from https://nexusipe-resource-exchange.s3.amazonaws.com/IPECP%20-%20Welcome%20to%20the%20New%2040-Year-Old%20Field%20-%20Brandt;%20The%20Advisor.pdf

Brian, J. W., Chetty, V. K., Anthony, D., Greenwald, J. L., Sanchez, G. M., Johnson, A. E., & Culpepper, L. et al. (2009). A reengineered hospital discharge program to decrease rehospitalization. *Annals of Internal Medicine*, *150*(3), 178–187. doi:10.7326/0003-4819-150-3-200902030-00007 PMID:19189907

Buring, S. M., Bhushan, A., Broeseker, A., Conway, S., Duncan-Hewitt, W., Hansen, L., & Westberg, S. (2009). Interprofessional education: Definitions, student competencies, and guidelines for implementation. *American Journal of Pharmaceutical Education*, *73*(4), 59. http://www.ncbi.nlm.nih.gov/pmc/articles/PMC2720355/ doi:10.5688/aj730459 PMID:19657492

Calvert, S. B., Kramer, J. M., Anstrom, K. J., Kaltenbach, L. A., Stafford, J. A., & Allen, N. M. (2012). Patient-focused intervention to improve long-term adherence to evidence-based medications. *American Heart Journal*, *163*(4), 657–665. doi:10.1016/j.ahj.2012.01.019 PMID:22520532

Canadian Interprofessional Health Collaborative. (2016). *CIHC overview*. Retrieved from http://www.cihc.ca/about/overview

Centers for Disease Control and Prevention. (2013). *Collaborative practice agreements and pharmacists' patient care services: A resource for pharmacists*. Retrieved from http://www.cdc.gov/dhdsp/pubs/docs/Translational_Tools_Pharmacists.pdf

Centers for Medicare & Medicaid Services. (2016a). *Community-based care transitions program*. Retrieved from https://innovation.cms.gov/initiatives/CCTP/index.html SG – change from 2016 to this.

Centers for Medicare & Medicaid Services. (2016b). *Readmissions reduction program (HRRP)*. Retrieved from https://www.cms.gov/Medicare/Medicare-Fee-for-Service-Payment/AcuteInpatientPPS/Readmissions-Reduction-Program.html

Centre for the Advancement of Interprofessional Education. (2002). *Defining IPE*. Retrieved from http://caipe.org.uk/resources/defining-ipe/

Centre for the Advancement of Interprofessional Education. (2016). *Welcome to CAIPE*. Retrieved from http://caipe.org.uk/

Coleman, E. A., & Boult, C. E. (2003). Improving the quality of transitional care for persons with complex care needs. *Journal of the American Geriatrics Society*, *51*(4), 556–557. doi:10.1046/j.1532-5415.2003.51186.x PMID:12657079

Davidson, R. A., & Waddell, R. (2005). A historical overview of interdisciplinary family health: A community-based interprofessional health professions course. *Academic Medicine*, *80*(4), 334–338. doi:10.1097/00001888-200504000-00005 PMID:15793015

European Interprofessional Education Network. (n. d.). *Our history*. Retrieved from http://www.eipen.eu/geschiedenis_9.html

Foster, A. J., Murff, H. J., Peterson, J. F., Gandhi, T. K., & Bates, D. W. (2003). The incidence and severity of adverse events affecting patients after discharge from the hospital. *Annals of Internal Medicine*, *138*(3), 161–167. doi:10.7326/0003-4819-138-3-200302040-00007 PMID:12558354

General Pharmaceutical Council. (2016). *What does a pharmacist do?* Retrieved from https://www.pharmacyregulation.org/raising-concerns/raising-concerns-about-pharmacy-professional/what-expect-your-pharmacy/what-does-0

Health Resources and Services Administration. (2016). *Health literacy*. Retrieved from http://www.hrsa.gov/publichealth/healthliteracy/

Institute for Healthcare Improvement. (2016). *IHI triple aim initiative*. Retrieved from http://www.ihi.org/engage/initiatives/TripleAim/Pages/default.aspx

Institute of Medicine. (1972). *Educating for the health team*. Retrieved from https://nexusipe-resource-exchange.s3.amazonaws.com/Educating_for_the_Health_Team_IOM_1972.pdf

Institute of Medicine. (2001). Crossing the quality chasm: A new health system for the 21st century. Retrieved from http://iom.nationalacademies.org/~/media/Files/Report%20Files/2001/Crossing-the-Quality-Chasm/Quality%20Chasm%202001%20%20report%20brief.pdf

Interprofessional Education Collaborative. (2016). *Resources*. Retrieved from https://ipecollaborative.org/Resources.html

Jacomino, M., Bamdas, J. M., Keller, K., Hamlin, E., Hawkins, M., Gordon, S., & Ouslander, J. G. (2015). An innovative interprofessional education program for university medical, nursing, and social work students learning in teams during sessions and visits with geriatric mentors. *Journal of Interprofessional Education & Practice*, *1*(3-4), 100–103. doi:10.1016/j.xjep.2015.10.003

Jencks, S. F., Williams, M. V., & Coleman, E. A. (2009). Rehospitalizations among patients in the Medicare fee-for-service program. *The New England Journal of Medicine*, *360*(14), 1418–1428. doi:10.1056/NEJMsa0803563 PMID:19339721

Kilcup, M., Schultz, D., Carlson, J., & Wilson, B. (2003). Postdischarge pharmacist medication reconciliation: Impact on readmission rates and financial savings. *Journal of the Journal of the American Pharmacists Association*, *53*(1), 78–84. doi:10.1331/JAPhA.2013.11250 PMID:23636160

Kohn, L. T., Corrigan, J. M., & Donaldson, M. S. (Eds.). (2000). *Institute of medicine: To err is human: Building a safer health system*. Washington, DC: National Academies Press.

McDaniel, A., & Robertson, K. (1995). Interdisciplinary professional education: A collaborative clinical teaching project. *American Journal of Pharmaceutical Education*, *59*(2), 131–136.

National Center for Education Statistics. (n. d.). *What is NAAL?* Retrieved from https://nces.ed.gov/naal/

National Center for Interprofessional Practice and Education. (2015). *About the national center.* Retrieved from https://nexusipe.org/informing/about-national-center

National Coordinating Council for Medication Error and Prevention. (2016). *About medication errors.* Retrieved from http://www.nccmerp.org/about-medication-errors

Naylor, M. D., & Keating, S. K. (2008). Transitional care: Movement from one care setting to another. *The American Journal of Nursing*, *108*(S9), 58–63. doi:10.1097/01.NAJ.0000336420.34946.3a PMID:18797231

Parker, R. (2000). Health literacy: A challenge for American patients and their healthcare providers. *Health Promotion International*, *15*(4), 277–283. doi:10.1093/heapro/15.4.277

Patient Protection and Affordable Care Act, 42 U.S.C. § 18001 (2010).

Payne, R. A., & Avery, A. J. (2011). Polypharmacy: One of the greatest prescribing challenges in general practice. *The British Journal of General Practice*, *61*(583), 83–84. doi:10.3399/bjgp11X556146 PMID:21276330

Pinquart, M., & Sorensen, S. (2003). Differences between caregivers and noncaregivers in psychological health and physical health: A meta-analysis. *Psychology and Aging*, *18*(2), 250–267. doi:10.1037/0882-7974.18.2.250 PMID:12825775

Project RED. (2014). *Project RED (re-engineered discharge).* Retrieved from http://www.bu.edu/fammed/projectred/

Rozich, J. D., & Resar, R. K. (2001). Medication safety: One organization's approach to the challenge. *Journal of Clinical Outcomes Management*, *8*(10), 27–34.

Schulz, R., Newsom, J., Mittelmark, M., Burton, L., Hirsch, C., & Jackson, S. (1997). Health effects of caregiving: The caregiver health effects study: An ancillary study of the cardiovascular health study. *Annals of Behavioral Medicine*, *19*(2), 110–116. doi:10.1007/BF02883327 PMID:9603685

Script Your Future. (2014). *Script your future program.* Retrieved from http://www.scriptyourfuture.org/wp-content/uploads/2014/11/lessons_learned.pdf

Script Your Future. (2016). *Tools.* Retrieved from http://www.scriptyourfuture.org/tools/

Sebaaly, J., Parsons, L. B., Pilch, N. A., Bullington, W., Hayes, G. L., & Easterling, H. (2015). Clinical and financial impact of pharmacist involvement in discharge medication reconciliation at an academic medical center: A prospective pilot study. *Hospital Pharmacy, 50*(6), 505–513. doi:10.1310/hpj5006-505 PMID:26405342

Silo Mentality. (2016). In *Business Dictionary.com.* Retrieved from http://www.businessdictionary.com/definition/silo-mentality.html#ixzz3yZpAGcrA

Society of Hospital Medicine. (2015). *Project BOOST® mentored implementation program.* Retrieved from http://www.hospitalmedicine.org/BOOST/

Stanton, M. P., & Lammon, C. A. (2008). The "wins" of change: Evaluating the impact of predicted changes on case management practice. *Professional Case Management, 13*(3), 161–168. doi:10.1097/01.PCAMA.0000319970.61358.9a PMID:18562911

Starr, B., & Sacks, R. (2010). *Improving outcomes for patients with chronic disease: The medication adherence project (MAP).* Retrieved from http://www.nyc.gov/html/doh/downloads/pdf/cardio/cardio-map-tools-manual.pdf

Tam, V. C., Knowles, S. R., Cornish, P. L., Fine, N., Marchesano, R., & Etchells, E. E. (2005). Frequency, type and clinical importance of medication history errors at admission to hospital: A systematic review. *Canadian Medical Association Journal, 173*(5), 510–515. doi:10.1503/cmaj.045311 PMID:16129874

The Joint Commission. (2016). *National patient safety goals effective January 1, 2016.* Retrieved from http://www.jointcommission.org/assets/1/6/2016_NPSG_AHC.pdf

The Joint Commission. Joint Commission Center for Transforming Healthcare, & Joint Commission Resources. (n. d.). *Transitions of care: The need for a more effective approach to continuing patient care.* Retrieved from http://www.jointcommission.org/assets/1/18/Hot_Topics_Transitions_of_Care.pdf

The University of Texas at Austin. (n. d.). *Physician role.* Retrieved from http://www.healthipe.org/healthcare-roles/physician

Think Florida. (n. d.). *Home page.* Retrieved from http://think-florida.org

University of Hawai'i at Hilo. (2012). *College of pharmacy awarded $14.3 million to develop system to save healthcare costs* [News release]. Retrieved from http://hilo.hawaii.edu/news/press/release/1196

University of Washington. (2016). *Center for health sciences interprofessional education, research, and practice.* Retrieved from http://collaborate.uw.edu/about/about-us.html

World Health Organization. (2010). *Framework for interprofessional education and collaborative practice.* Retrieved from http://apps.who.int/iris/bitstream/10665/70185/1/WHO_HRH_HPN_10.3_eng.pdf?ua=1

World Health Organization. (2016). *Patients for patient safety*. Retrieved from http://www.who.int/patientsafety/patients_for_patient/en/

Zillich, A. J., Snyder, M. E., Frail, C. K., Lewis, J. L., Deshotels, D., Dunham, P., & Sutherland, J. M. et al. (2014). A randomized, controlled pragmatic trial of telephonic medication therapy management to reduce hospitalization in home health patients. *Health Services Research*, *49*(5), 1537–1554. doi:10.1111/1475-6773.12176 PMID:24712335

KEY TERMS AND DEFINITIONS

Health Literacy: The degree to which individuals have the capacity to obtain, process, and understand basic health information needed to make appropriate health decisions (Health Resources and Services Administration, 2016).

Interprofessional Education: (IPE): Occurs when two or more professions learn with, from, and about each other to improve collaboration and the quality of care (CAIPE, 2002).

Medication Errors: "Any preventable event that may cause or lead to inappropriate medication use or patient harm while the medication is in the control of the healthcare professional, patient, or consumer. Such events may be related to professional practice, healthcare products, procedures, and systems including prescribing; order communication; product labeling, packaging, and nomenclature; compounding; dispensing; distribution; administration; education; monitoring; and use" (The National Coordinating Council for Medication Error and Prevention, 2016).

Polypharmacy: Concurrent prescribing of at least four or five drugs (Payne, & Avery, 2011).

Readmission: Admission to a subsection (d) hospital within 30 days of a discharge from the same or another subsection (d) hospital (CMS, 2016b).

Transitions of Care: Refers to the movement of patients between healthcare practitioners, settings, and home as their condition and care needs change (The Joint Commission, 2016).

Triple Aim: A framework developed by the Institute for Healthcare Improvement that describes an approach to optimizing health system performance (IHI, 2016).

Chapter 5
Humane Education:
A Call to Action for Elementary School Students

Cassandra M. Kenski
Florida Atlantic University, USA

Jaclyn N. Falcone
Florida Atlantic University, USA

ABSTRACT

The relationship between human and canine has long been a topic of interest, studied by many. It can be argued that the effect of a canine on their human is one of life's greatest and most impactful. Humane education recognizes this relationship and those of other animals in humans' lives. Humane education provides students with the background information necessary to properly treat animals, while simultaneously instilling a multitude of desired character traits that young people carry far into adult hood. During the 2014 and 2015 school year, an elementary school in The School District of Palm Beach County, Florida began implementing humane education in the classroom, as part of their environmental Green and School-wide Positive Behavior Support initiatives. Humane education curriculum implementation included visits from local author and President of The Little Blue Dog, a non-profit organization with humane treatment of animals at its core. A field trip to a Peggy Adams, a local, no-kill animal rescue was also provided for students in Grades 3rd and 4th, where students toured the facility and wrote haiku poetry about the pets that were up for adoption. Classrooms in Grades Pre-K through 5th were consistently exposed to topics and content pertaining to the proper care and treatment of animals, including critical character traits such as respect, empathy, responsibility, and kindness. As a result of the implementation of the humane education integration, the elementary school's student body further developed a culture in which the fore mentioned character traits (among others) were admired and adopted, creating a school environment in which respect and kindness were the expectation, and responsibility, a necessary must.

DOI: 10.4018/978-1-5225-0640-9.ch005

A BRIEF INTRODUCTION

Grassy Waters Elementary School is located in suburban West Palm Beach, Florida and serves students Grades Pre-K through 5 (J. Galindo, personal communication, December 5, 2015). A Title I campus with approximately 730 students in attendance, 75 percent of students on campus qualify for free or reduced lunch. Approximately 87 percent of the students on campus are minorities, with 9 percent identified as English Language Learners (ELL). Among the 730 students in attendance, a significant 21 percent qualify for Individualized Education Plans (IEP) (J. Galindo, personal communication, December 5, 2015).

During the 2014 and 2015 school year, Grassy Waters Elementary School began implementing humane education in the classroom, as part of their environmental Green and School-wide Positive Behavior Support Program initiatives. The humane education curriculum implementation included visits from local author and President of The Little Blue Dog, a non-profit organization with humane treatment of animals at its core. A field trip to a Peggy Adams Animal Rescue, a local, no-kill animal rescue was also provided for students in Grades 3rd and 4th, where they toured the facility and wrote haiku poetry about the pets that were up for adoption. Classrooms in Grades Pre-K through 5th were consistently exposed to topics and content pertaining to the proper care and treatment of animals, including critical character traits such as respect, empathy, responsibility, and kindness.

This chapter will walk you through the evolution of the human-canine relationship, bond, positive effects, history of humane education and finally an example in practice at Grassy Waters.

THE EVOLUTION OF THE HUMAN-CANINE RELATIONSHIP

In order to fully understand the significance of human-animal liaison, it is necessary to briefly review the evolutionary history of the human-animal relationship. Archeologists have found fossils showing people with canines since the dawn of humanity (Fawcett & Gullone, 2001). Most researchers agree that the mutually beneficial relationship between people and dogs has existed in history for thousands of years (Caspari, 2003; Clutton-Brock, 2006). Evidence of this companionship even pre-dates the agricultural revolution (Bradshaw, 2011; Hare & Woods, 2013).

The behavior and role of dogs has changed throughout history to adapt to the human social environment (Russack, 2000). Through the ages, dogs have guarded, herded, hunted for food, pulled sleds for transportation, sniffed out criminal cases and medical cases, and were the first animal to be domesticated (Dotson & Hyatt, 2008; Schaefer, 2002). Tales of the dog-human relationship date back to ancient Chinese, Greek and Egyptian societies. In his royal court, the Han Chinese emperor, Ling, was said to keep dogs as senior officials; aristocratic Athenians reportedly paid more for dogs than they did for human slaves; Mary, Queen of Scots kept a pack of little dogs adorned in velvet suits. (Schaffer 2009, p. 9)

In more recent history, The Society of Friends formed York Retreat in the 1790s to use animals to help asylum patients learn self-control and nurturing skills as a means to prevent drug use (Digby, 1984). In January of 1821, the domestic dog was first defined as "man's best friend" by an unknown author in a poem published in the *New-York Literary Journal*. In the early 1900's, Sigmund Freud discovered that when his Chow Chow, Jofi, was present during psychoanalysis sessions his clients felt comfortable and encouraged to confide (Beck, 2010).

By the 1950s and 1960s as families started to move away from cities and into suburbs, the idea of owning a home with two kids, a dog, and a picket fence became the quintessential American dream. An article from the Washington Post in the 1950s estimates the total number of dogs in America at the time to be between 12 and 15 million. By the mid-twentieth century dogs have made their way from outside in the doghouse to inside in the plush dog bed. By 1991 the American Veterinary Association released a report estimating the new total number of dogs to be about 51 million, rising to 68 million by 2002 according to the Humane Society (Katz 2003, p. 10).

In his book *One Nation Under Dog*, Michael Schaffer addresses the changes in this country: "In a relatively short period of time, the United States has become a land of doggie yoga (sic) and frequent-flier miles for traveling pets, a society where your inability to find a pet sitter has become an acceptable excuse to beg off a dinner invitation, a country where political candidates pander to pet owners and dog show champions are feted like Oscar winners." (Schaffer 2009, p. 8). The canine relationship has continued to expand and today we see the impact of dogs on elementary school children, as evidenced by the study at Grassy Waters to be explained later on in this chapter.

Human-Canine Bond

The American Veterinary Medical Association defines the human-animal bond (HAB) as a mutually beneficial, dynamic relationship between people and animals that is influenced by behaviors that were essential to the health and wellbeing of both (Olson, 2002; Schaffer, 2009). Research has suggested that the human-animal bond can have a strong influence as an intervention strategy with a variety of people (Valentine et al., 1993), this theory is being tested with the Mutt-i-gree program discussed below. To emphasize the Human-Animal Bond concept, *Chicken Soup for the Dog Lover's Soul* (Canfield, 1999) is a book of human-animal bond stories that sold over 1 million copies in the first year of publication. Here is a story excerpt titled "The Golden Years" from page 132-133 of this book:

My best friend, Cocoa, and I live in a senior citizen apartment complex in a lovely small town. Cocoa is a ten-year-old poodle and I am a sixty-nine-year-old lady, so you can see we both qualify as senior citizens. Years ago, I promised myself that when I retired I would get a chocolate poodle to share my golden years. From the very first, Cocoa has always been exceptionally well behaved. I never have to tell him anything more than once. He was housebroken in three days and has never done anything naughty. He is extremely neat—when taking his toys from his box to play, he always puts them back when he is finished. I have been accused of being obsessively neat, and sometimes I wonder if he mimics me or if he was born that way, too. He is a wonderful companion. When I throw a ball for him, he picks it up in his mouth and throws it back to me. We sometimes play a game I played as a child—but never with a dog. He puts his paw on my hand, I cover it with my other hand, he puts his paw on top, and I slide my hand out from underneath the pile and lay it on top, and so on. He does many amusing things that make me laugh and when that happens, he is so delighted he just keeps it up. I enjoy his company immensely. But almost two years ago, Cocoa did something that defies comprehension. Was it a miracle or a coincidence? It is certainly a mystery.

One afternoon, Cocoa started acting strangely. I was sitting on the floor playing with him, when he started pawing and sniffing at the right side of my chest. He had never done anything like this ever before, and I told him, "No." With Cocoa, one "no" is usually sufficient, but not that day.

He stopped briefly, then suddenly ran toward me from the other side of the room, throwing his entire weight—eighteen pounds at the right side of my chest. He crashed into me and I yelped in pain. It hurt more than I thought it should have. Soon after this, I felt a lump. I went to my doctors, and after X rays, tests and lab work were done, they told me I had cancer.

When cancer starts, for an unknown reason, a wall of calcium builds. Then the lump or cancer attaches itself to this wall. When Cocoa jumped on me, the force of the impact broke the lump away from the calcium wall. This made it possible for me to notice the lump. Before that, I couldn't see it or feel it, so there was no way for me to know it was there. I had a complete mastectomy and the cancer has not spread to any other part of my body. The doctors told me if the cancer had gone undetected even six more months, it would have been too late.

Was Cocoa aware of just what he was doing? I'll never really know. What I do know is that I'm glad I made a promise to spend my golden years with this wonderful chocolate brown poodle for Cocoa not only shares his life with me he has made sure that I will be around to share my life with him!

More than 63% of American households currently have at least one pet (Walsh, 2009); according to the Humane Society of the United States, 78.2 million dogs are owned. Today, most people consider canines to be a "part of the human family" (Risely-Curtis, 2010; Schvaneveldt et. al. 2001; Walsh, 2009; Wisdom, Saedi, & Green, 2009) supporting self-efficacy, strengthening sense of empowerment, and reinforcing self-worth (Beck & Katcher, 1996; Corson & Corson, 1980; Lott, 1988; Melson, 1991, 2003; Wisdom, Saedi, & Green, 2009). This extension of family includes allowing dogs to sleep in their owner's bed (Bradshaw, 2011), bathe in their sinks or tubs, carry their photographs, obtain medical insurance for them, treating dogs just like an equal member of the family.

PROFOUND EFFECTS OF THE HUMAN-CANINE RELATIONSHIP

Research has established that animals, particularly dogs, have positive effects on humans, both physiologically and psychologically (Albert & Anderson, 1997; Allen, Blascovich, Tomaka, & Kelsey, 1991; Arambašic, Kresteš, Kuterovac-Jagodíc, & Vizek-Vidovic, 2000; Beck & Katcher, 1996; Bryant & Donnellan, 2007; Charnetski, Riggers, & Brennan, 2004; Crawford, Worsham, & Swinehart, 2006; Wood, Giles-Corti, Bulsara, & Bosch, 2007). Futhermore, Weil (2003) found ten distinctive characteristics that humane individuals possess, including "the willingness to choose and change" (p. 12) how we treat others, kindness, compassion, generosity, trustworthiness, courage, perseverance and self-control, humor and playfulness, wisdom, and integrity. The humane educator seeks to foster these traits by encouraging personal responsibility (self-efficacy), developing emotional intelligence, challenging students to critically examine cultural values and personal ethics, increasing knowledge about the interdependence of all life, equipping students with the skills to humanely serve others, and building community within the classroom and in society (Institute for Humane Education, 2008; Thomas & Beirne, 2002).

Dogs can be our teachers in many ways as well. This excerpt from pages 103-104 from *Chicken Soup for the Dog Lover's Soul* (Canfield, 1999) from an unknown author lists 18 "Things We Can Learn from a Dog:"

1. *Never pass up the opportunity to go for a joy ride.*
2. *Allow the experience of fresh air and the wind in your face to be pure ecstasy.*
3. *When loved ones come home, always run to greet them.*
4. *When it's in your best interest, always practice obedience.*
5. *Let others know when they've invaded your territory.*
6. *Take naps and always stretch before rising.*
7. *Run, romp and play daily.*
8. *Eat with gusto and enthusiasm.*
9. *Be loyal.*
10. *Never pretend to be something you're not.*
11. *If what you want lies buried, dig until you find it.*
12. *When someone is having a bad day, be silent, sit close by and nuzzle them gently.*
13. *Delight in the simple joy of a long walk.*
14. *Thrive on attention and let people touch you.*
15. *Avoid biting when a simple growl will do.*
16. *On hot days, drink lots of water and lie under a shady tree.*
17. *When you are happy, dance around and wag your entire body.*
18. *No matter how often you are criticized, don't buy into the guilt thing and pout. Run right back and make friends.*

Identified below, are the positive effects of canines on humans in regards to the following areas: physical, physiological, psychological, family interaction, social catalyst, and child development.

Physical

The human-canine bond has been positive in the area of exercise (Cutt, Giles-Corti, & Knuiman, 2008). There have been a number of studies concerning the link between dog ownership and physical activity (Brown & Rhodes, 2006). In both the United States and Austria, dog owners were more likely to achieve the recommended amount of time of physical activity than non-dog owners (Brown & Rhodes, 2006; Cutt et al., 2008). In China, pets were banned from urban areas until 1992. Since then, studies have shown that dog ownership has spiked along with health related outcomes. Chinese owners reported exercising more, sleeping better, took fewer sick days and visited the doctor less often. Overall, they self-reported better fitness and health (Haedy, Na, & Zhueng, 2008).

Physiological

Even the simple act of petting an animal promotes relaxation by decreasing blood pressure (Friedmann, et al., 1983; Nagengast, et al., 1997) and increasing peripheral skin temperature (Velde, et al., 2005). The relaxation effect is said to be true in children and adults (Trivedi & Perl, 1995). Charnetski, Riggers, and Brennan (2004) demonstrated that petting a dog had a positive effect on immune system function, as measured by Immunoglobin A (IgA). The results from Odendaal's (2000) study suggested that physiological effects could be achieved within 5 and 24 minutes of positive dog interaction.

Zilcha-Mano, Mikulincer, and Shaver, (2012) found that when compared to no pet presence, the number of life goals generated and self-confidence in goal attainment increased by physical or even cognitive pet presence.

Psychological

Beck and Katcher (1996) presented the following research results: pet owners talk to their pets as if they were people and the way people talk to cats, dogs, and birds resembles the way we talk to infants; pets can coax smiles and words out of socially withdrawn institutionalized patients of all ages; pets can help psychotherapy progress faster; and, in children, carefully controlled studies have shown that contact with pets and nature can reduce symptoms of Attention Deficit/Hyperactivity Disorder (ADHD). Shiloh, Sorek, and Terkel (2003) suggested an "attentional shift hypothesis," in which pets distract attention from an anxiety-generating stimulus, helping alleviate the anxiety. A relationship with pets can decrease stress, depression, anxiety, and loneliness and increase self-esteem and general psychological wellness (Martin & Farnum, 2002, p. 658; Crawford, et al., 2006).

It was previously found that children developed a sense of security from an animal companion, stuffed animal, or fictional animal (Schaefer, 2002). At night, a small child may have received comfort from his pet dog sleeping by his bed, or by cuddling his stuffed dog (Martin & Farnum, 2002).

Family Interaction

Tannen (2004) reported that families use pets as resources in mediating interactions with each other, using their dogs to buffer criticism, effect frame shifts, deliver praise, teach values, mediate or avoid conflict, and both reflect and constitute familial identities. Here is an anecdotal story to provide an example of a dog's aid in mediating; when a wife is yelling at her husband in an argument, the husband turns to their dog and in a baby voice says "Mommy is upset right now, Daddy needs your help! Can you give her kisses so she can be happy again?" The obedient dog goes to the wife, kissing her face, causing the wife to laugh and the husband to breathe a sigh of relief. In this example the dog was able to mediate this situation, he provided comedic relief in a time of conflict, and shifted the frame to that of a family bond. Pets can become a resource for communication between families. They are able to buffer criticism and constitute family bond, especially for couples without human children because according to Bilger (2003), "Eighty-three per cent [of pet owners] refer to themselves as their pet's mom or dad" [p. 48].

Social Catalysts

Camp's research (2001) identified themes such as increased community participation, social contact, personal skill development, and a greater likelihood to have fun due to dog ownership. Messent (1983) found that, even when walking in an unfamiliar location, the presence of a dog significantly increases the likelihood of contact between a stranger and the dog owner. Veevers (1985) found that companion animals provide a medium of expression for the personality and preferences of the owner, for example think of Paris Hilton and her late Chihuahua, Tinkerbell. When walking a dog around the neighborhood, people often stop to ask about the dog and pet or play with the dog. This allows the dog owner the opportunity to interact and get to know the neighbors in a way that wouldn't otherwise be as easy.

Owners who bring their dogs to the dog park have an additional avenue for socialization. At most dog parks the owners will sit together and socialize while the dogs will run and play together. The common bond is dogs and stories and laughs of dog ownership. Most dog parks have separate sections for large and small dogs; this breaks down the group further into similar interests and preferences.

Child Development

Vygotsky's concept of cultural mediation (Cole & Wertsch, 1996), suggests that companion animals are likely powerful motivators for learning because children learn and retain more about subjects they are emotionally invested in and children's learning is most efficient when it occurs within meaningful relationships.

HUMANE EDUCATION'S BACKGROUND

The concept of humane education is not something new ("American Humane," 2010). In 1663, philosopher John Locke first recognized and documented the profound impact that the proper, kind treatment of animals has on a developing child's character. Locke commented that, "Children should from the beginning, be bred up in an abhorrence of killing, or tormenting any living Creature," ("American Humane," 2010).

Humane education first became accepted in the United States in the mid-1800s with the "kindness to animals ethic" (Unti & DeRosa, 2003). From this point, an awareness and need for the inclusion of humane education continued ("American Humane," 2010). Efforts to teach children animal kindness more than likely began with the development of the first human social groups (Ascione, 2015). Formalized programs intentionally aimed at fostering children's compassion and responsibility towards animals emerged in the United States about a century ago (Ascione, 2015). As of 1879, the American Humane Association embraced a resolution promoting human education in public schools ("American Humane," 2010). Three years later, George T. Angell began to organize groups of students known as "Bands of Mercy," where young people learned about and assisted animals. Within a year's time, American public schools housed 600 "Bands of Mercy" groups with approximately 70,000 members ("American Humane," 2010).

As of 1920, 20 states passed requiring humane education be part of their schools' curriculum ("American Humane," 2010). Unfortunately, the rise of humane education awareness came at a time when great change was happening in America. Automobiles replaces horse-drawn carriages, shifting the humane education focus to adaptation and evolution. Animal welfare organizations now focused their efforts on carriage horses. Political groups and changes in the "world of education," put added pressure on public schools. This strain ultimately resulted in two World Wars and the Great Depression. This eliminated any additional resources for humane education ("American Humane," 2010).

Throughout the 1900s the country recognized the discipline as a source for teaching values and positive behaviors in children. Organizations including the ASPCA, the American Humane Association (AHA), the Humane Society of the United States (HSUS), the National Association for Humane and Environmental Education (NAHEE), and the Latham Foundation were instrumental in advancing the discipline. Today, most humane education is centered around companion animals and Animal Assisted Therapy (AAT) and ebbs and flows depending on funding and national importance.

There are four main elements to humane education that The Institute for Humane Education (2008) identified, these include (a) the provision of accurate information about humane education topics so that learners can make informed choices; (b) the cultivation of curiosity, creativity, and responsibility; (c) the development of reverence, respect, and responsibility; and (d) the presentation of positive choices to learners that will enable them to create a more humane world. There is still much concern that the United States is far away from achieving widespread Humane Education. For example, there are several established procedures for pets that are not medically necessary, which may be called 'cosmetic' or 'convenience' surgeries (Swabe 2000). These include tail-docking, ear-cropping, de-clawing, and de-barking. Below are descriptions taken from the Canadian Federation of Humane Societies (CFHS) website, and declawing from the Humane Society of the United States (HSUS) website:

Ear cropping involves cutting off up to two thirds of the earflap and is done when the dog is 4-6 months old. After the procedure, which requires full anaesthesia, splints and tape are used to hold the ear in an upright position. Ear cropping is not always successful and at times only one ear will stand erect, while the other flops back. There is a risk of infection after the surgery, and the dogs' behaviour is sometimes negatively affected. The puppy will likely experience post-surgical pain.

Tail docking has also been performed for centuries and although it may cause pain, it is often done without any anaesthetic. Tail docking is performed when the puppy is only a few days old and involves removing the hair from the tail and then clamping the tail with a rubber band at the desired length, at which point it is cut with a scalpel or cutters, stitched up, and bandaged. In the process, muscles, tendons, nerves, bone, and cartilage is severed.

Declawing traditionally involves the amputation of the last bone of each toe and, if performed on a human being, it would be comparable to cutting off each finger at the last knuckle. Declawing can leave cats with a painful healing process, long- term health issues, and numerous behaviour problems.

During laser surgery, a small, intense beam of light cuts through tissue by heating and vaporizing it, meaning there's less bleeding and a shorter recovery time. But the surgical technique itself is similar to the traditional method (or "onychectomy"), with the laser simply replacing a steel scalpel blade. So while the use of a laser may slightly reduce the duration of the healing process, it does not change the nature of the procedure.

One more example of the long way we still have to go in the United States and the importance of humane education is this story from a dog owner in Palm Beach County: "When we selected the breed of dog that would be best for our family we researched breeders to ensure safe practices and not support a "puppy mill." We found a fantastic breeder with a love and respect for her profession and most of all her dogs. When we purchased our Cane Corso, Luna, the breeder had already cropped her ears and clipped her tail, saying it was breed standard and safe for the puppies. As dog owners, we were unaware of the welfare issues at stake. It is alarming to find research on such procedures that are simply unnecessary and cause pain and risk to the dogs."

Cox (2009) advocated an experiential approach to humane education when she stated,

Ultimately, the [humane education] programme should seek to inspire each learner to explore, understand and play their unique role in making the world a better place. Each learner will have their own gifts, skills and talents, which they can be helped to recognize and develop. They can also be encouraged to discover their own personal motivations, interests and beliefs, in order to inspire a sense of mission which will lead to right action. The methods used are designed to bring inspiration through the drawing out of each learner's intrinsic wisdom. It is not an instructional (didactic) process, but a facilitative one that provides a supportive atmosphere in which learners feels free to explore their beliefs and express themselves. (p. 3)

Grassy Waters provides students opportunity for immersive, hands on, student-driven experiential learning to grow their humane values. This learning is repetitive over an extended period of time, and the school has immersed their families and extra-curricular activities around this theme.

Fast-forwarding to current day, humane education has once again regained momentum ("American Humane," 2010). This includes public awareness and opportunities within American public and private school settings. The Association for Professional Humane Educators leads the way in providing professional development and networking opportunities for educators dedicating their lives' work to the promotion of humane attitudes toward the environment, animals, and people ("American Humane," 2010).

CHARACTER EDUCATION AND HUMANE EDUCATION

Character education (sometimes referred to as Values education), has been part of the American school system since the country's very first schools opened their doors (Loeser, 2014). The character component of a curriculum is an integral and vital part of the overall development of the students, as well as to the creation of the school culture, better ensuring a thriving learning environment (Elias, 2011). Character education not only encompasses personal values, but relational values as well (Loeser, 2014). Relationally, this includes attributes such as respect, fairness, civility, and tolerance towards others. Personal values within character education include topics including self-efficacy, self-disciple, effort, and perseverance (Loeser, 2014).

Aside from positively impacting the social and emotional growth and development of children, character education directly correlates to student academic performance and higher achievement (Loeser, 2014). For instance, if a student is unable to take responsibility for their schoolwork, they will likely struggle to stay academically afloat in the classroom (Loeser, 2014). A growing body of research supports character educations' overall effectiveness, citing changes for the better in students exposed to values education (Adams, 2013). Schools that implement a character education curriculum experience greater gains in academic achievement *and* standardized testing, compared to those schools that do not (Loeser, 2014).

THE BENEFITS OF HUMANE EDUCATION

Humane education plays an unmatched role in creating a more compassionate and caring society overall. This includes an accountability and responsibility for ourselves, each other, animals, and the Earth ("The Need, 2014"). Humane education fosters student empathy for *all* living beings on earth ("Parents and

Teachers," 2015). With regard to animals, humane education examines the root causes of human cruelty and abuse, working to prevent violence of all kinds. Research supports the value in humane education, citing individuals who abuse animals in their youth are five times more likely (as non-abusers) to commit violent crimes, four times more likely to commit property crimes (such as theft), and three times more likely to commit drug and/or disorderly conduct offenses ("Parents and Teachers," 2015). These numbers staggering but potentially preventable, with early intervention and the implementation of a humane education program ("Parents and Teachers," 2015). A main component of the humane education movement is the promotion of sentience, which is defined as the ability to experience consciousness including feelings and perceptions, such as suffering and the state of well-being ("The Need," 2014).

Humane education is often revered as, "the building block of a humane and ethically responsible society," ("The Need," 2014). The benefits of humane education are countless and the long-term effects immeasurable ("Humane Education for Kids," 2015). Humane education promotes animal safety and prevents animal overpopulation in communities. For children, humane education teaches desired character traits, such as compassion and responsibility, encouraging service to benefit others (community service) ("Humane Education for Kids," 2015). It helps young people to develop a personal understanding of themselves as individuals, recognizing their own unique attributes and fostering in them a sense of self-efficacy ("The Need," 2014). Humane education aids young people in developing a deep feeling for all living things, based on empathy and respect. Even more impressive, the provision of humane education shapes students' belief and value systems, helping them to develop desired traits such as wisdom and justice ("The Need," 2014). The inclusion of this type of education prevents animal cruelty and abuse, promoting pet health and responsible care ("Humane Education for Kids," 2015). What's more, the provision of humane education in the classroom may potentially solve young people behavior challenges, so that more pets are in happy, long-term homes versus shelters ("Humane Education for Kids," 2015).

The provision of humane education in the classroom ultimately provides students with a specific and essential skill set (Ortiz, 2015). This skill set includes the development of critical thinking skills and higher order thinking, as students question perspectives and examine their ability to make a change for the better (Ortiz, 2015). Humane education programs encourage students to make positive choices and challenge forms of oppression and abuse, in *all* areas of their lives (Ortiz, 2015). Students view themselves as "agents of change," fostering a sense of responsibility that calls them to action, as they take personal accountability for the proper care and treatment of animals and Mother Earth ("The Need," 2014).

Empathy is the ability to understand and share, identifying with the way another feels ("The Need," 2014). According to researcher Professor Baron-Cohen, empathy in individuals ranges from low to high. Low empathy causes individuals to think only of their own interests. Empathy is quite possibly the most valuable resource in the world today, as Baren-Cohen identifies the lack of society's empathy as the, "'critical, global issue of our time." Empathy relates to the state of health within our communities. A lack of empathy compromises the relationships within these communities, jeopardizing community cohesion which then results in violence ("The Need," 2014).

Compassion is like empathy, but with the added element of desire to take action ("The Need," 2014). Students who identify with an animal's pain and suffering, cannot only relate to that animal in some way, but also often times demonstrate compassion in becoming "part of the solution." Compassion in an emotion that demands action, motivating the individual to produce a solution and find a better outcome. The intent of humane education is to develop students' compassion, with empathy as part of the process ("The Need," 2014).

Ethics and values are those beliefs that are considered by most as "good" for the individual, society, animals, and the Earth overall ("The Need," 2014). Ethics also serve as a moral "compass" of sorts. As laws and social norms are ever-changing, it is necessary that individuals are capable of consistently examining and determining their own moral stance on various issues. Humans traditionally develop their strongest notions regarding ethics, as children. Human education works to influence these ethics and students' moral "compass" at an early age, better ensuring healthy ethics and values foundations long-term. Humane education promotes peaceful societies, in which ethics and values are implored ("The Need," 2014).

Humane education promotes happiness, including individual and overall ("The Need," 2014)! By deliberately teaching the fore mentioned, humane education has the potential to influence individuals both psychologically and ethically. This creates a feeling of emotional euphoria in participants. In other words, students and other individuals involved in the humane education implementation process often experience "emotional kick back." By becoming more aware of animal kindness, working together to create solutions, and simultaneously developing emotionally, happiness is a seemingly natural outcome of the humane education experience ("The Need," 2014).

HUMANE EDUCATION AT GRASSY WATERS ELEMENTARY SCHOOL

Grassy Waters Elementary School's community and faculty stakeholders bridged character education *with* humane education. By definition, humane education includes instructional approaches to teaching students how to be kind and properly treat animals (Ascione, 2015). At Grassy Waters Elementary School, humane education was strategically built into the curriculum, impacting students in Grade Kindergarten through Grade 5. Teachers were given access to a curriculum entitled *The Mutt-i-grees Curriculum*. Teachers used this curriculum as a "blue print" for implementing humane education lessons and activities in their classrooms.

The Mutt-i-grees Curriculum was intentionally designed and created to teach children social and emotional skills ("The Mutt-i-grees Curriculum," 2010). The development of the curriculum was a collaboration of efforts, including those of the *Petsavers Foundation,Yale University School of the 21st Century*, and the *Cesar Millan Foundation*. What makes the *Mutt-i-grees*' approach to character education unique, is that it teaches the fore mentioned skills through the intentional highlighting of the characteristics and needs of dogs awaiting adoption at shelters. The curriculum components teach empathy and the related social and emotional skills, to students in Grades Pre-Kindergarten through Grade 3 ("The Mutt-i-grees Curriculum," 2010).

The Mutt-i-grees Curriculum is packaged in a user friendly, sectioned binder. The binder sections include Introduction, Design, Implementation, Lesson Plans Pre-K/Kindergarten, Lesson Plans Grades 1/2/3, as well as the provision of a Resources section, allowing Grassy Waters Elementary School educators to continue character education upon the completion of the Lesson Plans ("The Mutt-i-grees Curriculum," 2010). This curriculum strategically incorporates five curricular themes. Each of the five themes are directly related to character development and creatively infused in lessons that span across a variety of subject areas ("The Mutt-i-grees Curriculum," 2010).

Additionally, school stakeholders at Grassy Waters Elementary School reached out to local members of the community, soliciting humane rights advocates to join in the school's efforts in positively impacting students. One such community member was Ms. Karen Roberts. Karen Roberts is a children's book author and President of *The Little Blue Dog, Inc*. Ms. Roberts mission through her books for children and community outreach is to provide young people with age-appropriate humane education. Ms. Roberts facilitated numerous field trips for students to a local animal rescue, *Peggy Adams Animal Rescue League*. During these field trips, students toured the rescue facilities, learning about proper care and treatment of animals, as well as how a rescue operates. Students were also active participants, participating in service learning projects during the field trip. Students created toys for the animals residing at *Peggy Adams Animal Rescue League*, such as catnip socks and toilet paper roll treat dispensers. What's more, Ms. Roberts bridged academic state standards and community service, as students interacted with the rescue's animals and later developed haiku poems featuring each animal's unique characteristics. These poems were displayed throughout the *Peggy Adams Animal Rescue League* facility.

Ms. Roberts also joined forces with Grassy Waters Elementary School's *Reading Buddies Program*. The *Reading Buddies Program* specifically targets struggling student readers who often feel intimidated reading to a student peer or adult. The program provides teachers the opportunity to identify and select students to instead read books of their choosing to K-9 Good Citizen dogs on campus. Ms. Roberts added her pups to the *Reading Buddies* mix, bringing Roxie and Cinnabon in on a regular basis as part of the *Reading Buddies Program*! Students enjoy reading to Ms. Roberts pups, often choosing a *Little Blue Dog* book to read aloud! Students who previously loathed reading aloud, embraced the opportunity to read to an author's dog! These same students who struggled with reading were inspired to "write a book like Ms. Karen," and immediately wanted to start writing their own "dog book" after participating in the *Reading Buddies Program*!

Previous research suggests that students reading to dogs simultaneously improves reading skills, while also stimulating social and emotional growth and development ("Reading to Dogs," 2015). Reading to dogs provides students an opportunity to practice their reading skills, motivating students who may be hesitant to read to a student peer or adult. Children are more likely to challenge themselves, selecting a book that may be a little more difficult when reading to a dog, as they are less intimidated. Historically, research also indicates that students participating in programs such as *Reading Buddies*, demonstrate improved reading fluency ("Reading to Dogs," 2015).

Just being in the presence of a dog and petting a pup is also associated with positive *physical* effects on both children and adult humans (Le Roux, Swartz, & Swart, 2014). In previous studies, students' blood pressure was lower when reading aloud in the presence of a dog versus when reading aloud to a fellow student or adult. Moreover, students' attention and academic performance motivation improved when animals were regularly present in the classroom learning environment. For hesitant student readers, anxiety lowered when in the presence of a dog (Le Roux et al., 2014).

Grassy Waters Elementary School also conducted a number of animal shelter supply drives on campus. This was done in effort to literally "drive home" the message of humane education, involving student families in gathering items for local rescue organizations. One such drive was entitled Pillowcases for Pups. Students and their families collected clean, gently used pillowcases to donate to animal rescues within Palm Beach County, FL. Animal rescues used these pillow cases inside of animal crates and runs, providing animals a "cozy spot."

After the first animal shelter supply drive, parents and families at Grassy Waters Elementary School were very much emotionally invested in the humane education initiative on campus. Administration received positive feedback and countless student family members demonstrating enthusiasm about the benefits of incorporating humane education within the curriculum. For example, one student's parent worked at a veterinarian's office and offered to visit classrooms and present information regarding the importance of pet care, including the imperativeness of the responsibility to spay and neuter pets. Another parent offered information regarding a local feral cat coalition. Grassy Waters Elementary School hosted another drive as a result of this connection, entitled *Cat Chow Round-Up*, collecting cat food for feral cats in need. The impact of the humane education initiative on campus was beyond impactful and seemingly boundless!

CONCLUSION

As a result of the implementation of the humane education integration, Grassy Waters Elementary School further developed a culture in which the fore mentioned character traits (among others) were admired and adopted, creating a school environment in which respect and kindness were the expectation, and responsibility, a necessary must. Animal welfare also came to light, as teachers and students delved further into humane education content. Students learned about the concept of animal rescue and the large number of animals in need. In doing so, students and teachers were inspired to take action locally at various animal rescues. Projects such as the drives "Newspapers for Cats" and "Pillowcases for Pups," involved school families in collecting newspaper for cat boxes and pillowcases, small blankets, and gently used towels for dogs. These items were then distributed to local animal rescues within Palm Beach County, Florida.

The history of the human-canine relationship and the human-canine bond is longstanding and has grown and developed throughout the years. Today, dogs are part of the family and are beneficial in impacting humans across the board. To take care of the pets across our country and learn valuable life-long lessons humane education is an important component that will surely enhance our country as a whole.

REFERENCES

Adams, C. (2013, February27). Character education seen as student-achievement tool. *Education Week*, 2013, 7.

Albert, A., & Anderson, M. (1997). Dogs, cats, and morale maintenance: Some preliminary data. *Anthrozoos*, *10*(2/3), 121–124. doi:10.2752/089279397787001193

Allen, K. M., Blascovich, J., & Mendes, W. B. (2002). Cardiovascular reactivity and the presence of pets, friends, and spouses: The truth about cats and dogs. *Psychosomatic Medicine*, *64*(5), 727–739. doi:10.1097/01.psy.0000024236.11538.41 PMID:12271103

Allen, K. M., Blascovich, J., Tomaka, J., & Kelsey, R. M. (1991). Presence of human friends and pet dogs as moderators of autonomic responses to stress in women. *Journal of Personality and Social Psychology*, *61*(81), 582–589. doi:10.1037/0022-3514.61.4.582 PMID:1960650

American humane operational guide. (2010). Retrieved from http://www.americanhumane.org/assets/pdfs/animals/operational-guides/op-guide-humaneed.pdf

Arambašic, L., Keresteš, G., Kuterovac-Jagodíc, G., & Vizek-Vidovic, V. (2000). The role of pet ownership as a possible buffer variable in traumatic experiences. *Studia Psychologica*, *42*(1-2), 135–146.

Ascione, F. R. (2015). 21st Century animal resource and educational services. Retrieved fromhttp://21stcenturycares.org/research.htm

Association of Professional Humane Educators. (2011, Summer). Is humane education an endangered species? *The Latham Letter*, *32*(3), 6–9.

Beck, A., & Katcher, A. H. (1996). *Between pets and people*. West Lafayette, IN: Purdue University Press.

Beck, M. (2010, December 21). Beside Freud's couch, a chow named Jofi. The Wall Street Journal. Retrieved from http://online.wsj.com/articles/SB10001424052748703886904576031630124087362

Bilger, B. (2003). the last meow. Conde Nast Publications, Inc.

Bradshaw, J. (2011). *Dog sense*. New York, New York: Basic Books.

Brown, S. G., & Rhodes, R. E. (2006). Relationships among dog ownership and leisure-time walking in western Canadian adults. *American Journal of Preventive Medicine*, *30*(2), 131–136. doi:10.1016/j.amepre.2005.10.007 PMID:16459211

Bryant, B. K., & Donnellan, M. B. (2007). The relation between socio-economic status concerns and angry peer conflict resolution is moderated by pet provisions of support. *Anthrozoos*, *20*(3), 213–223. doi:10.2752/089279307X224764

Camp, M. M. (2001). The use of service dogs as an adaptive strategy: A qualitative study. *The American Journal of Occupational Therapy*, *55*(5), 509–517. doi:10.5014/ajot.55.5.509 PMID:14601810

Canadian Federation of Humane Societies (CFHS) Ear cropping and tail docking. Retrieved from http://cfhs.ca/athome/ear_cropping_and_tail_docking Regarding Canadian Animal Law, see http://cfhs.ca/features/a_disappointing_day_for_animals_in_canada/

Canfield, J. (1999). *Chicken soup for the pet lover's soul: Stories about pets as teachers, healers, heroes and friends*. Deerfield Beach, FL: Health Communications.

Caspari, E. (2003). Animal life in nature, myth and dreams. Wilmette, EL: Chiron.

Charnetski, C. J., Riggers, S., & Brennan, F. X. (2004). Effect of petting a dog on immune system function. *Psychological Reports*, *95*(3, Pt. 2), 1087–1091. PMID:15762389

Clutton-Brock, J. (2006). Origins of the dog: Domestication and early history. In J. Serpell (Ed.), *The domestic dog: Its evolution, behaviour and interactions with people* (pp. 7–20). New York: Cambridge University Press.

Cole, M., & Wertsch, J. V. (1996). Beyond the individual-social antinomy in discussions of Piaget and Vygotsky. *Human Development*, *39*(5), 250–256. doi:10.1159/000278475

Corson, S. A., & Corson, O. E. (1980). Pet animals as nonverbal communication mediators in psychotherapy in institutional settings. In S. A. Corson & E. O. Corson (Eds.), *Ethology and nonverbal communication in mental health* (pp. 83–110). Oxford: Pergamon Press.

Cox, J. H. (2009). *Humane education: A guide on methodology for educators*. Prepared for the Humane Education Trust of South Africa. Retrieved from http://www.worldanimal.net/docs/HET%20Humane%20Education%20Methodology.pdf

Crawford, E. K., Worsham, N. L., & Swinehart, E. R. (2006). Benefits derived from companion animals, and the use of the term "attachment". *Anthrozoos*, *19*(2), 98–112. doi:10.2752/089279306785593757

Cutt, H., Giles-Corti, B., & Knuiman, M. (2008). Encouraging physical activity through dog walking: Why don't some owners walk with their dog? *Preventive Medicine*, *46*(2), 120–126. doi:10.1016/j.ypmed.2007.08.015 PMID:17942146

Digby, A. (1984). The changing profile of a nineteenth-century asylum: The york retreat. *Psychological Medicine*, *14*(4), 739. doi:10.1017/S003329170001970X PMID:6400132

Dotson, M. J., & Hyatt, E. M. (2008, May). Understanding dog-human companionship. *Journal of Business Research*, *61*(5), 457–466. doi:10.1016/j.jbusres.2007.07.019

Elias, M. J. (2011). The character of schools, the character of individuals, and the character of society: Creating educational policy to reflect inextricable interconnection. *KEDI Journal of Educational Policy*, 2011, 141-149.

Fawcett, N. R., & Gullone, E. (2001). Cute and cuddly and a whole lot more? A call for empirical investigation into the therapeutic benefits of human-animal interaction for children. *Behaviour Change*, *18*(2), 124–133. doi:10.1375/bech.18.2.124

Friedmann, E., Katcher, A. H., Thomas, S. A., Lynch, J. J., & Messent, P. R. (1983). Social interaction and blood pressure: The influence of animal companions. *The Journal of Nervous and Mental Disease*, *171*(8), 461–465. doi:10.1097/00005053-198308000-00002 PMID:6875529

Galindo, J. personal communication, December 5, 2015

Hare, B., & Woods, V. (2013). *The genius of dogs: how dogs are smarter than you think*. Penguin.

Headey, B., Na, F., & Zheng, R. (2008). Pet dogs benefit owners' health: A 'natural experiment' in china. *Social Indicators Research*, *87*(3), 481–493. doi:10.1007/s11205-007-9142-2

Humane education for kids. (2015). Retrieved from http://www.safehavenhumane.org/humane-education-kids

Humane Society of the United States (HSUS). Declawing Cats: More Than Just a Manicure, Retrieved from http://www.hsus.org/pets/pet_care/cat_care/declawing_cats_more_than_just_a_manicure/

Institute for Humane Education. (2008). What is humane education? Retrieved from http://humaneeducation.org/sections/view/what_is_humane_education

Katz, J. (2003). *The New Work of Dogs: Tending to Life, Love, and Family*. New York, NY: Random House Trade Paperbacks.

Le Roux, M. C., Swartz, L., & Swart, E. (2014, May30). The Effect of an animal-assisted reading program on the reading rate, accuracy, and comprehension of grade 3 students: A randomized control study. *Child and Youth Care Forum*, *43*(1), 655–673. doi:10.1007/s10566-014-9262-1

Loeser, J. (2014). Values, character, & moral education.

Lott, D. (1988). Feeding wild animals: The urge, the interaction, and the consequences. *Anthrozoos, 1*(4), 255–257. doi:10.2752/089279388787058326

Martin, F., & Farnum, J.Martin & Farnum. (2002, October). Animal-assisted therapy for children with pervasive developmental disorders. *Western Journal of Nursing Research, 24*(6), 657–670. doi:10.1177/019394502320555403 PMID:12365766

Melson, G. F. (1991). Children's attachment to their pets: Links to socioemotional development. *Children's Environments Quarterly, 82*, 55–65.

Melson, G. F. (2003). Child development and the human-companion animal bond. *The American Behavioral Scientist, 47*(31), 31–39. doi:10.1177/0002764203255210

Messent, P. R. (1983). Social facilitation of contact with other people with pet dogs. In A. H. B. Katcher & M. Alan (Eds.), *New perspectives on our lives with companion animals* (pp. 351–359). Philadelphia: University of Pennsylvania Press.

Nagengast, S. L., Baun, M. M., Megel, M., & Leibowitz, J. (1997). The effects of the presence of a companion animal on physiological arousal and behavioral distress in children during a physical examination. *Journal of Pediatric Nursing, 12*(6), 323–330. doi:10.1016/S0882-5963(97)80058-9 PMID:9420370

Odendaal, J. S. J. (2000). Animal-assisted therapy -- magic or medicine? *Journal of Psychosomatic Research, 49*(4), 275–280. doi:10.1016/S0022-3999(00)00183-5 PMID:11119784

Olson, P. N. (2002). The modern working dog: A call for interdisciplinary collaboration. *Journal of the American Medical Association, 221*(3), 352–355. doi:10.2460/javma.2002.221.352 PMID:12164529

Ortiz, A. (2015, February). Humane liberation: Incorporating animal rights into critical pedagogy. *The Vermont Connection, 32*, 67–77.

Parents and teachers. (2015). Retrieved from http://www.paws.org/kids/parents-and-teachers/

Reading to dogs: A library's guide to getting started. (2015). Retrieved from http://readingtodogs.weebly.com/research.html

Research Starters. (2010). *The mutt-i-grees curriculum*. Port Washington, New York: The Petsavers Foundation.

Risely-Curtiss, C. (2010). Social work practitioners and the human-companion animal bond: A national study. *Social Work, 55*(1), 38–46. doi:10.1093/sw/55.1.38 PMID:20069939

Russack, N. (2000). *Animal guides: In life, myth and dreams*. Toronto, Ontario, Canada: Inner City Books.

Schaefer, K. (2002, January). Human-animal interactions as a therapeutic intervention. *Counseling and Human Development, 34*(5), 1–18.

Schaffer, C. B. (2009, Winter). Animals connecting people to people: Insights into animal-assisted therapy and animal-assisted activities. *Reflections: The SoL Journal, 15*(1), 42–45.

Schvaneveldt, P. L., Young, M. H., Schvaneveldt, J. D., & Kivett, V. R. (2001). Interaction of people and pets in the family setting: A life course perspective. *Journal of Teaching in Marriage & Family*, *1*(2), 34–52. doi:10.1300/J226v01n02_03

Shiloh, S., Sorek, G., & Terkel, J. (2003). Reduction of state-anxiety by petting animals in a controlled laboratory experiment. *Anxiety, Stress, and Coping*, *16*(4), 387–395. doi:10.1080/1061580031000091582

Swabe, J. (2000). Veterinary dilemmas: ambiguity and ambivalence in human-animal interaction. In A.L. Podberscek, E.S. Paul, & J.A. Serpell (Eds.), Companion Animals and Us: Exploring the relationships between people and pets. Cambridge: Cambridge University Press.

Tannen, D. (2004). Talking the dog: Framing Pets as interactional resources in family discourse. *Research on Language and Social Interaction*, *37*(4), 399–420. doi:10.1207/s15327973rlsi3704_1

The Need for humane education. (2014). Retrieved from http://worldanimal.net/our-programs/humane-education/the-need-for-humane-education

Thomas, S. C., & Beirne, P. (2002). Humane education and humanistic philosophy: Toward a new curriculum. *The Journal of Humanistic Counseling, Education and Development*, *41*(2), 190–199. http://www.c-ahead.com/publications.htm doi:10.1002/j.2164-490X.2002.tb00142.x

Trivedi, L., & Perl, J. (1995). Animal Facilitated Counseling in the Elementary School: A Literature Review and Practical Considerations. *Elementary School Guidance & Counseling*, *29*(3), 223–234.

Unti, B., & DeRosa, B. (2003). Humane education: Past, present, and future. In D. J. Salem & A. N. Rowan (Eds.), *The state of the animals II: 2003*. Washington, DC: Humane Society Press.

Valentine, D. P., Kiddoo, M., & LaFleur, B. (1993). Psychosocial implications of service dog ownership for people who have mobility or hearing impairments. *Social Work in Health Care*, *19*(1), 109–125. doi:10.1300/J010v19n01_07 PMID:8296220

Veevers, J. E. (1985). The social meanings of pets: Alternative roles for companion animals. In M. B. Sussman (Ed.), *Pets and the family* (pp. 11–30). New York: Haworth Press. doi:10.1300/J002v08n03_03

Velde, B. P., Cipriani, J., & Fisher, G. (2005). Resident and therapist views of animal- assisted therapy: Implications for occupational therapy practice. *Australian Occupational Therapy Journal*, *52*(1), 43–50. doi:10.1111/j.1440-1630.2004.00442.x

Walsh, F. (2009). Human-animal bonds II: The role of pets in family systems and family therapy. *Family Process*, *48*(4), 481–499. doi:10.1111/j.1545-5300.2009.01297.x PMID:19930434

Weil, Z. (2003). *Above all, be kind: Raising a humane child in challenging times*. Gabriola Island, BC: New Society.

Wisdom, J. P., Saedi, G. A., & Green, C. A. (2009). Another breed of "service" animals: Stars study findings about pet ownership and recovery from serious mental illness. *The American Journal of Orthopsychiatry*, *79*(3), 430–436. doi:10.1037/a0016812 PMID:19839680

Wood, L. J., Giles-Corti, B., Bulsara, M. K., & Bosch, D. A. (2007). More than a furry companion: The ripple effect of companion animals on neighborhood interactions and sense of community. *Society & Animals*, *15*(1), 43–56. doi:10.1163/156853007X169333

Zilcha-Mano, S., Mikulincer, M., & Shaver, P. R. (2012). Pets as safe havens and secure bases: The moderating role of pet attachment orientations. *Journal of Research in Personality*, *46*(5), 571–580. doi:10.1016/j.jrp.2012.06.005

KEY TERMS AND DEFINITIONS

Character Education: A well-rounded approach to teaching youth to help them develop civic virtue and moral character.

Humane Education: A program intended to foster compassion, empathy, and respect for all living things.

Human-Animal Bond (HAB): A mutually beneficial, dynamic relationship between people and animals that is influenced by behaviors that was essential to the health and wellbeing of both.

"Part of the Family": The mindset that pet "parents" as opposed to pet "owners" see their pets as equal family members and viewed as their children.

Reading Buddies Program: Specifically targets struggling student readers who often feel intimidated reading to a student peer or adult. The program provides teachers the opportunity to identify and select students to instead read books of their choosing to K-9 Good Citizen dogs on campus.

Chapter 6
Preparing Future Physicians to Adapt to the Changing Health Care System:
Promoting Humanism through Curricular Design

Joanna Lauren Drowos
Florida Atlantic University, USA

Sarah K Wood
Florida Atlantic University, USA

ABSTRACT

One vital goal of medical education is to promote the development of desirable professional qualities among future physicians, such as compassion, empathy, and humanism. Future physicians must finish their training prepared to meet the changing health needs of society, yet in reality many students graduate from medical school more cynical and less empathetic than when they began. During clinical clerkships, many students experience an "ethical erosion" as they transition in to real world clinical settings. Through innovative longitudinal integrated curricular designs focusing on continuity, medical students participate in the comprehensive care of patients over time and have continuous ongoing learning relationships with the responsible clinicians. As patients place increasing importance on the doctor-patient relationship, learning models that foster stronger connections between medical students and their patients, as well as with their teachers and communities, are needed in order to better prepare the next generation of physicians to serve a changing health care system.

DOI: 10.4018/978-1-5225-0640-9.ch006

INTRODUCTION

As the health care system continues to evolve, medical education must advance to meet society's and patients' needs. As Cohen (2009) described, current trends in patient expectations for health care, requires the development of a patient-centered physician workforce, made up of individuals with good communication and teamwork skills. One essential goal of medical education is to promote the development of desirable professional qualities among future physicians, such as compassion, empathy, and humanism. Future physicians must finish their training prepared to meet the changing health needs of society yet in reality many students graduate from medical school more cynical and less empathetic than when they began. Students enter medical school with core values of altruism, humanism, and service, which may drive them toward medicine as their career choice in the first place. These traits, however, may actually erode during training, as students graduate feeling cynical and less connected to patients, as found by Coulehan and Williams (2001). The reasons for this transformation include changes in the learning environment, an evolving health care system, and traditional curricular designs that may promote a loss of empathy. In general, medical education has become more fragmented, with highly specialized physicians performing more specific tasks for each patient during brief encounters. During clinical clerkships that occur mostly in the third year of medical school, many students experience an "ethical erosion" or loss of empathy, as they transition from preclinical classroom learning experiences in to real world clinical settings. In response to these troubling trends, medical educators have been developing innovative educational models and curricula that can promote desirable professional traits among medical students. This first year of clinical learning is typically challenging and overwhelming, and for many students, moral and ethical development can be impacted negatively as they navigate their new role in providing patient care. In response to the often dehumanizing "hidden curriculum" that exists in health care delivery settings medical educators have begun to develop innovative clinical curriculum designs using continuity as the leading principle. One example of an educational innovation is longitudinal integrated clerkships (LICs), which allow students additional opportunities to participate in comprehensive care, while building relationships with both patients, faculty, and other health care professionals. This new integrated clerkship model, based on longitudinal exposure to physician preceptors and continuity with patients is being implemented across the nation and around the globe. These longitudinal integrated clerkships (LICs) vary in structure but have the central goals of continuity of care, continuity of curriculum, and continuity of supervision. Medical students participate in the comprehensive care of patients over time and have continuous ongoing learning relationships with these patients' clinicians. Expected changes from this model include enhanced clinical skills, more attention to values and ethics, improved quality of the learning experience, more meaningful direct clinical supervision and feedback, as well as a possible positive impact on career goals. Some LICs have outcome data suggesting a possible relationship between student participation in an LIC, and future interest in primary care or working with rural or underserved populations. Overwhelmingly, results from this model demonstrate students finish their education with strong clinical skills and more empathy than students who complete traditional block clerkship models (Norris et al., 2009). As patients place increasing importance on the doctor-patient relationship, learning models that foster stronger connections between medical students and their patients, as well as with their teachers and communities, are needed in order to better prepare the next generation of physicians to serve a changing health care system.

BARRIERS TO HUMANISM AND PROFESSIONALISM IN MEDICAL EDUCATION

Ethical Erosion Among Medical Students

The medical education process impacts student empathy. Deleterious changes in humanistic qualities have been described as students become "immunized" against these values after matriculation, particularly during the clinical years (Coulehan & Williams, 2001). Study results from one medical school, illustrate a significant decline in mean empathy scores during the third year of training. A research group led by Hojat et al. (2009) at Jefferson Medical College, administered the validated Jefferson Scale of Physician Empathy to students at five different times throughout their undergraduate medical education training. Statistical analysis revealed that empathy scores remained stable during the first two years, or preclinical portion of the curriculum. A significant decline in empathy scores was observed at the end of the third year, or clerkship year, which persisted until graduation. Students continue to perpetuate the behaviors learned during early clinical experiences as they are reinforced during continued training. These behavior patterns may persist during residency training and ultimately in to their future practices.

During clinical clerkships in the third year of medical school, many students experience an "ethical erosion" as they transition from preclinical classroom learning experiences into clinical settings. As described by Feudtener, Christakis, and Christakis (1994), ethical erosion refers to the progressive loss of professionalism occurring during medical training, particularly during the clerkship year. More recent studies confirm that ethical erosion continues to occur among medical students in current educational settings (Martimianakis et al., 2015). Clinical learning during the first year typically challenges and overwhelms, as students need to learn a significant amount of knowledge, as well as to understand the culture of their new profession. The patterns of decline observed in the Jefferson Medical College study were similar for men and women, and for those who pursued their medical training in people-oriented and technology-oriented specialties (Hojat et al., 2009). This significant observed deterioration in empathy levels occurs during the time when students are caring for patients they had, presumably, anticipated helping. In many academic tertiary care centers, the treatment focus turns toward technology, and it can be difficult to direct empathy toward a challenging patient (Newton, Barber, Clardy, Cleveland & O'Sullivan, 2008). Achieving empathy can also be hindered by cultural differences between physicians-in-training and their patients. The erosion of empathy in medical school can be attributed to several factors, including lack of role models, a high volume of material to learn, time pressure, and patient and environmental factors favoring fragmentation and specialization of care (Watson, 2003).

The Hidden Curriculum

The formal curriculum planned by medical educators holds the intention of instilling knowledge, skills, and certain desirable behaviors among students. However, medical student learning is highly impacted by both the informal and hidden curricula, particularly during the clinical years. Hafferty (1998) defined the informal curriculum as the "unscripted, predominantly ad hoc, and highly interpersonal form of teaching that takes place among and between faculty and students" (p. 404) outside of formal settings. An example of this includes conversations in the hallway or late night discussions in on-call rooms that may influence students in a powerful way. In settings like this, a student may appreciate what is really valued at their particular institution, such as a retelling of a story where one physician argued with another physician publicly, or a physician stood up to a patient in an argument. Medical students often witness or experience demeaning behavior at the hands of their physician supervisors or other health care personnel, and that humiliation reinforces blunted moral development and a loss of compassionate behavior. Students can be mocked for being too caring and empathetic with patients and told they will never survive in medicine if they are so "soft." Traditional teaching methods, such as "pimping" with questions may set students up for criticism and humiliation when they don't know correct answers. Patients are frequently dehumanized in clinical settings when they are identified by their room number or their diagnosis, such as "the asthmatic in bay 3." Referring to patients in this way has become so common in certain settings that individuals speak this way without even considering how a patient may feel if they heard this. Students may adopt these behaviors when they are modeled by residents or physicians so they "fit in," despite having been educated against this in the formal curriculum.

Beyond the extremely influential informal experiences that students have in clinical settings, the hidden curriculum is also defined by Hafferty (1998) on a larger scale as "a set of influences that function at the level of organizational structure and culture" (p. 404) that sometimes send conflicting messages from the intended educational focus. An illustration of this includes when a medical school proudly advertises the amount of research funding received as a quantitative reflection of the quality of the educational program. The message perceived by students becomes that basic science learning and research are truly valued at this particular medical school. Both the informal and hidden curriculum undermine medical student empathy because students easily recognize that campus policies and resource allocations are directed toward the true priorities of a medical school. Students may garner that "what is really important to learn" is based on these messages; for example, a focus on basic science courses over the need for humanities, which may conflict with the stated educational mission of the medical school. The hidden curriculum has been well described by Hojat et al. (2009), as typically it drives students' attention away from the humanities and patient's psychosocial needs, and toward more advanced medical care that may conflict with patient values. Ethical erosion is a serious, negative consequence of the hidden curriculum.

Increasing Fragmentation of the Learning Environment

The learning environment that medical students experience has changed in response to changes in the health care delivery system. Hirsh, Ogur, Thibault, and Cox (2007) described these patterns noting that nationwide there had been a dramatic decrease in the length of hospital stays, with the majority of care provided now occurring in the outpatient setting, rather than during hospital admissions. The demographics of the patients and problems encountered in the hospital has been altered also, limiting opportunities for the types of conditions seen, as well as the opportunity to observe disease progression. Most patients admitted are sicker now, presenting for an acute issue such that students frequently do not get to observe their illness as part of a continuum of care. Students only see patients for a moment in time and therefore they are unable to view the patient in a larger patient-centered humanistic context. Moreover, students have fewer opportunities for providing wellness or prevention-related services in the hospital setting.

Additionally, the growth in hospitalists, physicians who only provide care while patients are admitted as inpatients, has led to a separation between the inpatient and outpatient oversight of patients. Now primary care doctors have the option of continuing to follow their own patients while admitted, or to defer to the hospitalist who spends all of their time in the inpatient setting. The hospitalist model means also that several physicians, typically working in teams, share coverage for a particular population of patients during various shifts. Less continuous time is spent by any one attending in the inpatient setting, and there is often no integration with the care provided in the outpatient setting. This loss of continuity for the students and residents as they rotate through a variety of patients with a variety of attending physicians, is also compounded by work hour restrictions that limit the amount of time spent in the hospital. Students and residents work in teams, signing off care to one another at various points when their shifts are over. Therefore, typically medical students are unable to see the care of patients from a holistic viewpoint as they participate in only fragments of their care.

In recent years, the clinical learning environment has become increasingly fractured by growing specialization and demands for clinical productivity that has impacted the practice environment for many medical school faculty. Many academic medical centers offer advanced fellowship programs, where highly specialized physicians perform only a select group of procedures. Often patients see a variety of physicians who perform only one small role in their overall care. When students are assigned to these highly trained specialists for learning, this limits opportunities to see a variety of pathology, and limits the ability to develop relationships and interact with patients for longer than the brief intervention. Further, students miss the opportunity to see the progression of the patient's disease over time and to observe the comprehensive care that occurs beyond the small role played by their particular specialized attending physician (Hirsh et al., 2007). As patients struggle to navigate increasingly complex systems of care, the trainees and physicians who care for them often have less and less insight into the challenges they face.

As medical schools have faced declining budgets over time, there is increased pressure on faculty to be clinically productive and to obtain research funding. As described by Hirsh et al. 2007, the prevailing culture requires educational activities to compete with research and clinical practice needs for scarce medical school resources. Some medical schools are responding to this pressure by engaging volunteer, or sometimes paid, physician faculty from the community, or by relying on medical teams for teaching. Community faculty play an increasing role in educating medical students, however many of these individuals face competing pressure from their own clinical practices. These individuals may have varying skill levels and interest for teaching, and often only have limited time available. In most medical schools, students are assigned to specialty-specific teams of interns, residents, and supervising faculty physicians for relatively brief, arbitrarily sequenced rotations in acute care hospitals (Watson, 2003; Whitcomb, 2005).

Traditional block clerkship models place students on teams in a particular specialty, for a defined period of time. In this setting as described by Christakis and Feudtner (1997), students learn and perform various clinical duties for the patients admitted to the particular service where they are assigned. At the end of the rotation, the student will move on and repeat the cycle in a different specialty, with a new group of faculty and patients. Unfortunately, this system promotes students sequentially joining teams they are unfamiliar with, in new settings they are unaccustomed to, and providing care to patients with whom they have no relationship. Students are faced with having to develop many simultaneous new relationships with residents, attending physicians, nurses, staff, and patients, without having adequate time to devote to more meaningful long-term connections. Repeatedly students are subjected to constant time pressure to move on to learn something new. Just when a student begins to develop a sense of mastery with skills that are valued by the team, he/she must start over in a different setting with a new team and unknown patients. While this strategy offers certain benefits, such as prioritizing efficient practices, and promoting a focus on the medical issue at hand, this approach may differ from what the patients' ultimately value.

Consequences of this existing clinical clerkship rotation structure, include social isolation and estrangement from the medical team and from patients, as there is not time to develop meaningful relationships. Functioning as a team requires a certain level of trust and without this confidence in students' performance typical hierarchies and authority structures are reinforced. Students may not feel comfortable to ask questions, or challenge the care provided by the members of the team at a higher rank. Students may end up resenting and neglecting the psychosocial issues facing patients, as these also take time to uncover, and can be assigned to other members of the health care team to manage. Students may avoid intimacy as a result of this environment, and may fail to intervene on issues that do not relate to the direct medical care of their patients. Ultimately these learned habits may shape the types of physicians these students become, as well as their future interactions with patients (Christakis & Feudtner, 1997). Other potential factors impacting empathy, include fatigue or burnout, which are exacerbated also by a lack of continuity as students begin new challenging clinical rotations every few weeks.

Student Mistreatment and Burnout

Burnout is a measure of physical and psychological exhaustion, combined with mental and emotional distress, resulting primarily from occupational and professional demands. Among physicians practicing in the United States, studies estimate burnout to range between 40-70%. While the cause of burnout is complex and remains unclear, evidence suggests many students begin to experience burnout during medical school, with reports that it occurs in as many as 49% in the US, and 28-61% of medical students in Australia (Cecil, McHale, Hart, & Laidlaw, 2014). Burnout is characterized by a depersonalization, where emotional indifference or dehumanization of the patient may occur. Additionally, students may experience a lessened perception of their own accomplishments, which can interfere with their confidence and skill development. Medical school is known to be challenging time, with factors such as academic pressures, educational debt and personal life events contributing to the overall stress. Alternative curricular models have the potential to mitigate the effects of burnout, by providing an educational structure that is learner-centered and allowing students to contribute to patient care in meaningful ways.

Many studies demonstrate a lack of clinical role models, or specifically positive clinical role models that may also contribute to the decline in empathy and increased level of burnout during the clerkship years. While clinicians consider an empathic physician-patient relationship as one of the most important aspects of professionalism, these interactions are best demonstrated by physician role models at the bedside while caring for patients. Research shows that many medical students perceive themselves as being somewhat mistreated by their clinical supervisors and attendings, as the students are trying to move toward a role with more autonomy and responsibility, while simultaneously being subservient to their superiors who are evaluating them. Typical hierarchical medical team structures and extreme Socratic teaching methods can leave students feeling humiliated and demoralized. This student abuse or "traumatic de-idealization" combined with a shortage of positive role models, contributes to the ethical erosion experienced by medical students (Newton et al., 2008). Mentoring relationships between students and clinical faculty are hindered further by traditional block clerkship models, as students do not have the opportunity to develop meaningful relationships with their supervising physicians or to become comfortable in the roles they are playing. Also, the time-limited nature of block rotations diminishes the ability of students to demonstrate their skill and knowledge progression and receive more trust, autonomy, and responsibility from their supervisors.

THE CASE FOR CHANGE

Deficiencies in the Current Medical Education System

The Carnegie Foundation for the Advancement of Teaching in Stanford, California published results of a medical education study after reviewing the research on medical education and the learning sciences. As outlined by Cooke, Irby, and O'Brien (2010), the group completed 14 site visits, concluding that medical education is not learner centered, and that it tends to be long and inflexible. Additional findings in the report included an over-emphasis on inpatient medicine, with education occurring often in hospitals that lacked appropriate infrastructure to support educational activities. Poor linkages exist between the formal knowledge gained through didactics with the experiential learning taking place in clinical settings. Many medical school curricula fail to prepare students to work in complex health care delivery systems, or to address all patient populations. The characteristic of medical education described in the report that most supports the development of LICs is the lack of opportunity for students to engage in patient care longitudinally.

Four key recommendations are described in the Carnegie Foundation study, all of which support the development of longitudinal clinical experiences. The study suggests that medical education needs to better integrate the knowledge gained with clinical experiential learning, and to foster habits of inquiry and a desire for excellence among students. Another key recommendation involves standardizing expectations and assessments while allowing individualization within curriculum. This would allow for flexibility in learning while setting clear goals for outcomes. Lastly, designing curricula that foster identity formation for future physicians, through a focus on professional values, is deemed as a necessary change within the current medical education system. Longitudinal clinical experiences are recommended as a method to integrate formal didactic knowledge with experiential learning. These experiences also support professional identity formation through a commitment to values that are aligned with the current delivery system with a focus on community practice. They also allow observation of role models with the accompanying coaching, instruction, assessment and feedback (Poncelet et al., 2014).

Training Medical Students to Meet the Needs of a Changing Health Care System

As the health care system continues to evolve, medical education must also evolve to meet society's needs. To prepare graduates for medical practice in a changing system, medical schools have changed their curricula to focus on integration of basic and clinical sciences, health promotion and disease prevention, and interprofessional education. Students are taught to focus attention on the ethical, social, psychologic, and financial impact of disease upon the patient, family, and society. Patients and health care systems are expecting medical school graduates to have these skills as they enter practice (Hirsh et al., 2007). Medical school curricula now include courses that emphasize humanitarian values, empathic communication skills, as well as community engagement. Yet, it is still hard for students to focus on the humanities, critical communication skills, and professional identity formation in an already crowded traditional four-year curriculum with high-stakes assessments that emphasize only basic science learning, as described by Newton et al. (2008). Medical schools remain tasked with producing students who have a broad skill-set and certain core competencies that are applicable to all medical specialties.

A call has gone out to develop physicians who are empathic, humanistic, and strong communicators, through counteracting the often destructive "hidden curriculum." Medical educators have been innovative and have developed new curriculum designs using continuity as the leading principle. Integrated clerkship models, based primarily on longitudinal exposure to patients and physician preceptors are being implemented extensively in rural, tertiary care, and community based medical schools nationally and internationally. The concept of educational continuity emphasizes the complex cross-disciplinary skills of doctoring and professionalism, rather than preparing students solely for discipline-specific clinical and procedural skills (Hirsh et al., 2007).

Continuity as a Central Principle for Clinical Education

One of the benefits of these new educational models are that patient and learner centeredness are fostered by continuity within the learning environment, as students have opportunities to connect repeatedly with their own patients and experience true "continuity of care". As outlined by Hirsh et al. (2007), students in the longitudinal integrated clerkship model spend long periods of time, even up to a year, in the same clinical setting building relationships with their preceptor, their patients, and the healthcare team. The longitudinal nature of the experience allows students to develop skills, build trust, and be increase levels of responsibility and autonomy in the care of patients. "Continuity of curriculum" promotes connections between science and clinical medicine, and the developmental attainment of core clinical competencies, as important educational themes are integrated across clinical disciplines. This is important from the perspective of students learning how all specialties and care are integrated as they consider the global experience of the patient. "Continuity of supervision" enhances opportunities for role modeling and mentoring, limiting the "traumatic de-idealization" students may experience in more traditional supervisory structures. With additional time students can develop relationships with their instructors, giving the opportunity for raising questions and contributing ideas to the medical team. This emphasis on continuity of care, curriculum, and supervision provides a solid foundation for maintaining and enhancing an even more fundamental continuity: the continuity of idealism.

Continuity with patients is central to developing therapeutic relationships and understanding disease processes in an LIC, but other examples of continuity also contribute to the enhancement of the learning environment. Teherani et al. (2009) studied the process of continuity with preceptors that allows students to understand and experience the daily working life of the physicians with whom they are paired, as well as the rewards and challenges encountered on a day-to-day basis. Students observed firsthand the scheduling logistics, the management of patient care responsibilities, the essential collaboration with the healthcare team, the incorporation of technology, and the administrative burden that accompanies various medical specialties. This provided valuable insight into lifestyle considerations and assisted students with making better-informed career choices. Relationships with preceptors typically strengthen over time, allowing students to observe and participate in a wide variety of clinical and non-clinical situations under the guidance of an experienced physician. This includes exposure to managing uncertain situations, dealing with ethical challenges, and having difficult conversations with patients that students may not otherwise encounter. The ability to experience over time the ebbs and flows in the busy life of a practicing physician and observe directly the process by which critical communication skills, professionalism, and teamwork work in tandem in the care of patients becomes a true asset for students in LICs.

CHARACTERISTICS OF LONGITUDINAL INTEGRATED CLERKSHIPS (LICS)

Defining Longitudinal Integrated Clerkships (LICs)

According to the Consensus LIC definition developed by the International Consortium of Longitudinal Integrated Clerkships (Norris, 2009), LICs are characterized by being the central element of clinical education whereby medical students (a) participate in the comprehensive care of patients over time; (b) participate in continuing learning relationships with these patients clinicians; and (c) meet the majority of the year's core clinical competencies, across multiple disciplines simultaneously through these experiences. LICs are founded on the principle that when students are able to spend more time in a clinical setting they can become an integral, vital, and contributing member of the health care team. In this apprenticeship-type model, students learn by working closely with the same physicians, nurses, staff, and patients. Students can be advocates for their patients while simultaneously learning about all aspects of their care. Students may begin the year as information gatherers, then as their skills improve they will develop the ability to interpret the information they collect, and eventually contribute to developing patient management plans. This developmental type of learning, embedded in an authentic clinical context, hopefully will help create physicians that can meet the challenges of the current healthcare landscape. Certain medical schools that have adopted this model have the additional expectation that students will develop connections to the host community or site where students train. This occurs most commonly in rural settings, where students may spend significant amounts of time integrated in to the community where they train.

LICs have both a longer duration than traditional clerkships, and an integration of disciplines for purposes of continuity. This provides for an increased opportunity that faculty and students will become well acquainted with each other and have a much greater opportunity for students to participate in the continuity of patient care. Integrating disciplines such as medicine, surgery, pediatrics, obstetrics and gynecology, family medicine, and psychiatry, allows students to view the complexities of individual patients with multiple medical problems through a holistic, rather than discipline-focused, lens. Additionally, more opportunities emerge to view the patient through an entire illness process, for more teaching from faculty than house officers, and to exposure of a wider breadth of clinical problems across a variety of inpatient and outpatient settings (Strasser & Hirsh, 2011).

The History of Longitudinal Integrated Clerkships (LICs) in Medical Schools

The oldest known Longitudinal Integrated Clerkship program was started at the University of Minnesota, School of Medicine in 1971. As of 2012, medical schools using LIC programs reside in Australia, Canada, South Africa, and the United States. Since that time additional schools in all of these places, and in Europe, continue to launch and explore the possibility of training medical students in an LIC. The length of time and structure of each LIC program varies, as well as the balance between inpatient and outpatient training and the disciplines included. Most programs include the core clinical content of internal medicine, surgery, pediatrics, and obstetrics and gynecology. Other experiences may be included depending on the resources available in each community and the curricular requirements of the medical schools. Other specialty experiences incorporated in LICs include psychiatry, family medicine, and orthopedic surgery. Also LIC programs have been established in urban and rural sites successfully, most using ambulatory settings for the diversity of training.

LICs have succeeded with a variety of models and venues, including hybrid designs within highly specialized academic centers, academic urban community hospitals, and dispersed rural or remote clinics. Some medical schools are able to provide all their students with the ability to participate in an LIC program, while others offer it as an elective program for only a portion of the medical school class. In these schools there may be a special selection process for students, including an application or interview, that may consider learning style, motivations, as well as a career interest in primary care or rural care (Norris, et al. 2009).

Students in LIC models have the opportunity to benefit from longitudinal ambulatory care experiences, as more chronic diseases are managed now in the outpatient rather than inpatient setting. Over time, students develop effective relationships with patients, improve their insight into the psychosocial aspects of care, and gain a better understanding of the long-term management and progression of chronic diseases. These competencies are necessary for students to succeed in the modern practice environment. As of 2008 more than 2,700 medical students had completed an LIC program. Outcome data continues to demonstrate that LIC programs achieve their goals of providing continuity with patients and faculty and allow students to develop meaningful relationships during their training. The literature supports that this restructuring of clinical education is grounded in the science of learning, and LICs are already having a substantial impact on the medical education discourse. National as well as international programs are utilizing the LIC model successfully as an alternative to traditional or block rotation models (Hirsh, Walters, & Poncelet, 2012).

Students as Learners in LICs

Within Longitudinal Integrated Clerkships additional opportunities arise for student-centered learning to occur, beyond the experiences typically available in traditional block clerkships, as described by Stevens, Wilkerson, and Uijtdehaage (2014). While the overall clerkship objectives may be set by the faculty, students assume greater responsibility for their own learning in terms of structuring custom learning experiences based on their interests and what they feel they need to and want to learn. Preceptors can assist students with the development of these personalized learning plans, and at least at the start of the year, may strongly guide the use of their time until students are comfortable with the flexibility of the program. Typically, students are given the opportunity to explore a particular clinical area or work on solving a problem that may concern the community or health care system where they are linked for their training.

Furthermore, students benefit from being assigned faculty mentors and advisors who have an understanding of the overall structure, goals, and objectives for the comprehensive LIC curriculum. As described by Poncelet et al. (2011), usually the students' advisors serve for the entirety of the clerkship year in order to support the progression and development over time of the student's skills, knowledge, and behavior. LIC specific advising supplements but does not replace any existing advising or mentoring structures already in place in medical schools. Advisors who work closely with students across the clinical year are ideally suited to provide direct and specific feedback as to the process by which students can better meet curricular goals or remediate any deficiencies. In some cases, these advisors provide this feedback in place of community-based physician preceptors who may need assistance with this role. Regular meetings with clear agendas are appropriate, outlining specific progressive goals for the course of the year. Meetings ensure also that feedback is consistent, allowing time for reflection, as students consider how each need to improve their clinical skills.

Also learning theory helps provide insight into the motivation of students learning by considering self-determination theory. This theory describes three innate psychological needs that drive the motivation to learn; a sense of relatedness, a sense of autonomy, and a sense of competence. Relatedness denotes when a learner feels as if they are a member of a community or of a profession. These feelings are enhanced by building stronger relationships with team members, and by engaging junior learners in decision-making activities. Autonomy refers to the importance of a student feeling as if they have some control over their actions around learning. This is best achieved in situations when the student has earned the preceptor's trust, and the preceptor is able to allow the student's learning plan and goals to be implemented. A sense of competence becomes the third required need. This can be achieved when a student feels he or she has the knowledge or skills to accomplish a task. Even students who are early in their learning can experience this feeling, as long as the tasks to which they are assigned correlate with level of ability. This is best achieved when a faculty member has a developmental perspective on the current level of the learner as well as the long-term goal in mind of what they are striving to achieve (Schumacher, Englander, & Carraccio, 2013). The need to provide relatedness, autonomy, and competence are aligned clearly with the structure of the LIC model, as continuity over time with patients, faculty, and peers at a clinical site fosters these core values.

Additional factors impact a student's ability to learn that can be understood through the cognitive load theory, which considers the clinical working and learning environment that optimizes the ability to learn. When cognitive load is high, a student uses too much of their mental energy and working memory which decreases available space for learning. Schumacher, Englander, and Carraccio (2013), outlined cognitive load as being impacted by how difficult it is to develop a framework for understanding an idea, by how inherently difficult a concept is to grasp and by challenges that may arise because of the presentation of material. In considering the optimal context for learning, situated cognition suggests that all learning is based on the environment, situations and culture where students find themselves. This understanding of the learning environment considers both the formal, informal, and hidden curricula in shaping the messages students receive. The concept of situated cognition supports a cognitive apprenticeship model where students learn the thought processes of a profession in addition to the skills. This apprenticeship theory again supports an LIC model, where students have longitudinal continuity to see the patterns of their profession, and to develop the needed relationships with team members, to be able to ask questions and shape their own learning environment.

Patients as Teachers in LICs

As continuity is the primary goal of LIC programs, students are expected to develop ongoing relationships with patients, either through their preceptor's office or from an experience at the hospital. Cabana and Jee (2004), describe a process that students should follow with these patients through various health care settings, including both inpatient, outpatient and specialty care. Some students may have the opportunity to actively participate in patient care under the supervision of a faculty member, but in other cases students may be observing or may be involved as a support to the patient. In some instances, a student may be checking in with the patient and discussing what is going on, or even reviewing a chart in cases where they are unable to participate in a particular aspect of the patient's care. This requires initiative on the part of students, taking steps to check in and communicate with patients about how they are doing, and to make an effort to be involved in their care. In this relationship patients serve as teachers for the students they work with, with respect to the progression of their illnesses and in experiencing and navigating the health care system.

Preceptors can work with students to identify patients reflecting a range of core diagnoses in primary care and obtain each patient's consent to have the student involved in the patient's care. Students and preceptors will review the list periodically to ensure that the diagnoses of the patients represent those designated from the required list, and also common diagnoses seen in the outpatient primary care setting.

When possible, students will see these designated patients as they come for follow-up visits. If the student cannot be present for a visit of a patient, preceptors will try to update students on interim contacts and students will call patients to "check-in." When possible, students will be involved in significant consultations and admissions of their patients. Students are responsible for following up with records or contacts to be aware of what occurred and any changes in the management plan. Students should assist their preceptor with caring for a variety of patients with both acute and chronic problems that are not a part of their continuity experience. This will occur during the scheduled afternoons each week when panel patients may not be scheduled. In the event multiple patients require care, panel patients will always take priority. In order to increase learning opportunities in various settings, students are expected to check regularly and be responsive to their messages from patients. Students need understanding of professionalism, communication and accountability when dealing with patients. Students can offer to be advocates for their patients and help them navigate and communicate within the systems of care. Often students have more time to listen to patients than other busy health care professionals and this in itself can be comforting and helpful.

The most important aspect of the Longitudinal Integrated Clerkship experience is the continuity of caring between LIC students and the patients they follow over time. Through these multiple interactions, students gain exposure to different perspectives on illness as well as on health maintenance. Students develop the ability to better appreciate the process of diagnostic and therapeutic reasoning, the process by which illnesses evolve over time, as well as the development of therapeutic partnerships with their patients. Students are themselves able to better develop trusting relationships with patients, and can play a significantly more significant role in providing care. This provides additional learning opportunities, fosters greater caring and responsibility for patients, and a sense of professional duty. Then students empathize to a greater degree with the experience of patients, to understand the reasoning and roles played by various providers, and the interactions necessary with health care delivery systems. Soon students become better equipped to appreciate the connection between continuity of care and health outcomes, which ultimately improves patient satisfaction, decreases hospitalizations and emergency room visits, and makes receiving preventive and screening services likely. The relationship between socioeconomic factors, health care access and health outcomes, can also be better appreciated through LIC models (Cabana & Jee, 2004).

LICs are designed to allow students continuity with specific patients. In some cases this may be formalized through the development of a specific panel or cohort of patients to which the student follows over the course of the year. Some of these patients may be assigned to the student by their preceptor at the start of the year while others may be added in to achieve specific learning objectives as the year progresses. These individuals may be identified as students encounter patients in various settings, such as primary care or specialty clinics, emergency departments, or the inpatient setting. Then students provide care as these patients transition through the health care system across settings, while the number and types of patients selected may vary across the year. Additionally, students can have other assigned experiences, such as providing discrete care to a patient they are not going to follow longitudinally, for example, in a surgical case or during an assigned emergency department shift.

While the majority of patients are happy to have students involved in their care, patient acceptance of student involvement is required in an LIC model. To facilitate understanding of the student role, preceptors should emphasize that a student will never take the place of the attending physician, and that the attending physician will always be available and responsible to the patient. Students may add value by assisting with care coordination, providing communication with the attending physician, and providing additional education and support when appropriate. Student scheduling needs to provide flexibility where they can be available to a patient when they present or have a need arise (Gaufberg et al. 2008). Students need to understand their role and should maintain professional boundaries with the patients they follow. Students cannot provide medical advice by phone or email without first asking the responsible preceptor to guarantee that the advice offered is appropriate in scope and content.

Promoting Longitudinal Development in Longitudinal Integrated Clerkships (LICs)

Many medical schools use the preclinical years to teach students to perform history and physical examinations. Traditionally, during the third year clerkships students learn to apply these practices directly to patients and to develop the basic skills of clinical reasoning. In an LIC model, students learn the core knowledge, skills, and attitudes of multiple medical disciplines simultaneously. With a traditional block clerkship model, students spend time during the early rotations in the year mastering these more basic skills, in addition to obtaining the appropriate discipline-specific knowledge and skills. With the additional time built in to the LIC model, students have the opportunity to utilize their improving basic clinical reasoning as the foundation for more advanced learning across every medical subject. Students gain expertise and enhance their skills in each discipline over time, however in parallel (Hirsh et al., 2012). These learning experiences can occur through interactions with the same patient over time, as their illness changes, rather than by limited experiences with multiple patients. This opportunity is enhanced by having LIC students typically remain in the same health care system for the course of the entire year thereby allowing them to become familiar and comfortable with the patterns of patient care and the logistics at that clinical center. In traditional clerkship models, students are required to learn new systems each time they transfer to a new site. This can include learning new documentation systems, new policies and procedures, as well as understanding a new culture. All of this detracts from the opportunity to delve deeper into each subject and truly master the accompanying knowledge and skills. Also, continuity of setting allows students to play a more meaningful role on the health care team, including the development of interprofessional relationships, and to make better connections with available community resources. Community connections and relationships within a single setting introduces students to systems-based practice and its real world application (Armstrong, Mackey, & Spear, 2004).

Continuity with peers in an LIC also contributes to learning in important ways. Through exposure to the same group of peers over the year, students develop collaborative relationships that provide social support, allow sharing of best practices, and enhance group processes and reflecting. These peer networks allow a safe space where students can succeed in challenging experiences together, as well as confront and understand the hidden curriculum together.

The learning that occurs in LICs can also be tailored to meet the needs of each individual student. With the additional time provided to each preceptor, faculty can better judge each trainee and identify learning needs and goals that should be addressed over time. These goals can be monitored and reassessed for adjustment where appropriate. With enough time, and a supportive relationship that allows feedback, each student can better develop and achieve the goals of an individualized and customized learning plan (Wilkerson & Irby, 1998).

In both LIC and traditional block clerkship structures students can be challenged to gain exposure to certain types of illnesses. In an LIC faculty address partially this need through knowledge of their patients, knowledge of the learning needs of their students, and appreciation of the timing for when these experiences may occur in consideration of the student's educational trajectory. Faculty have opportunities to steer students towards intentional encounters that may achieve a particular learning objective, and foster a more deliberate and less random learning experience. In both LIC models and traditional block clerkships, students need to track the diagnoses and procedures encountered in clinical settings, which faculty should be monitoring regularly. Then, future clinical experiences can be tailored to address any learning gaps and better address individual student needs (Gaufberg et al. 2008).

LONGITUDINAL INTEGRATED CLERKSHIP (LICS) SUCCESS AND FUTURE DIRECTIONS

LIC Program Outcomes

While the total population of participating medical students in LIC curriculums remains small relative to the number of students completing traditional clerkship models, outcomes data has been encouraging. Students in LICs are able to see patients more frequently before their diagnosis is made, and after discharge from the hospital. The LIC model supports teaching by experienced faculty, more often than by residents as is the case in traditional structures, and can renew enthusiasm for teaching on the part of clinical faculty. Studies show that students completing longitudinal integrated clerkships performed as well as or better than their traditionally trained peers on measures of content knowledge and clinical skills. Also, LIC students expressed higher satisfaction with the learning environment, more confidence in dealing with numerous domains of patient care, and a stronger sense of patient-centeredness (Hirsh et al. 2012).

At Harvard Medical School (HMS), the Cambridge Integrated Clerkship (CIC) launched in 2004, and a pilot program of 8 students was created. As outlined by Ogur, Hirsh, Krupat, and Bor (2007), initial outcomes that were measured included tests of content knowledge, clinical skills, communication skills, content knowledge retention, student perceptions of experiences, and patient-centered attitudes of students. Subject exam performance, as measured by a standardized multidisciplinary assessment, supported that CIC students performed at least as well, and in some cases significantly better than traditional students at HMS, and had higher retention of material at the end of the year. Results from standardized clinical examination assessments, revealed that CIC students had significant improvements in communication skills at the end of the third year clerkships, as compared with traditional students.

Also, compared to traditional third year clerks, the CIC students described the third year as more rewarding and less marginalizing. The students felt better prepared to be truly caring physicians. CIC students felt better prepared also to deal with ethical dilemmas, to consider the social context impacting patients, to relate to patients of diverse backgrounds and to engage patients in shared decision-making. At the start and at the end of the clinical year, patient-centered attitudes of students were assessed through a validated measure, the Tasks of Medicine Scale (TOMS) (Schigelone, White, & Krupat, 2005). This scale asks students to rank order the importance of eight physician tasks, four biomedical, and four psychosocial. At the start of the year, all HMS students ranked the psychosocial concerns slightly higher. However, by the end of the year, HMS CIC students' scores had increased, while those of traditional students declined. Students participating in clinical learning within an LIC design at HMS appeared to be protected against the ethical erosion occurring among traditional students (Ogur et al., 2007).

Another medical school, the University of California San Francisco (UCSF) launched the UCSF Parnassus Integrated Student Clinical Experiences (PISCES) LIC in 2007. When evaluated by Mazotti, O'Brien, Tong, and Hauer (2011), the findings showed similar results to those of other LIC programs. Results from the evaluation of the PISCES LIC confirmed that LIC students performed as well or better on standardized exams and future clinical experiences, when compared with students trained in traditional block clerkships. More importantly, student perceptions of participation in the LIC rated higher in all evaluated domains. Students perceive a greater quantity and higher quality of observation and feedback provided from faculty, during clerkship training. Students and faculty also perceive the assessment process more positively, specifically in the areas of validity of the evaluation process, quality of clinical skills evaluation and willingness to provide constructive feedback.

Furthermore, faculty involved in PISCES described their perceptions of participating in the LIC positively. LIC preceptors reported a deep sense of reward gained through the long-term relationships with students and of having the opportunity to participate in their growth and development. LIC preceptors revealed also a sense of responsibility for teaching their discipline and a substantial commitment for insuring student learning. Over time, preceptors described the burden of teaching had diminished as students' clinical abilities improved as the year progressed. Perhaps even more importantly, patients who were surveyed appreciated student involvement in their care and preceptors did not feel challenged to integrate students into patient care experiences (Teherani et al., 2009).

In addition to improved student performance outcomes and faculty and patient satisfaction, the symbiotic relationships that develop between medical schools, communities, and health system partners are benefits of implementing LICs in medical schools, Institutional level support fosters leadership and high quality faculty development that enhances professional satisfaction among both university faculty and community based physician educators. Through an emphasis on the beneficial relationships LICs build for medical schools, as well as the health systems and communities served, these types of educational programs can continue to thrive, and successfully expand to other settings (Poncelet et al., 2014).

FUTURE OPPORTUNITIES AND CONSIDERATIONS

For a long time, leaders in medical education have long urged reforms of the principal clinical clerkship year to better align with the goals of humanistic patient-centered care and the needs of a changing health care system. Evidence confirms that the traditional, inpatient block clerkship model has significant limitations, and educational transformation is needed. Population needs and health system changes are poorly aligned with the block educational model. This model fosters a hidden curriculum that undermines the core values of professionalism that leads to ethical erosion and loss of empathy among medical students. Traditional time-limited, siloed, block clerkships do not align with modern educational principles, and may even hinder student learning. Learning theories like the self-determination theory and cognitive learning theories support that the learning environment plays a key role in shaping the experience and development of the learner. Also, learning in the workplace has also been well studied, and these principles should inform curricular design (Billett 2001). Areas such as personal change, leadership, and system change that have been described in the business and policy literature, as well as the education and social psychology literature should also be considered when designing new curricular models, such as LICs (Bruer 1993). Deficiencies in traditional block clerkship models, combined with the expectations of patients and populations, has generated support for new innovative curricular designs that benefit medical students, their future patients, and communities (Hirsh et al., 2007).

The LIC model offers one solution to address calls for medical education reform, by restructuring the third year clinical clerkship experience for students. Both a recent Carnegie Foundation Report and the Association of Faculties of Medicine of Canada's (n.d.), *The Future of Medical Education in Canada* report describe possible models that achieve needed reforms, including LICs as a potential solution. Because LICs align medical education with the delivery of health care, they are authentically embedding modern theories of adult learning into the medical education experience. Additionally, LICs offer an educational environment more consistent with future practice settings and strive to overcome the hidden curriculum that is prevalent in many medical schools. Data overwhelmingly supports that students who train in models that prioritize continuity, integration, and longitudinal experiences, develop less ethical erosion and even gain enhanced empathy, as compared against students completing traditional block clerkship models.

Medical schools considering the implementation of an LIC model need to engage stakeholders in understanding this model, to achieve buy-in early on from all collaborators. Most LICs require a partnership with community physician practices, hospitals and most importantly with the community itself. Many health care providers involved in traditional medical education may be unfamiliar with this model, or uncomfortable with change. Building a program like this requires developing appropriate alliances, and a strategic process with adequate financing and resources for sustainability and success (Ogur et al. 2007).

Longitudinal integrated clerkships are an example of a successful "disruptive innovation" and "translational educational science" by connecting educational principles to transform clinical education structure. The case for change stems from the desire to improve student learning, support medical student professional development, and to improve the delivery systems and communities where these future physicians will ultimately practice. LICs offer a complete restructuring of clinical education based on learning theory, with research that confirms their rationale and success in outcomes. LICs already have a significant impact on medical education and serve as an alternative to traditional block structures. The success of LICs persists across a variety of settings and community types, including highly specialized academic centers, academic urban community hospitals, and widely dispersed rural and remote clinics, all confirming the potential of students training in this model (Norris, 2009).

Implementing LICs within medical schools offers an opportunity for developing symbiotic curricula. A symbiotic curriculum requires a mutually reinforcing relationship, where both medical schools and the health systems they serve gain from the partnership. Medical schools and students will benefit from excellent learning opportunities in the community, and patients and health services are enhanced by the participation of learners. This symbiosis is founded on strong meaningful relationships between learners and patients, learners and clinicians, and learners and communities that are fostered through LICs. Curricula of this type requires that patients are willing to engage with medical students in their learning, to develop relationships, and to guide them to become the future physician they will ultimately trust and select for their own future medical needs (Prideaux, Worley, & Bligh, 2007).

REFERENCES

Armstrong, E. G., Mackey, M., & Spear, S. J. (2004). Medical education as a process management problem. *Academic Medicine*, *79*(8), 721–728. doi:10.1097/00001888-200408000-00002 PMID:15277126

Association of American Medical Colleges. (2004). *Educating doctors to provide high-quality medical care: A vision for medical education in the United States*. Washington, DC: Author.

Association of Faculties of Medicine of Canada. (n. d.). *The future of medical education in Canada (FMEC): A collective vision for MD education*. Retrieved from https://www.afmc.ca/medical-education/future-medical-education-canada-fmec

Billett, S. (2001). *Learning in the workplace: Strategies for effective practice*. Crows Nest, NSW, Australia: Allen & Unwin.

Bruer, J. (1993). *Schools for thought: A science of learning in the classroom*. Cambridge, MA: MIT Press.

Cabana, M. D., & Jee, S. H. (2004). Does continuity of care improve patient outcomes? *The Journal of Family Practice*, *53*(12), 974–980. Retrieved from http://www.jfponline.com/ PMID:15581440

Cecil, J., McHale, C., Hart, J., & Laidlaw, A. (2014). Behavior and burnout in medical students. *Medical Education Online*, *25209*(19). doi:10.3402/meo.v19.25209 PMID:25160716

Christakis, D. A., & Feudtner, C. (1997). Temporary matters. The ethical consequences of transient social relationships in medical training. *Journal of the American Medical Association*, *278*(9), 739–743. Retrieved from http://jama.jamanetwork.com/journal.aspx doi:10.1001/jama.1997.03550090063034 PMID:9286834

Cohen, P. (2009). Training for expertise: The Harvard Medical School Cambridge integrated clerkship tutorial. *The Clinical Teacher*, *6*(1), 28–33. doi:10.1111/j.1743-498X.2008.00260.x

Cooke, M., Irby, D., & O'Brien, B. (2010). *Educating physicians: A call for reform of medical school and residency*. San Francisco, CA: Jossey-Bass.

Coulehan, J., & Williams, P.C. (2001). Vanquishing virtue: The impact of medical education. *Academic Medicine, 76*(6), 598–605. Retrieved from:10.1097/00001888-200106000-00008

Feudtner, C., Christakis, D.A., & Christakis, N.A. (1994). Do clinical clerks suffer ethical erosion? Students' perceptions of their ethical environment and personal development. *Academic Medicine, 69*(8), 670-679. doi:10.1097/00001888-199408000-00017

Gaufberg, E., Shtasel, D., Hirsh, D., Ogur, B., & Bor, D. (2008). The Harvard Medical School Cambridge integrated clerkship: Challenges of longitudinal integrated training. *Clinical Teacher, 5(*2), 78-82. doi:10.1111/j.1743-498x.2008.00209.x

Hafferty, F.W. (1998). Beyond curriculum reform: Confronting medicine's hidden curriculum. *Academic Medicine, 73*(4), 403-437. doi:10.1097/00001888-199804000-00013

Hirsh, D., Gaufberg, E., Ogur, B., Cohen, P., Krupat, E., Cox, M., . . . Bor, D. (2012). Educational outcomes of the Harvard Medical School Cambridge integrated clerkship: A way forward for medical education? *Academic Medicine, 87*(5), 643-650. doi:10.1097/acm.0b013e31824d9821

Hirsh, D., Walters, L., & Poncelet, A.N. (2012). Better learning, better doctors, better delivery system: Possibilities from a case study of longitudinal integrated clerkships. *Medical Teacher, 34*(7), 548–554. doi:10.3109/0142159x.2012.696745

Hirsh, D.A., Ogur, B., Thibault, G.E., & Cox, M. (2007). "Continuity" as an organizing principle for clinical education reform. *New England Journal of Medicine, 356*(8), 858-866. doi:10.1056/nejmsb061660

Hojat, M., Vergare, M.J., Maxwell, K., Brainard, G., Herrine, S., Isenberg, G.A., . . . Gonnella, J.S. (2009). The devil is in the third year: A longitudinal study of erosion of empathy in medical school. *Academic Medicine*, *84*(9), 1182-1191. doi:10.1097/acm.0b013e3181b17e55

Martimiianakis, M.A., Michalec, B., Lam, J., Cartmill, C., Taylor, J.S., & Hafferty, F.W. (2015). Humanism, the hidden curriculum, and educational reform: A scoping review and thematic analysis. *Academic Medicine,* 90(11), S5-S13. doi:10.1097/ACM.0000000000000894

Mazotti, L., O'Brien, B., Tong, L., & Hauer, K.E. (2011). Perceptions of evaluation in longitudinal versus traditional clerkships. *Medical Education, 45*(5), 464-470. doi:10.1111/j.1365-2923.2010.03904.x

Newton, B.W., Barber, L., Clardy, J., Cleveland, E., & O'Sullivan, P. (2008). Is there hardening of the heart during medical school? *Academic Medicine, 83*(3), 244-249. doi:10.1097/acm.0b013e3181637837

Norris, T.E., Schaad, D.C., DeWitt, D., Ogur, B., Hunt, D.D., & Consortium of Longitudinal Integrated Clerkships. (2009). Longitudinal integrated clerkships for medical students: An innovation adopted by medical schools in Australia, Canada, South Africa, and the United States. *Academic Medicine, 84*(7), 902-907. doi:10.1097/acm.0b013e3181a85776

Ogur, B., Hirsh, D., Krupat, E., & Bor, D. (2007). The Harvard Medical School-Cambridge integrated clerkship: An innovative model of clinical education. *Academic Medicine, 82*(4), 397-404. Retrieved from:10.1097/acm.0b013e31803338f0

Poncelet, A., Bokser, S., Calton, B., Hauer, K.E., Kirsch, H., Jones, T., . . . Robertson, P. (2011). Development of a longitudinal integrated clerkship at an academic medical center. *Medical Education Online, 16*. doi:10.3402/meo.v16i0.5939

Poncelet, A.N., Mazotti, L.A., Blumberg, B., Wamsley, M.A., Grennan, T., & Shore, W.B. (2014). Creating a longitudinal integrated clerkship with mutual benefits for an academic medical center and a community health system. *Permanente Journal*, 18(2), 50–56. doi:10.7812/tpp/13-137

Prideaux, D., Worley, P., & Bligh, J. (2007). Symbiosis: A new model for clinical education. *Clinical Teacher, 4*(4), 209-212. doi:10.1111/j.1743-498x.2007.00188.x

Schigelone, A., White, C., & Krupat, E. (2005). *Medical students' attitudes toward the doctor-patient relationship: a cross-sectional study*. Madison, WI: Association of American Medical Colleges Central Group on Educational Affairs.

Schumacher, D. J., Englander, R., & Carraccio, C. (2013). Developing the master learner: Applying learning theory to the learner, the teacher and the learning environment. *Academic Medicine*, *88*(11), 1635–1645. doi:10.1097/ACM.0b013e3182a6e8f8 PMID:24072107

Stevens, C.D., Wilkerson, L., & Uijtdehaage, S. (2014). Longitudinal continuity experiences can repair disconnects in the core clerkships for medical students. *Academic Medicine, 89*(2), 205–207. doi:10.1097/acm.0000000000000108

Strasser, R., & Hirsh, D. (2011). Longitudinal integrated clerkships: Transforming medical education worldwide? *Medical Education*, 45(5), 436-437. doi:10.1111/j.1365-2923.2011.03939.x

Teherani, A., O'Brien, B.C., Masters, D.E., Poncelet, A.N., Robertson, P.A., & Hauer, K.E. (2009). Burden, responsibility, and reward: Preceptor experiences with the continuity of teaching in a longitudinal integrated clerkship. *Academic Medicine, 84*(10), S50-S53. doi:10.1097/acm.0b013e3181b38b01

Watson, R.T. (2003). Rediscovering the medical school. (2003). *Academic Medicine, 78*(7), 659-665. doi:10.1097/00001888-200307000-00002

Whitcomb, M.E. (2005). Redesigning clinical education: A major challenge for academic health centers. *Academic Medicine, 80*(7), 615-616. doi:10.1097/00001888-200507000-00001

Wilkerson, L., & Irby, D. M. (1998). Strategies for improving teaching practices: A comprehensive approach to faculty development. *Academic Medicine*, *73*(4), 387–396. doi:10.1097/00001888-199804000-00011 PMID:9580715

KEY TERMS AND DEFINITIONS

Attending Physician: A licensed practitioner of medicine who has completed their medical training and is certified by the appropriate specialty board, who is often giving supervising and teaching responsibility for medical students and residents.

Clerkships: The practice of medicine by medical students during their final year(s) of study, where they experience active learning in various clinical settings, under the supervision of more experienced clinicians.

Continuity: A general term for the uninterrupted management of a patient while transitioning between physicians or health care settings.

Curriculum: A statement of the intended aims and objectives, content, experiences, outcomes and processes of an education and training program that sets out the knowledge, skills, attitudes and behaviors the learner will achieve.

Empathy: The feeling of understanding and sharing another person's experiences and feelings.

Hidden Curriculum: The set of influences that function at the level of organizational structure and culture, and that communicate the unspoken rules and culture and assist students with professional identity formation.

Humanism: A focus of thought or action in which human interests, values, and dignity are prioritized.

Interprofessional Education: Learning that occurs when two or more professions learn with, from and about each other to improve collaboration and patient care.

Patient-Centeredness: The provision of care that is respectful of and responsive to individual patient preferences, needs, and values, and where clinical decisions are guided by patient values.

Preceptor: An experienced physician who works with a learner for a defined period of time, providing role modeling and learning experiences to assist the learner in acquiring new competencies required for safe, ethical and quality practice.

Symbiosis: A curriculum design based on a mutually reinforcing relationship between medical schools and health care providers, where both benefit.

Systems-Based Practice: The processes in the health care system that operate to provide cost effective care to individual patients and to populations.

Chapter 7
Mental Illness, Youth, and Lessons from Residential Treatment Centers

Krista Allison
University of Phoenix, USA

Chris Allison
Southwest Baptist University, USA

ABSTRACT

This chapter explores mental illness in children and youth. In addition to understanding who is affected, this chapter seeks to express a holistic and comprehensive approach to physical, mental, and spiritual health. Research in each of these areas is discussed and relevant stories are presented from the authors' combined 10 years of experience in various residential treatment centers. Additionally, practical tools for families, educators, and clinicians are discussed. The purpose of this chapter is to increase awareness of the struggles mentally ill children endure and equip families, educators, and clinicians with practical tools for assisting children with mental illnesses.

MENTAL ILLNESS AND YOUTH

The school bell rings. For most students, this sound signals a time to begin the school day or chat with friends between classes. The bell releases students to stretch their legs and scurry to the next class. Administrators might hear the final bell as the start of the work day. However, for some students with mental health issues, the sound of the bell ringing can cause additional anxiety or stress. For a student with early childhood trauma, a simple sound, like a bell, can even initiate a fight or flight response if the sound is associated with their trauma. Many daily sounds and experiences, which the mass of our population consider insignificant, can have significant impact on students dealing with a variety of mental illnesses and issues stemming from early childhood trauma.

DOI: 10.4018/978-1-5225-0640-9.ch007

In this chapter, we explore the growing concern of mental illness in children, youth, and college students and some holistic, comprehensive approaches that may help others in assisting students or clients struggling with mental illness. In recent years, clinicians are seeing more mental illness among students than in years past (NAMI, 2015). Throughout this chapter, findings from research will be discussed, leading practitioners to greater insights in working with students who have certain forms of mental illness. As parents, clinicians and educators, it is imperative to understand and equip others with some holistic approaches to assisting children and youth as they develop and cope with these issues.

WHO IS AFFECTED AND HOW?

Children and Youth

Depression, anxiety and mental illness has risen among children, adolescents and young adults in recent years. By some estimates, the number of high school and college students meeting the criteria for diagnosis of major depression and/or an anxiety disorder is five to eight times what it was a half century ago (Gray, 2010). Depression and anxiety often have side effects including irritability, restlessness, fatigue, physical ailments, and difficulty concentrating. With these side effects, learning and maturing may become unbearable.

In addition to depression and anxiety, the number of school age children diagnosed with Attention-Deficit/ Hyperactivity Disorder (ADHD), Conduct Disorder (CD) and Oppositional Defiance Disorder (ODD) is rising (CDC, 2015; Hamilton & Armondo, 2008). For instance, the diagnosis of ADHD rose from about 8 percent in 2003 to 11 percent in 2011 (CDC, 2015). In fact, the National Alliance on Mental Illness (NAMI) suggests one in five youth aged 13-18 has experienced a severe mental disorder (2015).

Children are directly affected by these mental illnesses. Disruptive behavior, outbursts, aggression, lying and stealing are some of the indicators of these disorders (CDC, 2015). As the number of students with these conditions rise, parents, clinicians and educators alike will face a great number of challenges. These challenges can result in a great number of opportunities to assist individuals and institutions seeking to meet the changing needs of our population.

Family and Friends

Family and friends with loved ones experiencing mental illness are often heavily affected. The illnesses of loved ones can be physically and mentally exhausting.

Physical exhaustion may play a role in family and friends' role with children who are mentally ill. Loss of sleep, worry, and efforts to comprehend children's behavior often require energy and can lead family and friends to feel tired and physically weary.

Mental illness in children can have psychological and social effects on family and friends. With 70% of youth in juvenile justice systems having at least one mental health condition and at least 20% living with a serious mental illness, parents and friends often face difficult decisions and can feel hopeless (NAMI, 2015). Serious mental illness costs America $193.2 billion in lost earnings per year, this figure illustrates the monetary difficulties involved with mental health which can often compound the issues of exhaustion surrounding a child or friend with a mental illness (NAMI, 2015).

Educators and Clinicians

Educators and Clinicians have a unique opportunity to assist children and youth by providing practical and holistic educational approaches for equipping those affected. The challenge of treating and coping with mental illness represents a chance for educators and clinicians to unite in an open-minded effort to provide physical, mental, and spiritual assistance for all involved.

Industry

Industries are also heavily affected by mental illness in children and youth. It is estimated approximately $4 billion is spent yearly on assisting mentally ill children through school-based programs in the United States (Sturm, Ringel, Stein, & Kapur, 2001). These programs come in the form of after-school care, school counseling, and other school-related services. This is the most popular of all methods for helping adolescents with mental illness and accounts for about 60% of all mental health expenditures for young people (Sturm, Ringel, Stein, & Kapur, 2001).

Community-based adolescent programs are also an option for those needing help. This includes independent organizations as well as churches, who offer counseling and programs to youth needing care. One popular organization, the Boys and Girls Club of America, offers programs and services which promote the development of boys and girls by instilling a sense of competence, usefulness, belonging, and influence (Boys and Girls Club of America, 2010).

Similar to the rise in mental illness, in recent years, residential care of adolescents has also increased. The Child Welfare League of America (CWLA) estimates there are approximately 10,000 public and private residential treatment centers in the United States (Drais-Parrillo, 2005). Although these environments provide a refuge for many individuals with moderate to severe mental health needs, most children and youth with a mental illness never seek medical attention (NAMI, 2015). With this being said, the families, educators, and clinicians who come into contact with these individuals daily can still equip them with a variety of skills to help them cope with mental illness and thrive in society.

THE IMPORTANCE OF ATTACHMENT AND LIFELONG LEARNING FOR THOSE STRUGGLING WITH MENTAL ILLNESS

Attachment and Lifelong Learning are two essential topics which will be discussed thoroughly throughout this chapter. These concepts affect every area of life. One's perceptions regarding attachment and lifelong learning will permeate daily interactions.

The process of attaching to other individuals is a basic, primary need. Everyone is born with this need and the way an individual connects becomes fundamental. The attachment process involves a variety of activities including provision of support, resources, affiliation, and care-giving behaviors (Mikulciner, Florian, Cowan & Cowan, 2002; Feeney & Collins 2003). Positive attachment experiences during infancy and adulthood are related to positive feelings such as joy, comfort, and contentment. Conversely, attachment experiences which are negative, hurtful, and traumatic can have negative effects on the individual's thoughts, emotions, mental, and physical health (Sable, 2007). The attachment process involves many components and is essential to the development and maintenance of close relationships, which help a mentally ill child successfully navigate towards healing.

Additionally, many youths who find themselves struggling with mental illness are in a state of substance addiction. Alcoholics Anonymous and similar programs typically encourage a healing process, which includes lifelong learning. Through this process, they are encouraged to work "one day at a time" with the notion that once they are an addict, they will forever be a "recovering addict" (Alcoholics Anonymous, 2001). Healthy attachment and a lifelong learning approach are critical components for youth as they cope with mental illness. These two components are necessary in order to take the knowledge and strategies gained and carry them into their adult life.

Throughout the world, lifelong learning has become a topic of interest in recent years. Lifelong learning is defined as a "process of gaining knowledge, and skills that continue throughout a person's life" (Macmillan Dictionary, 2011). In Thailand, the National Education Act BE 2542 of 1999 goes one step further and explains lifelong education "means integrating formal, non-formal and informal education so as to create ability for continuous lifelong development of quality of life" (Commission Office of the Prime Minister, 1999). In Europe, the European Commission defines lifelong learning as "all learning activity undertaken throughout life, with the aim of improving knowledge, skills, and competence, within a personal, civic, social, and/or employment related perspective" (European Commission, 2007).

In today's world of technological development and information overload, the ability to learn has become a key to personal success. Gross suggests instead of focusing on schools or colleges, education has to become a lifelong activity throughout society (1999). "In the world of the future, the new illiterate will be the person who has not learned how to learn" (Gross, 1999, p. 5).

The ideas of attachment and lifelong learning lead one to the notion that all areas of our life are interconnected and every learning activity is important. Likewise, it is imperative to continuously apply these principles in a holistic and comprehensive manner in order to improve our health.

A HOLISTIC AND COMPREHENSIVE APPROACH TO PHYSICAL, MENTAL, AND SPIRITUAL HEALTH

Merriam-Webster's dictionary defines holistic as "relating to or concerned with wholes or with complete systems rather than with the analysis of, treatment of, or dissection into parts" (2015). This concept is often used when referring to medicine or the human body. One cannot look at a human hand and know what makes it move without also acknowledging the arm, to which it is connected, the nerves and muscles working within it, and the brain sending signals to all parts involved in this system. Imagining the hand working by itself, without connection to everything else in the system, is like visualizing learning and educating without considering the impact of one's physical, mental, and spiritual health. Learning and educating will not be as successful without a holistic consideration of health included. Adopting a partial approach to learning and educating would be as effective as counting Thing from The Adam's Family a fully functioning person.

Similar to this notion, is the word comprehensive. As you think of car insurance, the idea of comprehensive coverage often comes to mind. When used in this context, the word comprehensive denotes complete or all-inclusive. If you have a new car which you value, you may desire comprehensive insurance coverage to ensure your car will be repaired, regardless of what issues arise. A comprehensive approach to mental health and education provides a similar assurance. Regardless of what area in the child's life may be hindering learning, a comprehensive approach would ensure needs are met, resources are provided, and knowledge is shared between various professionals within the system to assure the child is taken care of in the best possible manner.

Since so many children and youth with mental health concerns remain undiagnosed or untreated (NAMI, 2015), it is imperative for educators, administrators, and clinicians to remain vigilant and become informed so they may provide holistic and comprehensive care. Often this assistance is best practiced by involving various individuals from differing fields to best support children and youth.

An example of this type of support can be seen within residential treatment centers (RTC's). The practice of sharing knowledge and insights between and across professions occurs on a regular basis in this type of environment to assist individuals in their treatment. Direct care providers often find themselves in a supportive "parenting" type of role; therapists, counselors, and psychiatrists provide for the clinical well-being of the students; dieticians or chefs provide for the dietary needs; and educators provide academic instruction. Each of these professionals contribute to the overall health of the children in care. The combination of each department's care results in a holistic therapy environment which operates 24 hours a day. This constant, therapeutic approach to mental health care has proved effective for many who are dealing with some of the most difficult and intense mental illnesses (Allison, 2012).

A holistic and comprehensive approach to physical, mental and spiritual health is not only critical when considering those in residential treatment, but all children and youth. Most would agree health is not one dimensional. Instead, there are many areas of life that can be considered healthy or unhealthy. These areas could include physical fitness, mental health, and spiritual wellbeing. Health in one area does not necessarily constitute health in all areas. However, without health in all of these areas, learning can be impeded. If a single area of an individual's health struggles, the brain and body function differently and an individual's potential for growth and learning can be hindered.

Physical Health

Good health and good sense are two of life's greatest blessings. (Syrus, 1919)

Most who have experienced poor health or a common illness will agree with this quotation. In fact, as an effort to protect our health, look at the steps some Americans are willing to take. As the flu season approaches this year, people have become more vigilant regarding the precautions one can take to ensure a healthy season. Look around an office and you will probably see some anti-bacterial soap, tissues, and hand sanitizer. Most Americans have read news articles or studied signs of the flu in case an outbreak occurs. Some individuals have taken the initiative to be inoculated against the virus. The flu season creates a commotion in many locations and, according to the Center for Disease Control, caused nearly 300 deaths in 2008-2009 (CDC, 2009). This information may be alarming to some. However, when compared with the number of deaths caused by Diarrheal disease, the flue appears rather insignificant. Diarrheal disease kills approximately 1.5 million children every year (WHO, 2009).

So, why are most Americans more concerned about the flu than diarrheal disease? The answer to this question is most Americans have a clean source of drinking water and access to health services and information, if necessary. Diarrheal disease is both preventable and treatable. Because of the resources and infrastructure in America, most individuals never worry about diarrheal disease causing the death of someone they know.

Although America may not suffer greatly from diarrheal disease, the cost of medical care is staggering and the link between physical and mental health is undeniable. In our nation, cardiovascular disease alone is estimated to cost $503 Billion annually (CDC, 2012). This disease, and many like it, are closely associated with mental illness and spiritual health.

The CDC suggests the prevalence of diseases such as diabetes, asthma, obesity and arthritis are closely linked to mental health. These chronic illnesses account for approximately 75% of our national health expenditures making it important to address both the physical and mental health concerns facing our youth.

Mental Health

Study after study has illustrated one cannot consider the physical health without also considering the mental health of an individual. This concept is exemplified in many disheartening studies of Romanian children placed in orphanages from 1965 to 1989.

During this time, abortion was outlawed, contraception was banned and a celibacy tax was promoted. Ceauşescu, Romania's leader at the time, planned to develop "human capital" by increasing the birthrate. However, without proper finances to feed and care for these children, many families chose to leave their babies on the doorsteps of orphanages or sign them over to the state. By 1989, over 170,000 children were living in state run institutions. Infants coming to these state run facilities appeared healthy initially. However, as days went by, caregivers in the orphanage met the children's physical needs, but neglected their psychological and emotional needs. Whenever a child cried, their request for attention and care was unanswered. As days turned into weeks, infants stopped crying altogether and withdrew from learning and progressing. They ceased to thrive and began regressing. Many died. In one study, results showed 53 percent of the children who had lived in an institution received a psychiatric diagnosis before the age of four and a half. This is substantial when compared with the non- institutionalized children who had a diagnosis rate of 20 percent. Additionally, 62 percent of the children in the state's care had diagnoses by the age of five. These ranged from anxiety disorders (44 percent) to attention deficit hyperactivity disorder (ADHD) (23 percent) (Nelson, Fox, & Zeanah, 2013). When considering the research in this area, it becomes evident one cannot consider the physical health of an infant or individual without also considering their mental and emotional health. For these Romanian orphans, as their psychological and emotional needs were ignored, their likelihood of mental illness increased and their physical well-being subsequently decreased, even to the point of death.

The experience of Romanian orphans represents an extreme example, but the importance of mental health proves essential for all individuals. In fact, inexpressive people, those who avoid feelings and deny distress are more likely to suffer physical issues including cancer, asthma, and heart disease (Adler, Rosenfeld, Proctor II, 2015). Even the simple act of discussing a negative experience, rather than privately thinking about it, has been shown to improve life satisfaction, physical and mental health. For everyone, mental health represents a critical component to consider.

Spiritual Health

For those who practice in their field with the mind-body connection considered, spiritual health must not be overlooked. It is a critical component to holistic health. Spirituality is a widely accepted concept which typically involves the belief in a higher power, usually referred to as God. Recent research findings illustrate many patients find religion and spirituality to be resources which help them to cope with stress in their lives, including mental illness.

Research in this area is flooded with evidence supporting the importance of our spiritual health. One study followed up on 12 years of articles in the American Journal of Psychiatry and Archives of General Psychiatry, 72% of the religious commitment variables were found to benefit clients' mental health. In 92% of citations, items such as participation in religious services, social support, prayer and relationship with God were beneficial to those involved. The Journal of Family Practice reported similar findings. Verghese reports when considering those with mental illness, the "hope and spiritual support that patients get …help them to cope better" (Verghese, 2008, p.3.) With growing research in this area supporting the value of spiritual health, it is a critical component to consider in relation to creating a positive, holistic and comprehensive approach for working with mentally ill youth.

LESSONS FROM RESIDENTIAL TREATMENT CENTERS

In the US and abroad, engaging with mental illness in a holistic, comprehensive manner is gaining popularity. Residential Treatment Centers (RTC) represent one international industry which has grown from the notion of creating holistic, comprehensive care. RTCs, dedicated to the success of clients with moderate to severe mental illnesses, can provide a microcosm for studying holistic, comprehensive care. These environments often incorporate physical, mental, and spiritual components. Additionally, within a residential treatment center, adolescents have access to formal, informal, and non-formal educational activities. The combinations of these environments and activities allow these organizations to see great success, even with some of the most extreme cases. Because these facilities often represent a "last resort" for high risk youth, caregivers are often willing to pay high prices and do anything necessary to help their adolescent. These youths have been typically unsuccessful in other less restrictive settings and often need the structure a RTC can provide (Curtis, Alexander, & Lunghofer, 2001). Additionally, these programs are targeted towards adolescent individuals struggling with substance abuse, or who cannot form "age-appropriate relationships and those whose behavioral or emotional problems significantly affect daily functioning" (Curtis, Alexander, & Lunghofer, 2001, p. 380).

The price of residential treatment varies, as do the types of payments which are accepted at these facilities. Prices for residential treatment vary, but can cost upwards of $60,000.00 per month for full service programs (SEO Services, 2011). Additionally, a higher program cost does not necessarily correlate with the quality or success rate of a program. Many more expensive programs offer spa-like services, which do not necessarily produce better outcomes. Some programs accept insurance and some prefer payment for services up front. Often, the high costs of residential treatment make residential treatment options impractical for those who have less severe or undiagnosed mental illness. However, many of the effective approaches used within Residential Treatment Centers can be inexpensive and applied in non-residential situations.

Studying techniques and creating environments which are beneficial to those with more severe mental illness can better equip us with tools for assisting individuals in our immediate presence. Although it may be impractical for each of us to implement all the programs and techniques from the RTC environment into our daily practices and classrooms, some small changes may have large impacts for those in our care.

Throughout the past decade, the authors have worked with a variety of residential treatment centers. Working in several different capacities and environments has given the authors a fresh perspective on treating mental illness. The authors' aim is to convey some of the insights they have gained over their years in this industry and equip parents, educators, and clinicians who work with mentally ill youth. In the following pages, the authors will explore some effective and practical tools for engaging with students struggling with mental illness.

Focus on Attachment Style

One of the most important areas of interest when considering mental illness pertains to attachment. Attachment is critical for infants, as illustrated in the Romanian orphanages discussed earlier in the chapter. However, attachment styles continuously develop into adulthood. In 1987, Hazan and Shaver developed three categories to depict youth and adult attachment styles: secure, avoidant, and anxious/ambivalent. These styles were originally based on studies of infant attachment. Later studies revealed there are two fundamental dimensions involved in attachment. These dimensions include attachment related anxiety and attachment related avoidance (Brennan, Clark, & Shaver, 1998). As research has progressed, researchers have begun to adopt the idea of a two dimensional space which can be divided into four categories based on anxiety and avoidance (Schachner, Shaver, & Mikulincer, 2005).

This two dimensional model has become widely accepted with adult attachment researchers. Attachment avoidance, the first aspect of this model is typically referred to as the extent which an individual distrusts a relationship partner. This is usually characterized by a desire to maintain self-reliance and emotional distance. The second portion of this model, attachment anxiety, represents the amount an individual worrys that a partner will not provide comfort during times of need (Schachner, Shaver, & Mikulincer, 2005). These two dimensions create a continuum in which an adult individual may have an attachment style considered secure, preoccupied, dismissive avoidant, or fearful avoidant (Bartholomew, 1990). This notion led Bartholomew and Horowitz to create a four category model of attachment style (1991).

The categories are quite similar to the initial categories created for infants. Cell I represents a category in which a person may feel a sense of worthiness. These are individuals who generally feel others are accepting and responsive to their needs. Cell II symbolizes an individual who feels a sense of being unworthy of love. This individual has a positive view of others, but a negative view of self, creating an environment where the individual strives for self-acceptance by gaining the acceptance of others. Cell III is representative of an individual who has both a negative view of self as well as a negative view of others. This type of individual fears intimacy and distrusts others. They seek to protect themselves through distance and avoidance. Finally, in Cell IV, dismissive individuals are represented. Dismissive persons have a positive view of self; however, they have a negative view of others. They believe they deserve love, however, others will disappoint, and therefore, they protect themselves through avoidance of close relationships. Independence and invulnerability characterize these individuals (Bartholomew & Horowitz, 1991).

It is important to note the initial attachment of an infant has been linked to the attachment style of an adult. In fact, during a twenty-year longitudinal study, researchers found "individual differences in attachment security may remain stable throughout much of one's lifespan while remaining open to revision in light of experience" (Waters, Merrick, Treboux, Crowell, & Albersheim, 2000, p. 684). This study verified early attachment style was significantly associated with adult attachment style. 64% of adult participants involved in this study had an attachment style which corresponded to the same style of attachment during their infancy. This continuity suggests a possibility for attachment style to have a considerable impact upon many relationships throughout an individual's life.

Understand the Importance of Attachment

The process of attaching to other individuals consists of multiple dimensions. Attachment is created through activities including provision of support, resources, affiliation, and care-giving behaviors (Mikulciner, Florian, Cowan & Cowan, 2002; Feeney & Collins 2003). Positive attachment experiences during infancy and adulthood are related to positive feelings such as joy, comfort, and contentment. Conversely, attachment experiences that are negative, hurtful, and traumatic can have negative effects on the individual's thoughts, emotions, mental and physical health (Sable, 2007). The attachment process involves a variety components and is essential as we consider mental health.

Research illustrates the important role that attachment style plays in mental health and romantic relationships. Relationship partners often provide us with support during times of grief and distress. The presence, or absence, of social support during these times can determine our ability to cope with such situations and influence how these events affect us (Burleson & Goldsmith, 1998). In addition, some research suggests close relationships have the ability to increase perceived personal growth (Ruvolo & Brennan, 1997). With the aid of close relationships, one is able to better navigate tough times, as well as grow personally.

An individual's attachment style may play a considerable role in an individual's relationships. In a study conducted in 1987, Hazan and Shaver suggest romantic love is an attachment process and thus dependent on an individual's ability to connect. They conceptualize romantic love as a "biological process designed by evolution to facilitate attachment between adult sexual partners" (p. 523). The attachment style of an individual may determine one's desire to seek particular relationship partners. Attachment style may also determine the level of closeness pursued within these interactions which is often correlated with mental health (Adler, Rosenfeld, Proctor II, 2015).

Attachment also affects an individual's ability to connect with others and relational satisfaction. Researchers have found "one partner's attachment style was associated with the other partner's relationship satisfaction" (Kane, Jaremka, Guichard, Ford, Collins, & Feeney, 2007, p. 551). In fact, less support and less care were perceived by the partner of an insecurely attached individual. In other words, the quality of care-giving that is provided by insecure individuals impacts relationship outcome. In the end, research indicates individuals are more satisfied with relationships in which they feel "well cared-for" by their partners (p. 553).

Often, relationship development and satisfaction is impacted by typical characteristics associated with individual attachment styles (Brennan, Clark, & Shaver, 1998). For instance, an anxious ambivalent individual is usually characterized by a fear of independence and autonomy and a tendency to drink or binge under stressful situations. These individuals may fall in love at first sight or express jealousy, clinginess, or overdependence in romantic relationships. Emotional instability and lack of trust are also associated with anxious ambivalent individuals (Mikulincer, 1998). Characteristics associated with avoidant individuals include emotional distance and leaving in the midst of adversity (Brennan, Clark, & Shaver, 1998). These individuals are the least accepting of their partner's faults. However, secure individuals are the most accepting of and sensitive to their partner's needs. Secure persons tend to trust and share openly with relationship partners with a sense of flexibility. This often allows for deeper and more beneficial relationships which leads to better ability to cope with mental illness.

An individual's relationships and mental health may be impacted not only by the characteristics that are associated with his or her attachment style, but also by their ability to cope with distress. In a study conducted by Mikulincer (1998), attachment style was found to impact the way an individual deals with negativity. In this study, avoidant individuals were found to respond to insecurity by detaching, anxious ambivalent sought additional and excessive love and care. Conversely, secure persons' positive self-view remained unaffected by distress. An individual's ability to cope with negative distress impacts their relationships and mental health.

Research illustrates attachment style also plays an important role in the perceptions of relationship partners (Fraley, Niedenthal, Marks, Brumbaugh, & Vicary, 2006). In one study, individuals were shown movies of changing facial expressions. Anxiously attached individuals were more likely to perceive positive or negative changes of emotion earlier than other securely attached participants. The heightened sensitivity is thought to lead to inaccurate assumptions regarding judgment of emotion. Results from this study led researchers to conclude securely and insecurely attached individuals perceive visual emotional cues with differing levels of vigilance. This is important as loved ones seek to provide support for those dealing with mental illness. Keeping in mind that emotional cues play a large role in supporting individuals with differing attachment styles is critical.

Not only are close relationships important for the emotional and mental health of an individual, they also provide a source of feedback for the self. In close relationships, an individual may receive honest and accurate evaluations from relational partners. When this occurs, an individual receives verification of strengths and is better equipped to accept limitations (Katz & Joiner, 2002). However, research indicates insecurely attached individuals may not perceive the same cues as securely attached persons (Fraley, Niedenthal, Marks, Brumbaugh, & Vicary, 2006).

Research suggests attachment theory not only influences an individual's actions, but may also play a role in people's perception of messages (Fraley, Garner, & Shaver, 2000; Jones, 2005). Results indicate avoidant individuals are less perceptive and attentive during emotional events (Fraley, Garner, & Shaver, 2000). Therefore, avoidant individuals often encode less of the information available to them. In addition to this, Jones (2005) found dismissive and preoccupied individuals viewed low person-centered comforting messages more positively than secure or fearful, avoidant individuals. Avoidant individuals viewed effective communication skills as much more essential than non-avoidant individuals. In other words, research illustrates individuals perceive messages differently depending upon the attachment style the person employs. This is essential to keep in mind as one works with someone who may have a mental illness.

For nearly two years, the authors were directors in a residential treatment program working with students who have been diagnosed with Reactive Attachment Disorder (RAD). Each of these particular students had suffered some form of childhood trauma, which led to a RAD diagnosis. Trauma can come in the form of a divorce, adoption (even at birth), abuse, foster care transitions, childhood disease, or various other traumatic experiences. Focusing on the attachment issues first enabled these students to progress much further in treatment than would have been possible by solely treating their depression or ADHD diagnoses. If childhood trauma and/or attachment issues are operating at the core of a child's mental illness diagnoses, the information regarding a service animal (discussed later in this chapter) may be of interest.

Focus on Learning Environments

The idea of education only taking place in the classroom is an idea that permeates society. However, learning opportunities exist in every environment including formal, non-formal, and informal.

Learning environments can typically be evaluated as formal, informal or non-formal. Coombs and Ahmed (1974) suggest formal education pertains to the institutional, hierarchical structure typically observed in traditional grade schools. Informal education involves the process whereby an individual accumulates knowledge, skills, and attitudes from daily experiences such as conversations, reflection, reading, and exposure to the environment. Non-formal education is organized, systematic and occurs outside the framework of the formal system; such as 4-H, church, adventure therapy, or group therapy. When considering education, it is imperative to teach within each of these contexts, in order to better assist youth in the learning process.

A recent study at an RTC found nearly all participants in the study reported most of their learning occurred in the school or classroom environment; however, the school was frequently marginal in their recollections of profound learning experiences and participants often preferred alternate learning environments. Informal and Non-formal learning environments were declared as "more influential" learning environments than the Formal setting of the classroom (Allison, 2012). Recognizing and encouraging alternate learning environments may assist students struggling with mental illness and free them to invest in a variety of alternate locations for learning.

Many students in this study felt the need to justify or apologize for learning something new while in a recreational activity, sharing a hobby with a loved one, or simply reading alone. It is possible, due to the importance placed upon the school environment during the early childhood years, adolescents develop the notion that these formal experiences should have more value and are exclusive to learning. Unfortunately, this thought pattern may prevent individuals from more thorough understanding which may develop during the informal or non-formal interactions. For students struggling with mental illness, the compounded pressure of achievement comes from a formal environment may be less effective than meeting their needs through a more informal or non-formal approach.

Recreational Therapy, or adventure therapy, is one therapeutic approach established within Residential Treatment Centers (RTCs) to create alternate therapeutic and learning environments. The authors have been able to go on a few of these adventure therapy trips with students from RTCs. To be able to interact with students in the informal and non-formal environments often enhanced the students' learning in the classroom, even when the subject matter was unrelated. One such trip was a 100-mile bike ride along the Katy Trail in Missouri. The students trained for a couple months for this trip, while learning about the importance of goal setting and perseverance. To discuss goal setting and perseverance in regards to the classroom and educational achievement can be effective, but those discussions did not hold a candle to the inferno of perseverance we experienced on the bike trail.

About 75 miles into the ride, and the third day of the journey, one of the students decided they could go no further. This was a thought which had been in the back of most everyone's mind since around the 40th mile. The student pulled to the side of the trail, stepped off his bike, threw it in the bushes, and then sat down without a word. The group was about 10 miles from the nearest shred of civilization. Without much talking, the rest of the students sat down beside the discouraged teenager. One student spoke up, "We are not going to leave you. Once you are ready to go a little further, we want you to lead the way and set our pace. We will follow you."

This is the epitome of a therapeutic experience. Unplanned and unscripted, the student who had quit, now found he was capable of many more miles than he had ever imagined. He continued the rest of the day and finished 85 miles of the 100-mile trail with his peers. His sense of accomplishment and observance of his own perseverance was significantly impactful. This informal experience provided education he will long remember, many years past the classroom lesson on how to set goals.

Focus on Appropriate Adult Learning Principles: Especially for Older Youth and College Students

In the formal, pedagogical model of learning, teachers assume responsibility for making decisions about what will be learned, how it will be learned, and when it will be learned (Knowles, 1973). Teachers direct learning while students are passive recipients. Youth are required to adjust to an established curriculum based on the teacher's experience and knowledge. The pedagogical model often times inhibits the learner from making a contribution to the learning process. In Shaw's study with those in residential care, he concludes, "As a result, many learners leave school having lost interest in learning" (p. 138, 2004).

Even educators with good intentions can unknowingly suppress naturally inquisitive instincts of the students by controlling the learning environment. When this happens, some youth in transition to adulthood begin to view learning as a chore and a burden. By viewing youth in residential treatment through the lens of andragogy, some teachers have been more successful.

With the understanding youth in this environment may benefit from some adult learning principles, it is critical to examine some of the most influential individuals in this field. Knowles (1973), Rogers (1992), and Tough (1979) are three foundational individuals associated with developing the framework to support adult education. These views may help us in understanding how to incorporate some adult learning principles into our daily interactions with our children, clients, or students.

Knowles' research suggests adult individuals complete approximately eight learning projects per year (1973). Of these projects, only about 10% are associated with educational institutions. This means nearly 90% of educational experiences are taking place in non-formal or informal environments.

Rogers' views (1992) regarding learning are grounded in the belief that the facilitator is responsible for setting the initial climate. He expresses individuals are more likely to be motivated by things that have personal meaning, therefore, the facilitator asks about the general purposes of the group. Facilitators are resources for learning and make efforts to organize and make resources available for learning.

In 1979, Allen Tough wrote The Adult's Learning Projects. He explains how most adult learning takes place outside of institutional frameworks. Tough found the overwhelming majority (about 70%) of adult learning takes place outside institutional frameworks. About 20% of the learning projects are supported by others who are not professionals; these individuals included supervisors, colleagues, parents, friends, etc. Professional helpers, such as teachers, trainers, and counselors direct about 10% of our learning. This could be attributed to factors such as: the learner having a desire to control the learning process, non-institutional learning allowing for a flexible time commitment or non-institutional learning being attainable at a low cost.

Adult learning principles may be helpful in assisting students struggling with mental illness. Difficulties in school or learning may be eliminated by applying adult learning concepts and encouraging some alternative learning environments. Often in residential treatment, teachers and professionals dress in casual attire, set flexible time frames, allow for flexibility of assignment choices, and encourage active engagement from students. These efforts allow students to take more ownership of learning and utilize some adult learning principles. By promoting choice and providing options, we not only encourage adult learning concepts but also evade the region of the brain which signals the fight or flight response which is a common issue for those who suffer from mental illness. This leads us to the following section related to neurobiology.

Focus on our Knowledge of Neurobiology

Parents, clinicians and educators alike may find it beneficial to learn more about neurobiology and brain based practices in order to better assist children struggling with mental illness. The brain plays such a vital role in every area of an individual's health. It is imperative to consider as much neurobiological information as possible in our daily efforts to assist children, youth and students who may be struggling with mental health illness.

One myth, accepted by many educators pertains to the notion that brain parts work in isolation. The idea of having "language parts" or "mathematical parts" of the brain is inaccurate. Instead, the brain is a complex system and may use many pieces of different lobes (frontal, parietal, occipital and temporal) at one time. All skills require various sub-skills that draw from numerous areas of the individual's brain (Tokuhama-Espinosa, 2011). This knowledge leads one to a better understanding of the role stress hormones, such as cortisol, and dopamine, a neurotransmitter, play in the learning process.

Two efforts used to enhance neurobiological responses from students in residential treatment are Neurofeedback and binaural beats. Neurofeedback involves "retraining" the brain to utilize alternative pathways for carrying information based on consistent positive feedback. Binaural beats operate with a similar premise. Binaural beats are auditory brainstem responses which result from different frequencies provided to each ear. Regular listening is suggested to reduce stress and anxiety, and increase focus, concentration, motivation, confidence, and depth in meditation (Wahbeh, Calabrese, & Zwickey, 2007). Utilizing these two interventions with students struggling with mental illness in RTCs appears beneficial. Likewise, these efforts may prove beneficial for students in other communities, as well.

Focus on Play, Outdoor Activity, and Exercise

In our fast paced society of testing, achievement, and deadlines, it is easy to overlook playing, outdoor activities, and exercise. However, these are necessary components which may be lacking for those suffering from mental illness.

Research illustrates the importance of play. "More natural play may facilitate the growth of pro-social brains and minds and keep the incidence of ADHD to a minimum" (Panksepp, p.57, 2007). A Neuroscientist found play stimulates production of a protein, found in the amygdala and the prefrontal cortex, which are responsible for organizing, monitoring, and planning for the future. Another study found playing with objects for two hours a day produced changes in the brain weight and efficiency of experimental animals (Goldstein, 2012).

Similar to the importance of play is the significance of exercise. In his book, SPARK, Ratey explains the effect of exercise on the brain. He concludes exercise promotes brain growth, balances neurotransmitters, increases the proteins necessary for learning, and increases the electrical activity of the brain. He compares exercise to miracle-grow for the brain (2013).

In addition to play and exercise, outdoor activity holds a vital role in health. For example, researchers have discovered spending time outdoors can reduce the symptoms of ADHD (Godbey, 2009). In one study, researchers concluded even children whose ADHD symptoms had not responded to medication showed a definite behavioral improvement in outdoor settings. The symptoms were reduced most in green outdoor settings. In some children, medication was cut in half by spending time in nature.

Most residential treatment programs have recognized the need for play, exercise and outdoor activity. Programs may incorporate activities such as 4H, adventure therapy, wilderness curriculums, and fitness into the daily life of students in residential treatment, often observing great results. Incorporating these elements may be effective for the students struggling with mental illness.

Focus on Sensory Processing (Sensory Integration)

According to the Sensory Processing Disorder Foundation (SPD), sensory processing involves communication from the senses to the nervous system and one's ability to respond appropriately with the motor or behavioral response (2015). The foundation also suggests "1 in every 6 children experiences sensory symptoms that may be significant enough to affect aspects of everyday life functions" (2015). This can be illustrated in an individual who is oversensitive to touch. He or she may notice the clothing being worn and rather than being able to refocus on other important tasks, the feeling of the clothing may continuously register in the brain causing a "traffic jam" for the nervous system. Issues resulting from sensory processing can include motor clumsiness, behavioral problems, anxiety, depression, and school failure, among other impacts.

In some RTC's and clinical settings, sensory gyms have become useful tools for working students through this process. Some simple and inexpensive items, such as a weighted blankets or vests, can be used to calm anxiety and help students relax. This can be done in a professional setting or in the comfort of one's home.

Focus on Canines and Emotional Support Animals

Those of us who own a pet can most likely attest to the benefits they feel when their animal is present. The unlimited love, affection and companionship provided by animals also provides stability for those suffering from mental illness.

Research shows all animals possess the potential to improve an individual's psychological perspective. For instance, Cusack speaks of "zoo therapy" when discussing the diversity of animals used for therapeutic purposes (2014). Although this is may be the case, equine therapy and canine therapy seem to be the most prevalent among residential treatment centers.

The authors have had the opportunity to work in residential treatment centers which utilized a variety of animals. However, in the authors' experience, the greatest improvement therapeutically was with clients utilizing golden retrievers as support animals. These dogs' playful, energetic, and loving nature represent the perfect companion for many suffering from mental illness. In the RTC, therapists often referred to the golden retrievers as being the best therapists in the building. The canines often mimicked the student's behaviors, allowing staff to call attention to student behavioral issues without offending or shutting down the student.

One student the authors worked with was thoroughly frustrated with his canine. There was a particular day the student came forward complaining about his dog's impact on his day. His comment went something like this:

My dog woke me up this morning wanting his food, then made a mess AND pottied inside. I spent 20 minutes cleaning up after him, which made me late to my own breakfast. After I ate, my dog would not stop running around the building and I had to chase him for 10 minutes, which made me late to my recreation time. I was last in line for the ropes course and didn't get to go! Finally, now that I am in class, he keeps getting into everything he is not supposed to in the classroom and I can't get any work done!

The authors couldn't help but smile at him. Angered by the authors' obvious show of personal entertainment in hearing his story, the student asked "Why are you laughing?" One of the authors told him, "Because your dog has learned every single one of those things from you." This moment was transformational in the student's personal development.

Ideally, one would attain some clinical treatment alongside the support from the canine, creating a complimentary environment. For parents, educators and clinicians seeking an alternate method for reaching out to children, golden retrievers or emotional support animals may be an excellent choice.

Focus on Communication and Relationship

The same relational components we appreciate from animals can be even more critical from humans. Communication and relationship are critical to the education process. Research suggests when students reflect on education and lessons learned, it is often the relationship with the "teacher" which makes the lasting impact (Allison, 2012). These components are critical to physical health, mental stability and education.

The simple act of relating and communicating about an issue has the power to affect health. According to research, people who process a negative experience through conversation, rather than private reflection, reported a life satisfaction improvement and improved physical and mental health (Francis, 2003; Sousa, 2002). In extreme cases, this notion of communication and relationship can be a matter of living or dying.

For example, U.S. Senator John McCain was struck down over North Vietnam when he was a Navy pilot. Held as a prisoner of war (POW) for 6 years, he often found himself in solitary confinement. POWs would create covert codes by tapping on the walls in order to spell out words. In his book, he describes the risks and rewards involved with such behaviors:

The punishment for communicating could be severe and a few POWs, having been caught and beaten for their efforts, had their spirits broken as their bodies were battered. Terrified of a return trip to the punishment room, they would lie still in their cells when their comrades tried to tap them up on the wall. Very few would remain uncommunicative for long. Suffering alone was less tolerable than torture. "Withdrawing in silence from the fellowship of other Americans…was to us the approach of death." (McCain, 1999, p. 12).

Positive communication and relationships are not only critical for those living in peril, but also for those in residential treatment and environments all around us. For example, in a recent study regarding learning experiences at an RTC, Allison found the most memorable experiences and learning took place with staff who the student trusted and with whom they felt connected (Allison, 2012). Communication and relationship may represent the greatest need and most influential variable for those suffering from mental illness.

With estimates as high as 93% of our communication coming from non-verbal cues, the ability to communicate effectively with non-verbal means is imperative to successful communication and verbal de-escalation in moments of conflict (Adler, Rosenfeld, and Proctor II, 2015). Communication skills are easy to develop with some practice, cost nothing to implement, and are one of the most effective ways to improve our interactions with others who are upset or in a state of mental dysregulation.

AS YOU APPROACH A SITUATION OF CONFLICT

When trying to resolve conflict with others, the outcome of the conflict, be it beneficial or non-beneficial, is often determined before the first word is spoken. This is because individuals communicate to the other person throughout their entire approach. The individual's body posture communicates. Their speed with which they move communicates. Their facial expressions communicate. An individual can work to become aware of what they are communicating in these crucial moments leading up to our first words. A simple practice for controlling body language is called alignment. Consider engaging with an angry child. As one approaches, they can take a pace which matches the intensity of the situation they are entering. A quick pace can align with an intense student. A fast pace can overwhelm or set off an already angry student. A slow pace might communicate disinterest or an inability to hold one's ground. Now, apply those same three approaches to a student who is sad and isolating in a corner. The fast pace and quick pace approaches might cause the student to cower or further withdraw, while a slow pace might offer connection.

Once you are in the same space as the student, it is time to choose a posture from which you desire to communicate. Mirroring the student's physical position can create rapport and provide immediate connection. An example of this would be to sit down next to an isolating or depressed child and assume the same stance they are in. If the student is holding their knees to their chest, do the same.

Another way to create connection is to look in the same direction the child is looking. By sharing a focal point with the child, you can prevent yourself from becoming their focal point. Squaring off in front of a child face to face, even with a calm approach, can communicate a "me against you" demeanor. Stepping to their side can literally communicate you are on their side. If the situation is appropriate, a kind hand on their shoulder can further communicate alignment with their current position.

One of the authors once approached a conflict situation between two students. The students were standing face to face, yelling at each other. Not knowing the situation, the author needed to ask questions to understand the situation and help the boys move towards resolution. The author approached from their side and stepped next to one student, which placed the author looking face to face with the other. By choosing where to stand, the author had aligned himself with one student over the other. The previous argument between the boys was obsolete as the author now became the entire focus of the opposite boy's anger! All the author could constructively do was walk away from the situation and let a different staff learn from the author's mistake and approach from a more neutral position. It is extremely important to tailor your approach in a way that keeps you from becoming the target of the child's frustration. Once you have insulated yourself from their emotional lashing out, you can more effectively engage in exploring their source of frustration.

Ask Questions Before Making Comments

If you are being controlled by your emotions, this is one of the most difficult skills to effectively practice. If you are overly emotional, and another calm person is available, it could be best to let them engage with the dysregulated child. To engage in an empathetic exercise with a child, you must first explore and understand the emotions the child is feeling. This is done through asking a series of questions, chosen to explore the who, what, where, and when of the situation causing their emotion. For a student who has suffered early childhood trauma, is diagnosed with an attachment disorder, or has trouble regulating emotions, "why" questions should be off-limits. Often, these children become upset or emotionally dysregulated because they do not have the physical ability to emotionally regulate. We cannot expect these children to have the cognitive ability to reason themselves out of emotional stress. Asking "why" in regards to their emotion will often be met with, "I don't know." The truth is, these children realistically do not know what is causing their emotions. This is why they need empathetic experiences with adults to help them explore their own feelings. This will be explored in greater depth in the next section.

Bringing a Conflict to Resolution

Presuppositions and a "yes" set are two practical tools which can aid in the de-escalation of a conflict situation with a child who does not have the physical ability to emotionally regulate.

Presuppositions

There is no fool-proof way to resolve a conflict with any person, much less a child with mental illness. By being aware of your non-verbal communication, your approach, and seeking to understand the child, you greatly increase your chances of resolving the situation favorably. Here are some de-escalation tools which can help you move towards a favorable resolution.

"A presupposition is a structure of language that makes unverbalised assumptions" (Casale, 2015). Using presupposition statements can give the child choices, which gives them a feeling of control, while moving them towards a resolution you determine. Let's look at asking a child to clean their room as our situation which needs resolution. Telling our imaginary child, Johnny, to "Go clean your room" is often ineffective. A directive approach, like this one, is only effective when the authoritative speaker has some type of leverage which gives power to their statement. This power often is found in the ability to enforce consequences for lack of compliance. For a student with Reactive Attachment Disorder, who does not respond to punitive consequences, a directive approach is typically ineffective. Utilizing a presuppositional statement allows you to give the student some control, which can bypass the need for a consequence to reinforce the request.

Presuppositions of choice would allow the child to choose between two tasks needing to be completed. "Johnny, would you rather clean your room or do the dishes." We presuppose one of the two tasks will be completed and the other will not need to be.

Presuppositions of time allow a child to choose when they complete a task. "Johnny, would you like to clean your room before, or after, watching some television?" In my experience, a child will almost always agree to a task if they can delay it until later.

A key to successful presuppositions is subtlety. (Casale, 2015) declares presuppositions plus subtlety equals power. The less obvious the presupposition, the more likely a child will choose to engage with it and move towards a resolution. If a child refuses to engage with a presupposition, you have two options; engage in another de-escalation technique or state the impending natural consequence for non-compliance. Consistent use of natural consequences for non-compliance will help to improve a child's feeling of safety, because your actions and logic are predictable. If a natural consequence for non-compliance is proposed, you must be consistent with follow through, or your reliability and the safety of your relationship can be compromised.

A "YES" Set

Telemarketer research has shown you will have to ask for a sale at least three times in one conversation before a person responds with a "yes" answer (Goldstein, Martin, & Cialdini, 2008). Research has also shown once a person says "yes", they are more likely to say "yes" to subsequent questions. With this logic, you can ask a series of questions to the child, which will elicit an almost guaranteed "yes" response to each question. After you obtain three "yes" responses, you ask a question which you would like them to respond "yes" to.

The authors were once on a bus with about 50 students, all diagnosed with Reactive Attachment Disorder. The group was driving an hour to a parent-student retreat. As you can imagine, this is a very stressful weekend for students whose primary struggle is attachment to their parents. The students and staff were squished tightly onto the bus seats, to a point of discomfort. The air-conditioner stopped working. The music stopped working. The group was now sitting on a crowded, hot bus without any distraction from the discomfort. The angry comments began. Then, as if things could not get worse, the bus driver realized we had missed a turn and were momentarily lost. The students began to erupt and demands to unload were shouted. With the situation spiraling downward quickly, one of the authors chose to try a "yes" set. "Are you really uncomfortable right now", the author yelled. Unanimously, the students screamed, "Yes". Next, the author asked, "Are you angry there is no music and we missed our turn?". Once again, "Yes"! "Do you wish we had never gotten on this stupid bus?" the author questioned. "Yes" they replied a third time. Now it was time for the long shot. The author finally asked, "Can you commit to staying calm for 20 more minutes while we finish the drive to the retreat center?!" The authors could see the wheels turning in each of the students' heads. Some were silent while others mumbled a hesitant, "yes…". Miraculously, the students calmed down and were able to stay calm until the bus arrived at the retreat center!

Responding vs. Reacting

As you interact with a child dealing with mental illness during a conflict, you must maintain a correct mental frame. This mental frame will help you to keep your own emotions in check. The illustration of responding versus reacting offers clarity on your role in de-escalation. When you take a medicine, your bodies will experience one of three outcomes. Non-response to the medicine, which does not apply to the current discussion, a positive response, or a negative reaction. A positive response will result with the body changing in a favorable fashion and moving towards being well. A negative reaction will likely introduce new, sometimes more severe, symptoms. The same outcomes exist within our moments of conflict resolution. Everything you do and say will either elicit a reaction or a response. The goal is to minimize communication that elicits a reaction. If you receive a reaction to your communication, then you should evaluate your communication and determine if there is an alternate mode of communication which can bring about a more positive response. This diagnostic mindset can also be used to evaluate your non-verbal communication and how you have approached a situation and sought to understand the child's emotional state.

Focus on Emotional Intelligence and Empathy

Closely tied with communication and relationship is the ability to identify one's own emotions and perceive the feelings of those around them. Skills associated with this process are considered Emotional Intelligence. According to Goleman, five domains of Emotional Intelligence exist. These include: self-awareness, managing emotions, motivation, empathy, and social skills (Goleman, 1995).

The skills associated with emotional intelligence (EQ) have been shown to be more effective than those related to intelligence quotient (IQ). Unlike IQ, these skills are more easily improved. Developing our EQ may include activities such as practicing supportive feedback, analysis of emotions, or increasing vocabulary associated with feelings. These skills are not only effective in communicating with those suffering from mental illness, but they may also be helpful in identifying students who remain undiagnosed or will not seek medical attention.

Although greater emotional intelligence can assist in all interpersonal relationships, one of the keys for supporting those with mental illness is empathy. Empathy involves the ability to recreate someone else's perspective and experience life from another person's point of view (Adler, Rosenfeld, & Proctor, 2015). Some techniques which can be used to increase one's ability to show empathy include: reading about others' suffering, sharing personal narratives, and speaking with or visiting different people groups.

Developing skills such as open-mindedness, imagination, and commitment can help those who struggle with empathizing. Setting aside one's own thoughts and values and seeing those of the other person helps in understanding another's perspective. Additionally, being able to visualize and imagine how someone else is feeling represents another important skill. Finally, commitment ensures that even when empathizing may be difficult, the sincere desire to face the challenge will be worth the effort (Adler, Rosenfeld, & Proctor, 2015).

For those who have worked in residential treatment, empathy and emotional intelligence skills are critical. A day does not pass without utilizing these skills with clients. Beliefs such as "I'm worthless", "No one loves me" and "I can't do anything good" permeate the students' lives; therefore, empathy is critical in handling these difficult students. Establishing stability and relationship with the students is paramount.

Students struggling with attachment issues will often push the envelope in relationships while attempting to prove, or more often disprove, another's affection for themselves. The child will do something shocking, which likely will cause a break in the relationship, and then internally ask the question, "Do you still love me?" Obvious instances of this happen if a child is isolating or verbally or physically assaults an individual trying to care for them. Instances, like this next story, are much subtler.

Some residential treatments centers use time-outs to give a student time to reflect on their misbehavior or as a punitive consequence. In dealing with students suffering from attachment disorders, a time-in model has proved more clinically effective at one of the residential treatments centers the authors have worked with. Students needing time-in were given a different colored shirt from the other students, for safety, and one on one attention from a staff member. This provided an at-risk student with constant supervision and support. Time-in would persist until a student no longer needed the one on one attention from staff, which would sometimes take days or weeks, depending on the case.

One of the authors' former students was upset with his time-in on a particular occasion. Each night, as he got ready for bed, he would use his teeth to start small tears in his designated shirt. He would stare at the staff member sitting next to him and pull those tears, removing thin strips from his shirt until it looked like a mid-drift with no sleeves attached. The sight was a bit comical. What was not comical was the conversation happening inside of the student throughout this process. With each strip he removed, it was as if he was saying, "Do you still love me now? Are you going to take care of my needs when I don't have a shirt anymore?" The staff would sit by him until he tired enough to go to bed for the night. In the morning, the new staff would have a clean, whole shirt ready for the student. It was as if the staff's response was, "I do still love you and here is a new shirt to meet your needs for the day." This silent dance went on for near a week. Then, one day, without comment, the behavior stopped and the student's relationships strengthened with his staff. The behavior corrected and the relationships grew deeper without an intentional word being spoken. Trust was established and empathetic responses from the staff enabled the staff to persevere through the quiet conflict, instead of becoming frustrated and demanding the student simply stop ripping his shirt.

The ability to be empathetic is not only useful in the residential environment, but also in our work-places and schools. The key for parents, educators, and clinicians, is to recognize the poor behavior or difficulties that are generally seen coming from these students could be the product of deep, negative core beliefs, chemical imbalances in the brain, or various other issues. Our ability to empathize and walk with the students through their trauma and mental anguish can assist them as they cope with mental ill-ness. Increasing one's own emotional intelligence and ability to empathize can assist in understanding these difficulties and leading others to healthier lives.

Focus on Natural and Logical Consequences

Often punishment comes to mind when we think about consequences for our actions. We may visualize punitive punishments such as spankings or timeouts. However, often for those suffering from mental illness, particularly those with Reactive Attachment Disorder, this style of corrective behavior may exacerbate the outward behaviors of the child. A more effective approach to consequences would be to consider the wrongful action and provide natural and logical consequences.

For instance, a child may choose to draw on the wall or furniture with crayons. First, the child needs to understand this was not a proper decision. After this is established, the child may not be permitted to play with additional toys until the wall is clean (this is a logical consequence). If this cleaning takes some time and interferes with being able to go outside and play with his friend, this would be a natural consequence. The child also needs to understand how their actions affected you on an emotional level.

This manner of handling consequences is not always simple or efficient. Often, when handling students struggling with mental illness, the difficulties you run into are much more significant and involve some creativeness as you seek natural and logical consequences. For instance, while working in residential treatment, the authors once had a student who broke a fire sprinkler head in his bedroom, flooding his room and the entire school, which was located on the floor directly beneath his room. When overcome with anger, punitive consequences tend to be where the mind jumps to. Natural and logical consequences for this scenario are much more difficult to pinpoint when under stress and in the moment. Did the student help to clean up the situation? Yes, absolutely. In addition, the student helped with some of the construction and repair which needed to occur in the damaged facility. Financially, the student worked to repay parents (who initially footed the bill). Finally, and most importantly, the student met with every impacted staff and faculty in counseling sessions to hear about their feelings and frustrations. Understanding other's emotions and feelings helped with the student's ability to empathize and successfully prevented future issues of this nature. After experiencing empathy, the student was able to issue authentic apologies to each staff member of the treatment center which his actions impacted negatively. This process took weeks, but was invaluable for the student's growth.

All in all, it can be a great deal of work to come up with natural and logical consequences and there are times where sending a child to timeout may seem to be an easier choice. However, when it comes to lasting change, the time it takes to focus on natural and logical consequences, empathy, and debriefing after the event is well worth the commitment.

CONCLUSION

This chapter explores the impact of mental illness in children and youth on themselves, their loved ones, and those who interact with mentally ill children in various settings. In addition to understanding who is affected, this chapter seeks to express a holistic and comprehensive approach to the physical, mental, and spiritual health of mentally ill children.

After examining attachment styles, learning environments, and adult learning principles, we find there are many contributing factors to mentally ill children's ability to take in external stimuli, create long-term learning and knowledge, and find healing within their mental illness. A discussion of neurobiology, physical activity impacts, and sensory processing development reveals a biological factor in a mentally ill child's ability to regulate and relate to the world around them. Emotional support animals, as well as quality communication and your verbal de-escalation skills can assist a mentally ill child and move them toward regulation and compliance.

Two of the most beneficial practices, in helping mentally ill children to heal, are the practices of empathy and establishing boundaries with the use of natural consequences. One is able to connect on a deep level through empathy and establish a safe and reliable relationship through consistent communication and the enforcement of natural consequences, when necessary.

By walking along side, communicating effectively with, showing empathy to, and providing multifaceted support for children with mental illness, we can help them travel down the difficult road towards healing. While we might only hear a school bell ringing to start the day, these practices enable us to experience the bell as each child experiences it; giving us valuable insight and a deeper relationship through which we can facilitate healing.

REFERENCES

Adler, R., Rosenfeld, L., & Proctor, I. I. R. (2015). *Interplay*. New York, NY: Oxford University Press.

Alcoholics Anonymous. (2001). Alcoholics Anonymous (4th ed.). New York, AA. World Services.

Allison, K. (2012). Experiences and perceptions as expressed by adolescent females at a residential treatment center (RTC) [Unpublished Doctoral Dissertation]. Florida Atlantic University, Boca Raton, FL, USA.

Bartholomew, K. (1990). Avoidance of intimacy: An attachment perspective. *Journal of Social and Personal Relationships*, *7*(2), 147–178. doi:10.1177/0265407590072001

Bartholomew, K., & Horowitz, L. (1991). Attachment styles among young adults: A test of a four category model. *Journal of Personality and Social Psychology*, *61*(2), 226–244. doi:10.1037/0022-3514.61.2.226 PMID:1920064

Bartlett, J. (1919). Bartleby Quotations. Retrieved from http://www.bartleby.com/100/707.html

Boys & Girls Club of America. (2010). *Who we are.* Retrieved from http://www.bgca.org/whoweare/

Brennan, K. A., Clark, C. L., & Shaver, P. R. (1998). Self report measure of adult attachment. In J. A. Simpson & W. S. Rhodes (Eds.), *Attachment theory and close relationships* (pp. 46–76). New York, NY: Guilford Press.

Burleson, B. R., & Goldsmith, D. J. (1998). Handbook of Communication and Emotion: Research, Theory, Applications, and Contexts.

Casale, P. (2015). Presuppositions in linguistics and NLP. Retrieved from http://www.nlp-secrets.com/nlp-presuppositions.php

Centers for Disease Control and Prevention CDC. (2009). Flu Information Sheet. Retrieved from http://www.cdc.gov/flu/weekly/weeklyarchives2008-2009/weekly39.htm

Centers for Disease Control and Prevention- CDC. (2012). Heart Disease Facts. Retrieved from http://www.cdc.gov/heartdisease/facts.htm

Centers for Disease Control and Prevention- CDC. (2015). Mental health data and statistics. Retrieved from http://www.cdc.gov/mentalhealth/data-stats.htm

Commission office of the Prime Minister. (1999). *National Education Act of BE 2542.* Retrieved from http://planipolis.iiep.unesco.org/upload/Thailand/Thailand_Education_Act_1999.pdf

Coombs, P. H., & Ahmed, M. (1974). *Attacking rural poverty: How nonformal education can help.* Baltimore, MD: Johns Hopkins University Press.

Curtis, P. A., Alexander, G., & Lunghofer, L. A. (2001, October). A literature review comparing the outcomes of residential group care and therapeutic Foster care. *Child & Adolescent Social Work Journal*, *18*(5), 5. doi:10.1023/A:1012507407702

Cusack, O. (2014). *Pets and mental health.* Routledge.

Drais-Parrillo, A. (2005). The Odyssey Project: A descriptive and prospective study of children and youth in residential group care and therapeutic foster care. *Child Welfare League of America.* Retrieved from http://www.cwla.org/programs/research/odysseyfinalreport.pdf4

European Commission. (2007). *Making a European Area of Lifelong Learning a Reality.* Retrieved from http://eurlex.europa.eu/LexUriServ/LexUriServ.do?uri=COM:2001:0678:FIN:EN:PDF

Feeney, B. C., & Collins, N. L. (2003). Motivations for caregiving in adult intimate relationships: Influences on caregiving behavior and relationship functioning. *Personality and Social Psychology Bulletin*, *29*(8), 950–968. doi:10.1177/0146167203252807 PMID:15189615

SPD Foundation. (2015). About Sensory Processing Disorder. Retrieved from: http://www.spdfoundation.net/about-sensory-processing-disorder/

Fraley, R., Garner, J., & Shaver, P. (2000). Adult attachment and the defensive regulation of attention and memory: Examining the role of preemptive and postemptive defensive processes. *Journal of Personality and Social Psychology*, *79*(5), 816–826. doi:10.1037/0022-3514.79.5.816 PMID:11079243

Fraley, R., Niedenthal, P., Marks, M., Brumbaugh, C., & Vicary, A. (2006). Adult attachment and the perception of emotional expressions: Probing the hyperactivating strategies underlying anxious attachment. *Journal of Personality*, *74*(4), 1163–1182. doi:10.1111/j.1467-6494.2006.00406.x PMID:16787432

Francis, L. E. (2003). Feeling good, feeling well: Identity, emotion and health. In Advances in identity theory and research (pp. 123-134). Springer US.

Godbey, G. (2009). Outdoor recreation, health, and wellness: Understanding and enhancing the relationship.

Goldstein, J. (2012). *Play in children's development, health and well-being*. Brussels: Toy Industries of Europe.

Goldstein, N. J., Martin, S. J., & Cialdini, R. B. (2008). *Yes!: 50 scientifically proven ways to be persuasive*. New York: Free Press.

Goleman, D. (1995). *Emotional Intelligence*. New York, NY: Free Press.

Gray, P. (2010). The decline in play and rise in children's mental disorders. *Psychology Today, Blog*. Retrieved from https://www.psychologytoday.com/blog/freedom-learn/201001/the-decline-play-and-rise-in-childrens-mental-disorders

Gross, R. (1999). *Peak Learning*. New York, NY: Penguin Putnam Inc.

Hamilton, S. S., & Armando, J. (2008). Oppositional Defiant Disorder. *American Family Physician*, *78*, 861–867. PMID:18841736

Hazan, C., & Shaver, P. (1987). Romantic love conceptualized as an attachment process. *Journal of Personality and Social Psychology*, *52*(3), 511–524. doi:10.1037/0022-3514.52.3.511 PMID:3572722

Jones, S. M. (2005). Attachment style differences and similarities in evaluations of affective communication skills and person-centered comforting messages. *Western Journal of Communication*, *69*(3), 233–249. doi:10.1080/10570310500202405

Kane, H., Jaremka, L., Guichard, A., Ford, M., Collins, N., & Feeney, B. (2007). Feeling supported and feeling satisfied: How one partner's attachment style predicts the other partner's relationship experiences. *Journal of Social and Personal Relationships*, *24*(4), 535–555. doi:10.1177/0265407507079245

Katz, J., & Joiner, T. (2002). Being known, intimate, and valued: Global self-verification and dyadic adjustment in couples and roommates. *Journal of Personality*, *70*(1), 33–58. doi:10.1111/1467-6494.00177 PMID:11908534

Knowles, M. J. (1973). *The modern practice of adult education: From pedagogy to andragogy*. New York, NY: Cambridge Book Company.

Lifelong Learning. (n.d.). In *Macmillan Online Dictionary*. Retrieved from http://www.macmillandictionary.com/dictionary/british/lifelong-learning

McCain, J. (1999). *Faith of my fathers*. New York, NY: Random House.

Memorandum on Lifelong Learning. (2007). *European society of association executives*. Retrieved from http://www.esae.org/articles/2007_08_005.pdf

Mikulciner, M., Florian, V., Cowan, P. A., & Cowan, C. P. (2002). Attachment security in couple relationships: A systematic model and its implications for family dynamics. *Family Process*, *41*(3), 405–434. doi:10.1111/j.1545-5300.2002.41309.x PMID:12395567

Mikulincer, M. (1998). Attachment working models and the sense of trust: An exploration of interaction goals and affect regulation. *Journal of Personality and Social Psychology*, *74*(5), 1209–1224. doi:10.1037/0022-3514.74.5.1209

National Alliance on Mental Illness- NAMI. (2015). Mental health by the numbers. Retrieved from https://www.nami.org/Learn-More/Mental-Health-By-the-Numbers

Nelson, C., Fox, N., & Zeanah, C. (2013). The Anguish of the abandoned Child. Retrieved from http://www.adoptionpolicy.org/sad0413Nels3pRV.pdf

Office of the National Education Commission. (1999). *National Education act BE 2542. office of the prime minister Kingdom of Thailand*. Retrieved from http://www.onesqa.or.th/en/publication/nation_edbook.pdf

Panksepp, J. (2007). Can PLAY Diminish ADHD and Facilitate the Construction of the Social Brain? *Journal of the Canadian Academy of Child and Adolescent Psychiatry*, *16*(2), 57–66. PMID:18392153

Ratey, J. (2013). *Spark*. Boston, MA: Little, Brown and Company.

Rogers, A. (1992). Adults Learning for Development. Cassell Educational Limited, 387 Park Avenue South, New York, NY.

Ruvolo, A. P., & Brennan, C. J. (1997). What's love got to do with it? Close relationships and perceived growth. *Personality and Social Psychology Bulletin*, *23*(8), 814–823. doi:10.1177/0146167297238003

Sable, P. (2007, December). Accentuating the positive in adult attachments. *Attachment & Human Development*, *9*(4), 361–374. doi:10.1080/14616730701711573 PMID:18049933

Schachner, D., Shaver, P., & Mikulincer, M. (2005). Patterns of nonverbal behavior and sensitivity in the contest of attachment relationships. *Journal of Nonverbal Behavior*, *29*(3), 141–169. doi:10.1007/s10919-005-4847-x

Sensory Processing Disorder Foundation SPDF. (2015). About sensory processing disorder. Retrieved from http://www.spdfoundation.net/about-sensory-processing-disorder/

SEO Services. (2011). *Residential Treatment Center*. Retrieved from http://www.residentialtreatmentcenter.net/

Sousa, L. A. (2002). The medium is the message: The costs and benefits of writing, talking aloud, and thinking about lifes triumphs and defeats. *Dissertation abstracts International: Section B. The Sciences and Engineering*, 62(7-B), 3397.

Sturm, R., Ringel, J. S., Stein, B. D., & Kapur, K. (2001). Mental health care for youth who gets it? How much does it cost? Who pays? Where does the money go? *Rand.* Retrieved from http://www.rand.org/pubs/research_briefs/RB4541/index1.html

Syrus, P. (42BC). Found in *Familiar quotations.*

The Big Book Online (4th ed.). (2001). Retrieved from http://www.aa.org/bigbookonline

Tokuhama-Espinosa, T. (2011). *Mind, brain, and education science: A comprehensive guide to the new brain-based teaching*. WW Norton & Company.

Tough, A. M. (1979). *The adult's learning projects: A fresh approach to theory and practice in adult learning*. Toronto, Canada: Ontario Institute for Studies in Education.

UAMS. (2015). Spiritual Wellness. Retrieved from http://medicine.uams.edu/faculty/current-faculty/faculty-wellness-program/spiritual-wellness/

Verghese, A. (2008). Spirituality and mental health. *Indian Journal of Psychiatry*, *50*(4), 233–237. doi:10.4103/0019-5545.44742 PMID:19823605

Wahbeh, H., Calabrese, C., & Zwickey, H. (2007). Binaural Beat Technology in Humans: A Pilot Study To Assess Psychologic and Physiologic Effects. *Journal of Alternative and Complementary Medicine (New York, N.Y.)*, *13*(1), 25–32. doi:10.1089/acm.2006.6196 PMID:17309374

Waters, E., Merrick, S., Treboux, D., Crowell, J., & Albersheim, L. (2000). Attachment security in infancy and early adulthood: A twenty-year longitudinal study. *Child Development*, *71*(3), 684–689. doi:10.1111/1467-8624.00176 PMID:10953934

World Health Organization- WHO. (2009). Diarrheal Disease Factsheet. Retrieved from http://www.who.int/mediacentre/factsheets/fs330/en/index.html

KEY TERMS AND DEFINITIONS

Formal Education: Pertains to the institutional, hierarchical structure typically observed in traditional grade schools.

Informal Education: Involves the process whereby an individual accumulates knowledge, skills, and attitudes from daily experiences such as conversations, reflection, reading, and exposure to the environment.

Mental Health: Is "a state of well-being in which the individual realizes his or her own abilities, can cope with the normal stresses of life, can work productively and fruitfully, and is able to make a contribution to his or her community (WHO, 2015)

Mental Illness: Is a "condition that impacts a person's thinking, feeling or mood and may affect his or her ability to relate to others and function on a daily basis. Each person will have different experiences, even people with the same diagnosis" (NAMI, 2015).

Non-Formal Education: Is organized and systematic and occurs outside the framework of the formal system, such as 4-H, church, and group therapy. When considering education, it is imperative to consider all of these contexts to better understand the learning process.

Physical Health: Relates to the overall well-being of the body itself pertaining to human anatomy.

Residential Treatment Center: Generally, refers to congregate care for treatment services in a non-medical environment. Adolescents live together as "residents" or "students" and treatment methods often include a combination of therapeutic activities.

Spiritual Health: Is defined by the University of Arkansas for Medical Sciences (UAMS) as a "personal matter involving values and beliefs that provide a purpose in our lives. While different individuals may have different views of what spiritualism is, it is generally considered to be the search for meaning and purpose in human existence, leading one to strive for a state of harmony with oneself and others while working to balance inner needs with the rest of the world" (2015).

Chapter 8
Culture of Learning Cities:
Connecting Leisure and Health for Lifelong Learning Communities

Ebbin Dotson
University of Illinois at Chicago, USA

Dan K. Hibbler
DePaul University, USA

Leodis Scott
Columbia University, USA

ABSTRACT

This chapter contributes a conceptual framework for addressing the health of communities through the synergy of leisure, public health, and continuing education systems at a localized city level. The culture learning cities offers a broader setting and case for implementing solutions that increase the overall health of communities. Key built environments within learning cities, such as parks, can serve as nontraditional continuing education structures, where people can learn and share their differences and experiences that continually improve qualities of the individual, community, and society.

INTRODUCTION

Synergy across professions represents a creative solution to complex problems in society. The culture of learning cities is an authentic example of such synergy and collaboration across diverse communities. Learning cities can describe extensions of education and learning beyond schools, colleges and universities for addressing the overall life, health and well-being of citizens. Two aspects that can be advanced are public health and leisure within a culture of learning cities. A practical U.S. example of learning cities involves strategic land-usage, from the historic land-grant legislation of American colleges and universities to the significant allocation of parks and recreation areas. This chapter will consider a comprehensive role for promoting learning cities for building healthy and healthful communities including

DOI: 10.4018/978-1-5225-0640-9.ch008

enhanced relationships among professionals and practitioners, scholars and researchers, also citizens and lifelong learners for improving our community, our health, and our overall quality of life.

Learning cities describe an emerging concept about how communities can collectively support multiple, even conflicting initiatives for the good of all citizens. Such collaboration considers how environmental structures, such as parks, serve as nontraditional systems for leisure, public health, and lifelong learning. Professionals interested in advancing environments should consider diverse leisure activities that account for differences in age, race, and other societal identities, and incorporate such diversities into community education and broader notions of ecological health, social justice, and collective participation. Thus, healthy parks within healthy community synergism exemplify an important function within the context of learning cities.

This chapter contributes a conceptual framework for addressing the health of communities through the synergy of leisure, public health, and continuing education systems at a localized city level. We attempt to highlight the importance of health in advancing environments and contextualizing social concerns. We introduce conceptual models for leisure and recreation issues to account for tensions, conflicts, and negative aspects of shared experiences in communities. Race and culture differences have also been considered through the context of community education and lifelong learning-for-all. Within a comprehensive framework of learning cities, diversity and differences have been surveyed and addressed, which may lead toward every person's quality of life being enhanced.

Thus, learning cities can offer a broader setting and case for implementing solutions that increase the overall health of communities. In this chapter, the framework of learning cities describes parks, as nontraditional continuing education structures, where people can learn and share their differences and experiences that continually improve qualities of the individual, community, and society. Given that there is no one-size-fits-all conception of health, professionals and practitioners, along with park and recreation managers, even public health and continuing education practitioners, must begin reconstructing parks for the multiple concerns and challenges for becoming healthy communities.

THE IMPORTANCE OF HEALTH IN ADVANCING ENVIRONMENTS

Learning cities can harness collaborative synergy when combining public health and built environment perspectives to address complex problems in society. Formed to increase public health, the collaborations across communities and professions are among the best examples of advancing environments through multifaceted approaches. At individual and societal levels, individuals exercise personal care and social responsibility towards healthy outcomes. Figure 1 shows a conceptual framework for the drivers and burdens of health in a learning city. Among some of the most complex problems facing individuals and communities are the environmental burdens of confronting obesity, violence, and health care access. At the community level, education, lifestyle, and the built environment are shared resources driving positive health outcomes. In this framework, community level drivers are necessary to overcome and combat individual level burdens. Increases in community health status, or comparative health status between communities, are conceptualized as a function of the advancement of these drivers. This chapter will use parks and recreational initiatives to exemplify this function in action.

In this age of population health, learning cities incorporate education and justice into a broad notion of ecological health in which the built environment is as important to health status as the provision

Figure 1. Health status conceptual framework for learning cities

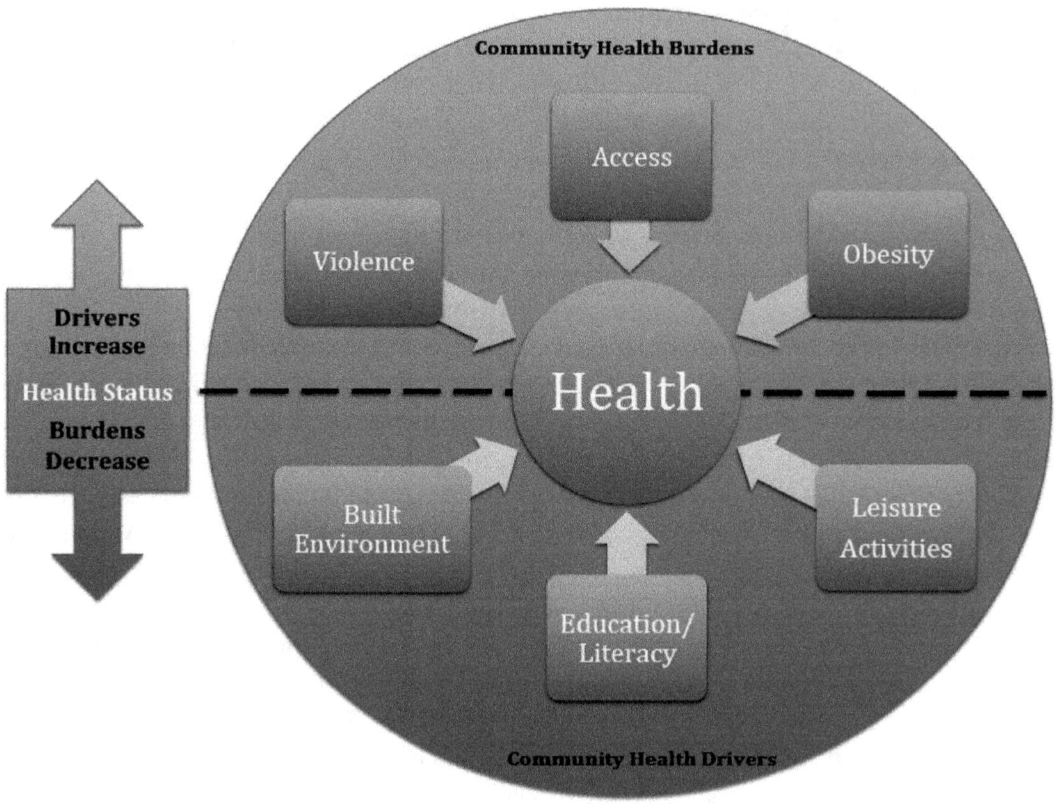

of care. Public health system goals directly impacted by the various drivers and burdens shown in the conceptual framework. The development of locally adjusted solutions that are also beneficial to the environment is therefore also dependent on the inclusion of environmental interests and the incorporation of environmentally relevant lay knowledge (Drazkiewicz et al., 2015). For example, urban green space provides a wide range of ecosystem services that could help combat many urban ills and improve life for city dwellers—especially their health (Maas et al., 2006; Wolch et al., 2014; van den Bosch et al., 2015).

To solve societal problems, identifying theoretical levels of engagement is an important concept towards understanding the impact of public health and its role for communities. Initiatives that draw upon ecological models for rationalization emphasize individual characteristics and environmental space as drivers of personal behavior (Sallis et al., 2008). Because environmental levels of influence do not explicitly consider the broader community, organizational, and policy influences on health behaviors, researchers suggest multilevel interventions based on ecological models and targeting individuals, social environments, physical environments, and policies being key to achieving population change in physical activity (Sallis et al., 2006).

This section will focus on the importance of health in advancing environments of learning cities. First, personal care and social responsibility to healthy outcomes will be discussed. Whereas ecological theories dominate behavioral health, institutional theory will be introduced as an alternative theoretical basis from which to better understand health-seeking behavior at the individual and community nexus. Second, obesity, violence, and health care access are described as complex societal issues. Both violence and obesity have downstream effects on individual and community health (Plichta, 2004). Lesser known are the implications that one has on the other, as well as the moderating effects that the built environment has in the context of access to health care.

PERSONAL CARE AND SOCIAL RESPONSIBILITY TO HEALTHY OUTCOMES

It is a tough assignment for researchers to connect community and individual health statuses with quality of life indicators in the public health arena. It is an unfair proxy because much of the environmental complexity that influences quality factors relating to healthy outcomes are outside the span of control of pubic health professionals and practitioners. Ecological modeling addresses some of the contextual issues that impact individual and community health seeking behavior. We introduce institutional theory as a way to bridge the gap and discuss the impact that organizations within various professions can have on quality of life at the city level. Institutional theory focuses on the behavior of organizations in a field or environment, and emphasizes that organizations are open systems, strongly influenced by their environments. The strength of the theory is the connectedness and structural equivalence of organizational responses to environmental constraints, both individual and community level. In this section, we further discuss constraints as complex issues associated with health outcomes.

Our [health and leisure] environments include socially constructed belief and rule systems that exercise enormous control over organizations, both how they are structured and how they carry out their work (Scott, 2003). Here, social factors manifest themselves as processes that create action or behave in response to environmental changes. Institutional theory, through the process of institutionalization, provides a foundational context to view these factors (Dacin, Goodstein, & Scott, 2002). In institutional theory, structuration is the change process by which organizations seek to exploit the most efficient available form of management, thus constantly making decisions to become more like the dominant set of successful organizations. Organizations facing the same set of environmental constraints, competition, and available resources become rational actors that find similar solutions. The environmental complexity during this decision process and conformity period includes social, economic, and political factors; such factors surface each time the linkage between the environment and interdependence of organizations comes into play.

The synergy between professions focusing on health and leisure can be exemplified in the interplay between organizations supporting health and education. Across learning cities in the United States, there are similarities in the health and educational frameworks for infrastructure and organizational policies, financial and legal resources, and human resource planning (Howard et al., 2015). Institutional theory provides a way to explain these similarities. For example, many existing health systems structure their organizations by anchoring patient care to a flagship hospital with several efficient referral hospitals and clinics within a geographical catchment area. To generate a financially viable patient population, access points straddle affluent and impoverished zip codes. Each of the systems' smaller hospitals and clinics are set up to capture the same categorical patients, with budget forecasting built on poisson distribution patient flow patterns, similar reimbursement, and patient mix schemes.

Comparing health and education, the convergence of school districts and decision-making around school closings mirror historical reductions in hospitals as well proliferation of the flagship-anchoring networked health systems. Several population-dense metropolitan areas in the United States remain carved into a racially and economically segregated mosaic of local public school districts, which in some cases enroll only a few hundred students and lie immediately adjacent to other tiny local public school districts that can seem a world away (Baker, 2014). The access to high performing schools, feeder patterns for resource rich student pools, and the mix of public and private schools are examples of the structuration process in institutional theory. Furthermore, social justice issues have captured political attention, making race, ethnicity, culture, and poverty essential components of these debates.

In short, one might ask what does this really have to do with health status and quality of life? Well, the ability to accurately predict which hospital is better, based on organizational characteristics or the viability of certain schools within districts, will be the same process organizational planners use to try and determine how health status and quality of life are significantly associated with the built environment. What predictive mechanisms used to address health and educational factors tell about institutional theory is that organizational behavior is based on environmental and interdependent factors. The challenge for social activists, health practitioners, urban planners, and education professionals is that organizational forms do not change often, and when they do change, the environment selects the dominant organizations. And because most organizations are competing for finite geographical resources, the diversity of organizational forms is isomorphic or in similar form to the diversity of environments.

To advance solutions for health in the environment, a learning city will need to explore the opportunities to create strong collaborations between successful organizations in each of its main professional fields. Health systems can learn about stability from school districts. Parks and recreation departments can learn about capacity-building and program efficiency from federally qualified health centers. Institutional theory suggests the iterative processes of learning cities will create convergence on optimal organizational forms. Ideally, this type of mimetic or imitative processes will generate stable convergence around one or a few forms, independent of competitive and efficiency imperatives (Strang & Macy, 2001).

CONFRONTING OBESITY, VIOLENCE, AND HEALTH CARE ACCESS

Confronting complex issues such as the interconnectedness between obesity, violence, and health care access requires both ecological and institutional theories. While it has been long understood that violence has implications for emotional and physical injury, it is only relatively recently that we are beginning to recognize the longer-term effects that reap an extensive toll on the broader health status of individuals, families and communities (Prevention Institute, 2011). The notion that violence is a contagion in public health allows organizations to develop institutionalized solutions to address it. In families, violence between partners increases the risk of violence directed at children and increases the risk of the children behaving violently themselves. Having one violent individual in a family makes it more likely there will be others (Huesmann, 2012).

Violence and chronic disease patterns are also linked. There is a significantly higher likelihood of engaging in behaviors known to contribute to chronic illness behaviors (smoking, eating disorders, substance abuse, decreased physical activity) for those who have been exposed to one or more of the range of types of interpersonal violence (e.g., child abuse, sexual assault, family violence, and community violence) (Prevention Institute, 2011).

Obesity is another synergistic topic in which its complexities also spill into violence and contagion. While genetic factors probably contribute, rapid increases in obesity suggest that individual behavior patterns, including low levels of physical activity, appear to powerfully influence obesity trends (Wolch et al., 2014). Children of women who report chronic intimate partner violence are 1.8 times more likely to be obese than other children; the effect is magnified for families living in unsafe neighborhoods (Kendall-Tackett & Marshall, 1999). Mothers with high exposure to neighborhood violence were twice as likely to report never exercising (Lumeng et al., 2006).

The sheer cost of violence and obesity, not to mention lost productivity, create economic dearth within communities and cities. Considerable portions of the costs of violence are paid by public sources and thus represent a cost to society in general (IOM & NRC, 2012). A study at the University of Southern California Medical Center found that 87 percent of the costs of treating gunshot wounds of the trunk were paid with public funds—with average hospital stays of 6.8 days and costs of $10,600 per patient (IOM & NRC, 2012). Chronic illness resulting from unhealthy eating and activity account for a growing percentage of escalating costs in the health care system (Hogan et al., 2003; Huang et al., 2009; Prevention Institute, 2010; Prevention Institute, 2007; Thorpe et al., 2004).

Furthermore, violence and fear of violence are significant barriers to healthy eating and active living for built environment researchers. People are less likely to use local parks or walk to school when they do not feel safe in their neighborhood, and violence reduces investments in communities—for example, grocery stores (Bennett et al., 2007; Shaffer, 2002; Zenk et al., 2005). Women who perceive their neighborhoods to be unsafe are 25 percent more likely to be obese, and children of parents who perceived their neighborhood as unsafe were 4 times more likely to be overweight than those of parents who perceived their neighborhood as safe (Boynton-Jarrett et al., 2010; Burdette et al., 2006; Rohrer et al., 2004).

LEISURE ENGAGEMENTS

Leisure engagement is the second conceptual driver of community health. Much has been written about the benefits of leisure and the overall positive outcomes of leisure participation. Kelly and Godbey (1992) have indicated the positive impact that leisure activities have on the family, individual development, and personal health. They also suggest that much of our leisure is experienced through a myriad of social groups, from the family to special interest clubs. Such social experiences shape not only our life satisfaction and self-definition; they also fundamentally affect family relations, friendships, and the environment. These leisure engagements are vast with different participation patterns, preferences, and politics.

Leisure may be crucial to persons in many periods of life. Research on leisure, stress, and coping is important within a broad spectrum of leisure scholarship, especially since it can be potentially integrated with research constraints and negotiations, lifespan development, diversity, and lifestyle (Iwasaki & Schneider, 2003). In fact, Ponde and Santana (2000) found that participation in leisure activities are a protective factor for women's mental health in Salvador Brazil indicating that the health benefits of leisure is not only an American phenomenon, but also have international implications. Later-life adults often focus on leisure investments and priorities, as well as work and significant relationships, making leisure more often central than peripheral though the journey of life. (Kelly & Godbey, 1992).

This section will focus on the interrelated aspects of leisure engagement activities impacting health in advancing environments of learning cities. First, the negative aspects of leisure will be discussed. Second, we will identify racial differences in leisure activities, and the downstream disparities produced by these differences. And third, the connection to healthy communities will be exemplified again using violence and obesity issues.

Negative Aspects of Leisure

Scholars and practitioners must also remain cognizant of the leisure tensions, conflicts, and potential negative aspects of the leisure experience. Over the course of debate, an a priori belief in the innate goodness of leisure has prevented leisure scholars from exploring its negative aspects (Jacobson & Samdahl, 1998). The classical term "purple recreation" refers to the recreational activities that challenge societal norms and expectations (Curtis, 1979), taking on a more socially negative description in recent times, especially among youth and violence researchers (Caldwell & Smith, 2007). For example, Robertson (1994) reported that people who participate in negatively considered activities, such as socially inappropriate actions, may achieve the same positive feelings and benefits. Some of these benefits include self-validation, which is typically associated with more acceptable forms of recreational activity, often referred as so-called, "good leisure." However, studies conducted in the past 20 years suggest that so-called descriptions of both "bad" and "good" leisure benefit all those who engage and participate in them (Robertson, 1999; Shinew & Parry, 2005; Shores et al., 2007).

According to Jacobson and Samdahl (1998), contemporary leisure theorists have emphasized ways that leisure can enhance or reaffirm one's sense of self, but they have not effectively acknowledged that leisure can be a context for negative messages about the self. Further, this possibility becomes particularly germane for individuals or groups who are subject to stigma and negative sanctions in other domains of their lives. Any person or group may experience stigma based on ascribed attributes that society views as important (such as age, gender, race, or ethnicity). Discriminatory practices and oppressive ideologies may typically result in reduced opportunities, in negative impacts on health, and in restricted or blocked access to resources, activities, and other opportunities (Germain, 1991). If these reactions occur in other aspects within the lives of people and groups who are "different," then it is feasible to assume that they will occur in leisure as well (Jacobson & Samdahl, 1998). Therefore, the investigation of disempowered groups, such as ethnic and racial minorities, provides the opportunity to examine, and perhaps challenge, assumptions about the innate goodness of leisure and its impact on health.

Black and White Differences of Leisure Behavior

Various studies have been conducted on Black/White differences in leisure behavior and preferences. For example, Washburne's (1978) seminal work found that Blacks participated in different types of leisure activities than Whites. He found that Blacks preferred sports and fitness-related activities more than Whites. Stamps and Stamps (1985) also compared the leisure preferences of Blacks to Whites. However, they took the examination one step further by looking at the influence of both race and social class on leisure participation. They concluded that race seemed to be more important than class in determining leisure participation and the impact on well-being. Philipp (1995) has looked at the concept of leisure constraints and race and found that Blacks were constrained in various leisure activities because of the lack of comfort and appeal associated with specific activities.

Additionally, Shinew, Floyd, McGuire, and Noe (1995; 1996) examined the association of gender, race, and social class with leisure preferences. This study utilized the multiple hierarchy stratification perspective, which assisted in explaining the findings of varied leisure preferences based on race, gender, and social class. Inasmuch as the leisure, race, and ethnicity literature has provided insights into the leisure habits of European-Americans and African-Americans (Philipp, 1997; Riddick & Stewart, 1994; Shinew et al., 1996; Woodard, 1988), there still remains a paucity of research outlining how all community organizations can collaborate in utilizing leisure to educate our citizens and provide leisure opportunities to promote health for all, even those who have been marginalized. Presently, there are no published studies in the leisure literature that address the emerging and important concept of "learning cities" as a vehicle to promote community learning and foster greater community and societal health. Longworth (1999) offers a basic description of learning cities that implement plans and strategies that function in the following ways: 1) encouraging wealth creation, personal growth, and social cohesion; 2) developing human potential of all citizens; and 3) creating working partnerships of all organizations. This basic description of learning cities underscores key principles regarding leisure activities as well as broader conceptions of health, education, lifelong learning and collaboration among all citizens.

There have been scholars and practitioners who have made attempts at strong collaborations between community organizations in an effort to improve leisure service access with the goal of creating healthy parks and healthy people. For example, Dustin, McKenney, Hibbler, and Blitzer (2004) advocate for the collaboration between public schools and park and recreation professionals, which is at the core of the learning cities description and idea. The authors suggested that park and recreation professionals be added to the staff (or faculty) of public schools to aid in the education of public school children. This idea may expand across an entire citizenry based on their proposal related to several facts that public schools facilities are grossly under-utilized; that most of life takes place outside the classroom; that park and recreation programs hook and hold attention for educational purposes; that park and recreation professionals have substantial teaching and counseling experience having an understanding about the importance of educating the whole child (or citizen); all of these facts having extensive synergistic possibilities. Dustin et al (2004) have been thinking at the heart of the learning cities concept where all city organizations collaborate to educate all members of the community, which would ultimately impact the overall health of individuals and our society as a whole.

IMPACT OF LEISURE IN HEALTHY COMMUNITIES

When thinking about the impact of leisure, the notional of an overall state of well-being comes into question. Although there is much academic debate over how to define well-being, there tends to be agreement that it is related to overall health and a movement toward life satisfaction. For the purposes of this chapter, well-being is defined as the dynamic process that ensures that people possess a sense of individual vitality; are able to undertake activities that are meaningful, are engaging, and are making them feel competent and autonomous. Moreover, people have a stock of resources to help them become resilient to change circumstances not within their immediate control (New Economic Foundation, 2012).

Social network theory provides a context to understand that individuals who have positive links and ties to others within our society tend to acquire higher levels of well-being and are overall more successful in modern life. This is primarily due to the multitude of resources available to them through their social networks. Also, it suggests that individuals with high levels of well-being and life satisfaction are in a position to contribute more positively to their community and make the world a better place for others to live (Russell, 1996). It is also worth noting social network theory, as a variant of network theory, is also linked to institutional theory. Almost all of the major perspectives in organizational theory, such as resource dependency and institutional theory, have incorporated or independently invented key elements of network theory (Borgatti, 2005).

HEALTHY EXAMPLES OF YOUTH DEVELOPMENT AND CRIME PREVENTION

Violence and obesity are also serious issues in the realm of leisure programming. During the 1990s, the National Recreation and Parks Association launched a "Benefits Are Endless" campaign to demonstrate the importance of parks and recreation to individuals, community, and to our environment. The campaign was also an attempt to reposition parks and recreation to a safe, and more significant, level in the minds and hearts of U.S. citizens. The research that resulted from the benefits movement demonstrated that parks, recreation and leisure services play a significant role in personal development (e.g., physical, emotional, intellectual and spiritual). It was also demonstrated that parks and recreation efforts made a community a more attractive place to live by acting as a catalyst for business and employment opportunities. Adding parks made neighborhoods even more desirable to live.

Leisure services have been successful at not only enriching the culture of the community such as providing arts programming, but also it has been successful at improving intercultural and intergenerational relations, which has decreased tensions among various groups. For the purposes of advancing the importance of leisure in the discussion of healthy communities, especially related to learning cities and metropolitan areas, there are a few examples within youth and crime prevention. These include "Play for Peace," "Midnight Basketball," and "Academic Cultural Enrichment."

Play for Peace

Play for Peace is a nonprofit organization that promotes peace, nonviolence, and fosters young leaders through children's play. The program, which receives funding from the U.S. Department of Education and the United Nations, has sites in areas where cross-cultural tensions are common: United States, Guatemala, India, Northern Ireland, South Africa, and the Middle East. With over 1.5 million children having participated so far, Play for Peace is open to children and youth from different cultural backgrounds who work together to create their own play activities. There is only one rule: Every activity is nonviolent and noncompetitive.

Midnight Basketball

Midnight basketball was a 1990s initiative to curb inner-city crime in the United States by keeping urban youth off the streets and engaging them with alternatives to drugs and crime. G. Van Standifer originally founded it in the late 1980s in the United States. Youth were provided with a safe haven to the inner city streets to play basketball after hours. However, basketball was only the marketing hook and promotion. Young people were offered opportunities to receive counseling, education and job training, addiction services, and even tattoo removal in an effort to disassociate them from gang affiliation. Empirically, a 2006 study of the 1990-1994 period during which rates of most crimes in the United States peaked, and when urban midnight basketball programs were first initiated as a crime-prevention strategy, found that—while confounding factors were likely involved—property crime rates fell more rapidly in cities that were early adopters of the original midnight basketball model than in other American cities during that same period.

Academic Cultural Enrichment

In 2000, the Champaign Park District in Illinois sponsored a program called the Academic Cultural Enrichment (ACE) Mentorship Program. It was an after-school program designed to meet the specific needs of African American youth. The program provides students with the competencies and skills needed to be involved, resilient, and successful. The ACE program sought to foster positive Black identities in the participants, and develop strong math, reading, oratorical, and analytical thinking skills. The program has a strong African cultural component, as well as academic and recreation components. Three research questions guided the program's evaluation project: 1) Are the program goals being achieved; 2) Do the parents and leaders perceive a positive change in the participant's behaviors and attitudes as a result of their participation in the program; and 3) What are the salient program aspects of the ACE Mentorship Program.

Program evaluation took place over a two-year period. Pretest and posttest survey data were collected from the participants for two consecutive years. At the end of the second year, interviews were conducted with leaders, parents, and participants. Additionally, the participants' academic grades were also examined. The information collected from the surveys indicated that the pretest and posttest scores on the Protective Factors Scale and Harter's Self-Perception Scale were not significantly different. The academic grades did indicate positive changes for most of the participants. Further, the information received from the interviews with the parents, leaders, and participants consistently indicated that the program is meeting its goals and is having a positive impact on the children. The salient program elements that seemingly contribute to the positive outcomes include effective and consistent leadership, parental involvement, and innovative programming.

The key point to remember is that the impact of leisure in changing communities involve personal, professional, and social development, as well as social networks, families, and communities. Existing programs can be further enhanced by taking on the consideration of leisure for healthy communities, and more importantly, the concept of learning cities.

ENVIRONMENTS OF HEALTH THROUGH PARKS

Public health, as a discipline, is taught as a flow chart of environmental issues that impact whole communities, which in turn differentially condition people for better or worse health statuses. Public open spaces, such as parks and green spaces, appear to be a key built environmental setting that provide opportunities for a variety of physical activity behaviors, such as recreational walking and playing sports (Koohsari et al., 2015; Bedimo-Rung et al., 2005; Kaczynski & Henderson, 2007). Given the limited success of individually-based approaches to behavior change, public health researchers have increasingly used socio-ecological models to further understand determinants of physical activity (Sallis et al., 2008). Within active living research, public open space is mainly conceptualized as park and greenspace, with less focus on other types of public open space (e.g., public plazas, nature reserves, and greenways). Building health environments can include park facilities and services through offering various opportunities to fulfill individual, social, economic, and environmental benefits (Bedimo-Rung, 2005).

This section details a few of the key components that tie health, leisure, and education. It first describes the community level characteristics of parts from a public health perspective. Next it layers a quality of life perspective on the availability of parks in communities. Lastly, it invites a broader discussion on how professionals collaborate to solve urban health and built environment issues preventing an interdisciplinary approach at increasing community health.

COMMUNITY CHARACTERISTICS OF PARKS

Focusing on parks over the past decade, researchers have paid a considerable amount of time establishing a link between park characteristics specifically related to community impact, obesity factors, and healthy living. Even as the health professions and design professions diverged, the built environment remains a key determinant of health (Jackson et al., 2013). It is no coincidence that in 1872 the seven founders of the American Public Health Association, now one of the most prominent associations for public health professions, included both an architect and a housing specialist (Jackson et al., 2013). Now described as biophilic designing, a growing body of research points to the health benefits of parks, green space, and other forms of nature contact for communities (Louv, 2008).

Public health often takes on the responsibility to address societal, environmental, and social initiatives around health. In an organizational set, identifying levels of engagement is an important concept to understand the impact of public health and its role for communities. Theoretically, the development of locally adjusted solutions that are also beneficial to the environment is therefore also dependent on the inclusion of environmental interests and the incorporation of environmentally relevant lay knowledge as discussed above (Drazkiewicz et al., 2015). For example, Checker's (2011) analysis of park development in Harlem found that efforts to address environmental justice issues linked to park availability had stalled because residents recognized that park development was primarily a strategy for real estate development and gentrification (D'Haee et al., 2015). Also, the theoretical perspectives of ecological models emphasize the fact that a person's behavior is not only affected by individual characteristics, but also by the environment in which he or she lives (Sallis et al., 2008).

To promote community engagement, public health practitioners rely upon the built environment to provide activity-based solutions for active/lifestyle issues. Arguably, the success of participation measured in environmental terms depends on various aspects of the wider context within which processes are situated and, importantly, on characteristics of participatory processes themselves, such as inclusion and influence of different interest groups (Drazkiewicz et al., 2015). For example, neighborhood physical resources, environmental threats and collective efficacy associated with children's general health status are mediated by family functioning (Fan & Chen, 2012; Christian et al., 2015).

QUALITY OF LIFE AND PARK ACCESS OF USE

Public health researchers often argue that quality of life is directly related to park access and use. Parks often serve as sites of physical activity, which is associated with enhanced health and reduced risk for all-cause mortality and many chronic diseases (Wolch et al., 2014). Combating obesity, reviews of the correlates of children's physical activity and outdoor play indicate that built environment features such as walk/bicycle paths, presence of cul-de-sac roads, access to parks, recreational facilities, and other local destinations or public transport are positively associated with children's physical activity, while high traffic exposure and crime are negatively associated (Christian et al., 2015). Mounting evidence is available to support a positive association between young children's outdoor play and physical activity and the presence of safe and green neighborhood places to be active (Christian et al., 2015). For example, living near (within 1 kilometer from home) recreation spaces was associated with walking in 5–8 year olds (Frank et al., 2007; Kerr et al., 2007).

Contrastingly, access and use are not always directly related. Researchers argue that parks also have reputations reflecting their use, repute, upkeep, and design quality (Byrne, Wolch, & Zhang, 2009). Furthermore, within cities, green space is not always equitably distributed and access is often highly stratified based on income, ethno-racial characteristics, age, gender, (dis)ability, and other axes of difference (Byrne, Wolch, & Zhang, 2009; McConnachie & Shackleton, 2010). While parks differ in terms of size, quality, range of facilities, availability of organized recreation, or perceptions of safety among actual or potential users, they are designed to serve diverse communities and wide-ranging recreational needs.

Thinking Outside the Box

In promotion of healthy parks, healthy communities, education, and urban planning, public health experts will need to think outside the box for solutions. The best solutions for leading to healthy communities will emerge from the learning cities framework that designates areas a continuing education structures. Many of the concerns about residential or commercial zonings have been the result of limited policies not viewing those same areas as larger zones for learning and continuing education, which contribute to the health of communities. It still remains challenging to develop specific policies and guidelines to (re) design these areas to support such learning and physical activity (Koohsari et al., 2015). This is mainly because there is a lack of prescriptive evidence for urban designers and policy makers for optimal amounts (also known as thresholds) of specific public open space attributes (such as attractiveness or proximity) needed to influence physical activity (Koohsari et al., 2013; Sugiyama et al., 2012).

Advancing health in environments is a challenge for learning cities. Those that are able to leverage the synergy between professions will fare better than those with limited cohesion. Institutional theory as an explanatory factor for why we see certain interventions lends itself to this discussion. In this chapter, the argument has been complementing an ecological modeling of behavioral health with a rationalization of how organizations within learning cities decide on the best infrastructure. Furthermore, when addressing complex issues such as violence and obesity, health care organizations are a reasonable example to elucidate environmental obstacles facing communities and individuals. Here, the benefits of preventing violence are multiplied because violence prevention generates a ripple effect and a slew of positive health outcomes (Davies, 2012). The downstream impact on health status and economic savings has the potential to be monumental.

The imperative to address such environmental injustices and related public health disparities, as well as enhance urban ecologies, has led planners to focus on both traditional parkland acquisition programs and innovative strategies for expanding green space resources (Wolch et al., 2014). In addition, community-based organizations, often aided by environmental groups, are refocusing urban brownfield remediation projects on urban green space to address public health and environmental justice concerns (Barnett, 2001). The public health community has reached across sectors to establish relationships with other professionals who are directly involved in decisions about the design of the built environment, and major national conferences in public health, planning, transportation, smart growth, parks and recreation, and related fields now routinely have included sessions on health and built environment issues (Jackson et al., 2013).

CONTINUING EDUCATION: COMMUNITIES OF LIFELONG LEARNING

What makes discussions about advancing healthy communities so inviting is that it reintroduces individuals to considering how their environment can be conducive to their own well-being. This requires a level of learning and engagement where the structures of education can support communities, but never dominate them. Current traditional higher education has dominated the opportunities of learning that exists beyond the structures of education. The underlying connection of the built environment contributing to the health, well-being, and overall quality of life for all people cannot be overstated. This discussion promotes parks in their broadest sense, serving communities with societal benefits and opportunities. It is also important to emphasize that there are different views and experiences among all people in society related to the essential conditions for positive and sustainable health outcomes.

Parks, again as an example, set in isolation from the context of family, community, even a city of individuals, may send a blind message: Simply that parks, and the discussion of park visits, activities, or innovations toward healthcare, are one-size-fits-all. The more insightful message embraces the diversities and complexities that parks must address in servicing healthy communities. But before the health impact of parks can reach its full potential, there must be some consideration given to the continual education and learning of citizens in the community: Those diverse individuals, who the parks are intended to serve. Given the matters of diversity related to gender, age, race, religion, sexual orientation, and other considered identities, such as social class, educational level, even health disparity, parks must consider how communities learn together and share diverse experiences of living. This section will focus on the concept of lifelong learning as a mechanism for communities to integrate leisure activities, the built environment, and educational practices to advance healthy communities. First, community education is outlined to provide a basis for discussion. And second, the impact of education on lifelong learning are highlighted to bridge the notion of increasing community drivers in the face of community burdens.

Community Education

The support of lifelong learning as a way to advance environments in healthy communities would bring about a *community education* that advances a multifaceted agenda, ranging from educational development and health quality to collective action and social justice (Jarvis, 2004). Community education is multifaceted partly due to the multiple definitions of community. Most scholars mention the work of Tönnies in comparing *community* versus *society* (Jarvis, 2004). In essence, *community* is an intimate and closer form of human relation than *society* (Hunt, 2005). The sense of community is further highlighted through the term commerce, which features the process of communication and exchange among individuals.

Moreover, when community modifies the term education, the meanings vary worldwide. In the U.S., community education is usually reserved to public schools. Others mention community-based learning occurring in libraries, churches, and community centers. However, the importance of community education in the context of our parks' discussion is in its collective focus to bring about solidarity and collective action. As Clark (1987) adds, "The primary aim of community education is to enable the members of any collective to become increasingly ecumenical and autonomous…a total process enabling individual and society to become more fully human (p. 62)."

It is the notion of becoming fully human, which drives the importance of considering community education and lifelong learning for our overall quality of life. Placing education and learning in a broader context of society, has led to a consideration of another concept we have reflected as "learning cities." Here, learning cities are rebuilt based on supporting lifelong learning and community education for all its citizens (Scott, 2015). Such a reconstruction will require the role of leisure in humanizing learning cities, socializing common experiences (Hibbler & Scott, 2015), and constructing the health and educational frameworks for infrastructure and organizational policies (Howard et al., 2015). Ultimately, learning cities would provide us the humanity, community, and policy for developing supportive structures, such as parks and recreation areas in nurturing our overall quality of life, health, and community education.

The potential for parks to play a role in community education and lifelong learning brings to life the newer idea of learning cities. Arguably, learning cities could be the 21st century version that traces back to the century-old land-grant idea and its institutions dedicated to provide land and resources for their citizens. The institution of land-grant colleges was an experiment in higher education in the U.S., but the individual states decided upon their respective establishments. As a result, various official establishment years of land-grant colleges existed according to the First Morrill Land-Grant Act of 1862. These land-grant colleges were presumably open to the public, becoming less prestigious than their older counterpart colleges that offered education for a privileged few (McDowell, 2001; Williams, 1991). The faculty of traditional education taught liberal arts and classics, while the land-grant colleges required an industrial new education acting as the national schools of science in agriculture, mechanics, and polytechnics. The key point has been that the original establishment of land-grant colleges has remained an experiment in transition, reinforced by the Hatch Act of 1887; the Second Morrill Act of 1890, and Equity in Educational Land-Grant Status Act of 1994 (McDowell, 2001).

The importance of land-grant institutions in this chapter is that they serve as a forerunner for the future of learning cities that expands education and learning to the public community. What is also important to note is that the land-grant idea and its institutions have been instrumental in promoting engaged scholarship through the trifold mission of teaching, research, and service: Now a hallmark of American higher education.

The practice of transforming urban space into urban greenspace, within the context of learning cities, takes on diverse concerns of communities. Still there remains a need to consider the social, political, even educational concerns for serving the good of humanity and community. For example, a significant organization that signaled an important movement in community education is the Highlander Folk School (1932-1961), which Myles Horton founded that served people struggling for social and economic justice (Stubblefield & Keane, 1994). Horton and Highlander represented a nontraditional view of education and social analysis to understand societal power in order to change it (Peters & Bell, 2001). The Highlander School and its social-educational activities developed into a radical institution and environment attracting a wide variety of visitors, writers, ministers, musicians, labor and political leaders, students, educators, government officials, and social reformers (Horton, 1989). The work of Horton and Highlander, as highlighted by the civil rights movement, was "toward a 'complete' democracy in all sectors of society; economic, political, industrial, and family" (Peters & Bell, 2001). Addressing the build environment as a way to increase the health and well-being for individuals will undoubtedly have to address the power that confronts these ambitions. Using environments to advance healthy communities must empower individuals, through community education and lifelong learning, to collectively act to bring about sustainable social justice and change.

Literacy Impact of Lifelong Education

The major lessons from such nontraditional sources of education and learning feature the expansive opportunity of the build environment to supporting collective and cooperative action. Educational organizations, must not only develop individuals, but also change communities to address the literacy power and problems that lie within them. Also, such organizations must collaborate with every sector of society to support a diversity of concerns such as health disparities. Developing initiatives in these ways would advance the notion of learning cities that allow people to work together toward a comprehensive democracy, where all voices are welcomed, heard, and appreciated.

In adopting a broader view of community education, it seems vital to remember the seminal writings of early 20th century thinker, Basil Yeaxlee and his thoughts about lifelong education and learning. Yeaxlee introduced learning and education as a lifelong enterprise (from cradle to the grave), integrating learning across work, leisure, and community (Cross-Durrant, 2001). Now almost every OECD country, from South Korea to Canada, makes reference to lifelong learning and the knowledge society in its education policies and its concepts now constitutes a meta-discourse in policy terms (Green, 2002). In wide agreement, lifelong learning promotes a transformation of education that fully develops individuals for perpetual growth, harmony, and the "wholeness" of humanity (Cross-Durrant, 2001).

More recently, lifelong learning has been further advanced referring to both individual and institutional forms of learning (Jarvis, 2004). Individual in that lifelong learning occurs throughout a person's entire lifespan, while institutional where lifelong learning occurs in formal educational settings. This explains how it involves formal, non-formal, and informal learning situations (Jarvis, 2004; Livingston, 2002). Compared with the strands of lifelong education, resemblances occur where informal learning situations are connected to expressions of community education, and non-formal learning situations are connect to expressions of continuing education. However, formal learning, which usually refers to institutional schooling, does not resemble expressions of recurrent education. In fact, formal learning has often ignored the intent to provide education as a public good for all (Chapman & Aspin, 1997; Jarvis, 2004).

Many would agree that any phrase claiming "lifelong learning for all" involves an individual and private expression of learning coupled with an institutional and public application of education. In this way, learning and education are distinct properties that are combined to form a new meaning for lifelong learning: A meaning that engulfs past differences into future roles and responsibilities; aims and aspirations; performances and outcomes for a larger learning-knowledge society (Yorks & Scott, 2013). Because lifelong learning is both private and public, it must extend itself within the context of economic and social change (Chapman & Aspin, 1997). The most pressing issue in the current century involves work and employment in a knowledge economy (Chapman & Aspin, 1997; Livingston, 2002).

In current times, it would be a similar mistake to view education only for the sake of attaining employment or for the sake of acquiring social skills. These are equally essential, but still overlook the importance of developing ones' community and collective society. The significance of including health and health services into the discussion of worldwide systems, bring about new ways of viewing education. These new ways would view parks, as nontraditional systems of continuing education, for the sake of understanding health and healthy communities. One major distinction about parks, although it may not offer accredited courses or guaranteed paying jobs, is that parks do offer the spaces for reinventing and prioritizing important needs. For what good is it to acquire a degree, if the knowledge obtained have not improved real lives; how long can we really work effectively, if our health undermines that work, jobs, and employment? The overall health that we are considering is not only individual, but also social; and the ultimate life we are promoting continues at every stage, lasting across generations.

Community education, lifelong education, or lifelong learning are different terms, but with similar meaning in its role for improving individuals' health, life, and well-being. However, it is important to note that lifelong learning is interpreted and practiced differently across areas of the United States, North America, and Europe in addition to South American, African, Australian, and Asian countries. These different interpretations will influence how lifelong learning policies are introduced and how learning cities will be advanced in respective communities. Yet, an overall common theme could describe lifelong learning that occurs throughout an entire lifetime, "from the cradle to the grave." It could address the distinctions regarding where this learning-for-a-lifetime may take place, which would bring about the meaning of learning in its relation to education, and other associated expressions such as community, continuing, and lifelong education. For the purposes here, we express lifelong learning in its broadest view that aligns with many nontraditional systems of continuing education, namely parks, or fundamental policies, specifically revisiting legislation of the Lifelong Learning Act, which further describes the societal impact and practice of learning cities in America (Scott, 2015).

DISCUSSION OF LIFELONG LEARNING, LEARNING CITIES, AND HEALTHY COMMUNITIES

Adopting a more comprehensive view of education and learning, from the start, resolves ongoing philosophical debates that span several decades (Jarvis, 2004). For instance, learning has been often attached to its immediate and practical activities, the acts of doing and achieving a list of goals and objectives. Likewise, education has been associated with its formal systems and structures insofar as producing and rewarding credentials and degrees, not for the purpose of improving the health and quality of life of human beings. In other words, education and learning have often been overlooked in considering the overall health of our society. The role of parks as educational structures can change the way education is viewed, such that the phrase, learning cities could become a common expression shared by all. Key expressions to underscore this renewed language of education and learning relating to healthy parks and people include "the giving of self in service" and individuals being "in perpetual living relationship to the whole." Both expressions describe education and learning as a continual process of connecting individuals to helping the entire community. In this way, lifelong learning takes on a greater purpose for everyone without exception, in the overall health, life, and learning-for-all.

Thinking about lifelong learning, as an all-inclusive education, may mistakenly suggest a distinction among individuals in our community, between adults and children, or different persons and their reasons for knowledge and skills. For some, it may be lifelong learning to work for everyone in a health community. For others, it must remain an all-inclusive concept that respects individual differences, yet remain a concept that does not divide others by their differences. By promoting learning cities, social unity is being argued for through the practice of lifelong learning. Within nontraditional continuing education structures, learning occurs outside of schools, colleges, and universities; in healthy communities, interaction among individuals takes place for other reasons than work, especially for reasons of recreational leisure, public health, and lifelong learning.

Augmented by meanings of community education and lifelong education, lifelong learning serves as another point into describing learning cities and the diverse individuals within communities. Exploring the wonderfully inexhaustible realms of collective knowledge signals the continuing process of inquiry and discovery that defines lifelong learning. Learning cities would allow lifelong learning to be cultivated, where humans can learn, personally and collectively, to live healthy lives and share spaces for continual development.

Just as land-grant institutions advanced the trifold mission of teaching, research, and service, Chapman and Aspin (1997) describe lifelong learning for three central elements: 1) economic progress; 2) personal development and fulfillment; and 3) social inclusiveness and democratic understanding. Economic progress has been closely associated with jobs and employment. Simply, earning a living wage has been an issue that cuts across social concerns of poverty and lower-economic classes. Personal development underscores the role of individuals to pursue their happiness and to take care of their personal health through actions, such as exercise, recreation, and nutrition. Social inclusiveness takes on a collective purpose that seeks compromise among individuals and reaches self-governing, democratic solutions for honoring humanity. Lifelong learning, in respect to these central elements, involves the responsibility of everyone to continually change by learning from one another. We continually learn through telling our experiences, revealing our issues, and sharing our solutions to common problems.

The synergy required in developing healthy communities point towards the need for implementing the elements of lifelong learning. We believe that the most productive steps involve the further inclusion of social leisure, public health, and continuing education structures. Such inclusion are the components of healthy parks, healthy communities, and ultimately, learning cities. In short, learning cities brings about a culture of collaboration required for addressing the importance of healthy and healthful communities. The slight distinction between *healthy* and *healthful* is the difference between showing good signs *of health* versus having what is beneficial *to health.* Adding parks show good signs of health in a community, and also applying lifelong learning is beneficial to this health, which becomes apparent in the implementation of learning cities.

FUTURE ARRIVAL OF LEARNING CITIES FOR HEALTHY PARKS

In our view, the future arrival of learning cities describes the support of government, organizations, and institutions in the collective development of education and learning. Thus, the challenge for any definition and description of lifelong learning, especially in regards to others, is how individuals continue to develop their quality of health, life, and well-being. The answer to this question may lie in rethinking lifelong learning and the implementation of parks and recreation areas within a learning cities framework. Since many historical accounts of education have been associated with individuals' preferences, parks are challenged to shift individuals' mindsets to think of a larger collective purpose, such as a healthy society. We contend that lifelong learning can support such an assessment. Supporters of lifelong learning must begin to notice its universal and absolute properties for the collective development in our freedom of expressions, which are in accordance to our community and humanity.

As a result, it would be paramount to consider implementing concepts of lifelong learning and learning cities within parks and communities. In our view, advancing learning cities is the most viable option. In the context of learning cities, education is expanded and learning would continuously happen at every stage of life. Both children and adults, whether across classrooms, parks, or cities would educate, learn, and interact together. The most immediate opportunity that parks and recreation administrators can promote is the need for individuals to continue learning throughout their lives from sharing experiences of different social identities, diverse cultures, and distinct challenges. The role of parks, recreation, and leisure, in partnership with other continuing education structures, will help contribute to lifelong learning on a broader scale. Such potential community collaboration reveals what is essential about learning cities, that they bring populations together through the synergy, health and well-being of a fully-diverse society.

REFERENCES

Baker, B. D. (2014). *America's most financially disadvantaged school districts and how they got that way: How state and local governance causes school funding disparities*. Washington, DC: Center for American Progress.

Barnett, H. (2001). The Chinatown cornfields: Including environmental benefits in environmental justice struggles. *Critical Planning*, *8*, 50–60.

Bedimo-Rung, A. L., Mowen, A. J., & Cohen, D. A. (2005). The significance of parks to physical activity and public health: A conceptual model. *American Journal of Preventive Medicine*, *28*(2), 159–168. doi:10.1016/j.amepre.2004.10.024 PMID:15694524

Bennett, G. G., McNeill, L. H., Wolin, K. Y., Duncan, D. T., Puleo, E., & Emmons, K. M. (2007). Safe to walk? Neighborhood safety and physical activity among public housing residents. *PLoS Medicine*, *4*(10), 1599–1607. doi:10.1371/journal.pmed.0040306 PMID:17958465

Borgatti, S. P. (2005). *The state of organizational social network research today* [Working paper]. Boston, MA: Department of Organization Studies, Boston College.

Boynton-Jarrett, R., Fargnoli, J., Suglia, S. F., Zuckerman, B., & Wright, R. J. (2010). Association between maternal intimate partner violence and incident obesity in preschool-aged children: Results from the fragile families and child well-being study. *Archives of Pediatrics & Adolescent Medicine*, *164*(6), 540–546. doi:10.1001/archpediatrics.2010.94 PMID:20530304

Burdette, H. L., Wadden, T. A., & Whitaker, R. C. (2006). Neighborhood safety, collective efficacy, and obesity in women with young children. *Obesity (Silver Spring, Md.)*, *14*(3), 518–525. doi:10.1038/oby.2006.67 PMID:16648624

Byrne, J., Wolch, J., & Zhang, J. (2009). Planning for environmental justice in an urban national park. *Journal of Environmental Planning and Management*, *52*(3), 365–392. doi:10.1080/09640560802703256

Caldwell, L., & Smith, E. (2007). Leisure as a context for youth development and delinquency prevention. In *Pathways and Crime Prevention* (pp. 271-296).

Chapman, J. D., & Aspin, D. N. (1997). *The school, the community, and lifelong learning*. London, UK: Cassell.

Checker, M. (2011). Wiped out by the Greenwave: Environmental gentrification and the paradoxical politics of urban sustainability. *City and Society*, *23*(2), 210–229. doi:10.1111/j.1548-744X.2011.01063.x

Christian, H., Zubrick, S. R., Foster, S., Giles-Corti, B., Bull, F., Wood, L., & Boruff, B. et al. (2015). The influence of the neighborhood physical environment on early child health and development: A review and call for research. *Health & Place*, *33*, 25–36. doi:10.1016/j.healthplace.2015.01.005 PMID:25744220

Clark, D. (1987). The concept of community education. In A. Garth, J. Bastiani, I. Martin, & K. Richards (Eds.), *Community education: An agenda for educational reform*. Philadelphia, PA: Open University Press.

Cross-Durrant, A. (2001). Basil Yeaxlee and the origins of lifelong education. In P. Jarvis (Ed.), *Twentieth century thinkers in adult education* (pp. 31–48). London, UK: Croom Helm.

Curtis, J. E. (1979). *Recreation: Theory and practice*. St. Louis, MO: Mosby.

D'Haee, S., De Meester, F., Cardon, G., De Bourdeaudhuij, I., Deforche, B., & Van Dyck, D. (2015). Changes in the perceived neighborhood environment in relation to changes in physical activity: A longitudinal study from childhood into adolescence. *Health & Place*, *33*, 132–141. doi:10.1016/j.healthplace.2015.03.004 PMID:25840351

Dacin, M. T., Goodstein, J., & Scott, W. R. (2002). Institutional theory and institutional change: Introduction to the special research forum. *Academy of Management Journal*, *45*(1), 45–56. doi:10.5465/AMJ.2002.6283388

Davies, R. A. (2012). The value of prevention. In *IOM (Institute of Medicine) & NRC (National Research Council), Social and economic costs of violence: Workshop summary*. Washington, DC: The National Academies Press.

Drazkiewicz, A., Challies, E., & Newig, J. (2015). Public participation and local environmental planning: Testing factors influencing decision quality and implementation in four case studies from Germany. *Land Use Policy*, *46*, 211–222. doi:10.1016/j.landusepol.2015.02.010

Dustin, D., Mckenney, A., Hibbler, D., & Blitzer, L. (2004). Thinking outside the box: Placing park and recreation professionals in K-12 schools. *Journal of Physical Education, Recreation & Dance*, *75*(1), 51–54. doi:10.1080/07303084.2004.10608542

Fan, Y., & Chen, Q. (2012). Family functioning as a mediator between neighborhood conditions and children's health: Evidence from a national survey in the United States. *Social Science & Medicine*, *74*(12), 1939–1947. doi:10.1016/j.socscimed.2012.01.039 PMID:22465381

Frank, L., Kerr, J., Chapman, J., & Sallis, J. (2007). Urban form relationships with walk trip frequency and distance among youth. *American Journal of Health Promotion*, *21*(4), 305–311. doi:10.4278/0890-1171-21.4s.305 PMID:17465175

Germain, C. B. (1991). *Human behavior in the social environment: An ecological view*. New York, NY: Columbia University Press.

Green, A. (2002). The many faces of lifelong learning: Recent education policy trends in Europe. *Journal of Education Policy*, *17*(6), 611–626. doi:10.1080/0268093022000032274

Hibbler, D. K., & Scott, L. (2015). Role of leisure in humanizing learning cities. In L. Scott (Ed.), *Learning cities for adult learners* (pp. 73–82). San Francisco, CA: Jossey-Bass. doi:10.1002/ace.20124

Hogan, P., Dall, T., & Nikolov, P. (2003). Economic costs of diabetes in the US in 2002. *Diabetes Care*, *26*(3), 917–932. doi:10.2337/diacare.26.3.917 PMID:12610059

Horton, A. I. (1989). *The Highlander folk school: A history of its major programs, 1932-1961*. New York, NY: Carlson Publishing.

Howard, J., Howard, D., & Dotson, E. (2015). A connected history of health and education: Learning together toward a better city. In L. Scott (Ed.), *Learning cities for adult learners* (pp. 57–72). San Francisco, CA: Jossey-Bass. doi:10.1002/ace.20123

Huang, E. S., Basu, A., O'Grady, M., & Capretta, J. C. (2009). Projecting the future diabetes population: Size and related costs for the U.S. *Diabetes Care*, *32*(12), 2225–2229. doi:10.2337/dc09-0459 PMID:19940225

Huesmann, L. R. (2012). The contagion of violence: The extent, the processes, and the outcomes. In *IOM (Institute of Medicine) & NRC (National Research Council), Social and economic costs of violence: Workshop summary*. Washington, DC: The National Academies Press.

Hunt, C. (2005). Community education. In L. English (Ed.), *International encyclopedia of adult education* (pp. 131–136). New York, NY: Palgrave Macmillan.

Institute of Medicine (IOM) & National Research Council. (NRC). (2012). Social and economic costs of violence: Workshop summary. Washington, DC: The National Academies Press.

Iwasaki, Y., & Schneider, I. E. (2003). Leisure, stress, and coping: An evolving area of inquiry. *Leisure Sciences*, *25*(2-3), 107–113. doi:10.1080/01490400306567

Jackson, R. J., Dannenberg, A. L., & Frumkin, H. (2013). Health and the built environment: 10 years after. *American Journal of Public Health*, *103*(9), 1542–1544. doi:10.2105/AJPH.2013.301482 PMID:23865699

Jacobson, S., & Samdahl, D. M. (1998). Leisure in the lives of old lesbians: Experiences with and responses to discrimination. *Journal of Leisure Research*, *30*(2), 233–255.

Jarvis, P. (Ed.). (2001). *Twentieth century thinkers in adult education* (2nd ed.). London, UK: Croom Helm.

Jarvis, P. (2004). *Adult education and lifelong learning: Theory and practice* (3rd ed.). New York, NY: RoutledgeFalmer.

Kaczynski, A. T., & Henderson, K. A. (2007). Environmental correlates of physical activity: A review of evidence about parks and recreation. *Leisure Sciences*, *29*(4), 315–354. doi:10.1080/01490400701394865

Kelly, J. R., & Godbey, G. (1992). *The sociology of leisure*. State College, PA: Venture.

Kendall-Tackett, K., & Marshall, R. (1999). Victimization and diabetes: An exploratory study. *Child Abuse & Neglect*, *23*(6), 593–596. doi:10.1016/S0145-2134(99)00033-2 PMID:10391516

Kerr, J., Frank, L., Sallis, J., & Chapman, J. (2007). Urban form correlates of pedestrian travel in youth: Differences by gender, race-ethnicity and household attributes. *Transportation Research Part D, Transport and Environment*, *12*(3), 177–182. doi:10.1016/j.trd.2007.01.006

Koohsari, M. J., Badland, H., & Giles-Corti, B. (2013). (Re) Designing the built environment to support physical activity: Bringing public health back into urban design and planning. *Cities (London, England)*, *35*, 294–298. doi:10.1016/j.cities.2013.07.001

Koohsari, M. J., Mavoa, S., Villianueva, K., Sugiyama, T., Badland, H., Kaczynski, A. T., & Giles-Corti, B. (2015). Public open space, physical activity, urban design and public health: Concepts, methods and research agenda. *Health & Place*, *33*, 75–82. doi:10.1016/j.healthplace.2015.02.009 PMID:25779691

Livingston, D. W. (2002). Lifelong learning and underemployment in the knowledge society: A North American perspective. In R. Edwards, N. Miller, N. Small, & A. Tait (Eds.), *Supporting lifelong learning* (Vol. 3, pp. 50–75). New York, NY: RoutledgeFalmer.

Longworth, N. (1999). *Making lifelong work: Learning cities for a learning century*. Sterling, VA: Kogan Page.

Louv, R. (2008). *Last child in the woods: Saving our children from nature-deficit disorder*. Chapel Hill, NC: Algonquin Books.

Lumeng, J., Appugliese, D., Cabral, H. J., Bradley, R. H., & Zuckerman, B. (2006). Neighborhood safety and overweight status in children. *Archives of Pediatrics & Adolescent Medicine*, *160*(1), 25–31. doi:10.1001/archpedi.160.1.25 PMID:16389207

Maas, J., Verheij, R. A., Groenewegen, P. P., De Vries, S., & Spreeuwenberg, P. (2006). Green space, urbanity, and health: How strong is the relation? *Journal of Epidemiology and Community Health*, *60*(7), 587–592. doi:10.1136/jech.2005.043125 PMID:16790830

McConnachie, M. M., & Shackleton, C. M. (2010). Public green space inequality in small towns in South Africa. *Habitat International*, *34*(2), 244–248. doi:10.1016/j.habitatint.2009.09.009

McDowell, G. R. (2001). *Land grant universities and extension into the 21st Century: Renegotiating or abandoning a social contract*. Hoboken, NJ: Wiley-Blackwell.

New Economic Foundation. (2012, November). *Well being patterns uncovered* [Report]. London, UK: New Economic Foundation.

Peters, J. M., & Bell, B. (2001). Horton of Highlander. In P. Jarvis (Ed.), *Twentieth century thinkers in adult education* (pp. 242–257). New York, NY: Croom Helm. doi:10.3998/mpub.16549

Philipp, S. F. (1995). Race and leisure constraints. *Leisure Sciences*, *17*(2), 109–120. doi:10.1080/01490409509513247

Philipp, S. F. (1997). Race, gender, and leisure benefits. *Leisure Sciences*, *19*(3), 191–207. doi:10.1080/01490409709512249

Plichta, S. B. (2004). Intimate partner violence and physical health consequences: Policy and practice implications. *Journal of Interpersonal Violence*, *19*(11), 1296–1323. doi:10.1177/0886260504269685 PMID:15534333

Ponde, P. M., & Santana, S. V. (2000). Participation in leisure activities: Is it a protective factor for women's mental health? *Journal of Leisure Research*, *32*(4), 457–472.

Prevention Institute. (2007). *The California Endowment: Reducing health care costs through prevention*. Oakland, CA: The Prevention Institute.

Prevention Institute. (2010). *Addressing the intersection: Preventing violence and promoting healthy eating and active living*. Oakland, CA: The Prevention Institute.

Prevention Institute. (2011). *Unity fact sheet: Violence and chronic illness*. Retrieved from www.preventioninstitute.org/unity

Riddick, C. C., & Stewart, D. G. (1994). An examination of the life satisfaction and importance of older female retirees: A comparison of blacks to whites. *Journal of Leisure Research*, *26*(1), 75–87.

Robertson, B. J. (1994). An investigation of leisure in the lives of adolescents who engage in delinquent behavior for fun, thrills, and excitement. *Dissertation Abstracts International. A, The Humanities and Social Sciences*, *54*(12-A), 4587.

Robertson, B. J. (1999). Leisure and family: Perspectives of male adolescents who engage in delinquent activity as leisure. *Journal of Leisure Research*, *31*(4), 335.

Rohrer, J. E., Arif, A. A., Pierce, J. R. Jr, & Blackburn, C. (2004). Unsafe neighborhoods, social group activity, and self-rated health. *Journal of Public Health Management and Practice*, *10*(2), 124–129. doi:10.1097/00124784-200403000-00006 PMID:14967979

Russell, R. (1996). *Pastimes: The context of contemporary Leisure*. Madison, WI: Brown & Benchmark.

Sallis, J. F., Cervero, R. B., Ascher, W., Henderson, K. A., Kraft, M. K., & Kerr, J. (2006). An ecological approach to creating active living communities. *Annual Review of Public Health*, *27*(1), 297–322. doi:10.1146/annurev.publhealth.27.021405.102100 PMID:16533119

Sallis, J. F., Owen, N., & Fisher, E. B. (2008). Ecological models of health behavior. *Health behavior and health education: Theory, research, and practice, 4*, 465-486.

Scott, L. (Ed.). (2015). *Learning cities for adult learners. New Directions for Adult and Continuing Education, 145*. San Francisco, CA: Jossey-Bass.

Scott, W. R. (2003). *Organizations*. Upper Saddle River, NJ: Prentice Hall Press.

Shaffer, A. (2002). *The persistence of L.A.'s grocery gap: The need for a new food policy and approach to market development*. Los Angeles, CA: Center for Food and Justice, Urban and Environmental Policy Institute.

Shinew, K. J., Floyd, M. F., McGuire, F. A., & Noe, F. P. (1995). Gender, race, and subjective social class and their association with leisure preferences. *Leisure Sciences*, *17*(2), 75–89. doi:10.1080/01490409509513245

Shinew, K. J., Floyd, M. F., McGuire, F. A., & Noe, F. P. (1996). Class polarization and leisure activity preferences of African-Americans: Intragroup comparisons. *Journal of Leisure Research*, *28*(4), 219–232.

Shinew, K. J., & Parry, D. C. (2005). Examining college students' participation in the leisure pursuits of drinking and illegal drug use. *Journal of Leisure Research*, *37*(3), 364.

Shores, K. A., Scott, D., & Floyd, M. F. (2007). Constraints to outdoor recreation: A multiple hierarchy stratification perspective. *Leisure Sciences*, *29*(3), 227–246. doi:10.1080/01490400701257948

Stamps, S. M., & Stamps, M. B. (1985). Race, class and leisure activities of urban residents. *Journal of Leisure Research*, *17*(1), 40–56.

Strang, D., & Macy, M. W. (2001). In search of excellence: Fads, success stories, and adaptive emulation. *American Journal of Sociology*, *107*(1), 147–182. doi:10.1086/323039

Stubblefield, H. W., & Keane, P. (1994). *Adult education in the American experience: From the colonial period to the present*. San Francisco, CA: Jossey-Bass.

Sugiyama, T., Neuhaus, M., Cole, R., Giles-Corti, B., & Owen, N. (2012). *Destination and route attributes associated with adults' walking: a review* [Doctoral dissertation]. American College of Sports Medicine.

Thorpe, K. E., Florence, C. S., & Joski, P. (2004). Which medical conditions account for the rise in health care spending? *Health Affairs*, *23*(5), W437–W445. PMID:15451978

van den Bosch, M. A., Mudu, P., Uscila, V., Barrdahl, M., Kulinkina, A., Staatsen, B., & Egorov, A. I. (2015). Development of an urban green space indicator and the public health rationale. *Scandinavian Journal of Public Health*.

Washburne, R. F. (1978). Black under-participation in wildland recreation: Alternative explanations. *Leisure Sciences*, *1*(2), 175–189. doi:10.1080/01490407809512880

Williams, R. L. (1991). *The origins of federal support for higher education: George W. Atherton and the land-grant college movement*. University Park, PA: Penn State University Press.

Wolch, J. R., Byrne, J., & Newell, J. P. (2014). Urban green space, public health, and environmental justice: The challenge of making cities 'just green enough'. *Landscape and Urban Planning*, *125*, 234–244. doi:10.1016/j.landurbplan.2014.01.017

Woodard, M. D. (1988). Class, regionality, and leisure among urban Black Americans: The post-civil rights era. *Journal of Leisure Research*, *20*(2), 87–105.

Yorks, L., & Scott, L. (2013). Lifelong tools for the learner, educator, and worker. In V. C. X. Wang (Ed.), *Handbook of Research on Technologies for Improving the 21st Century Workforce: Tools for Lifelong Learning* (pp. 42–55)., doi:10.4018/978-1-4666-2181-7.ch004

Zenk, S. N., Schulz, A. J., Israel, B. A., James, S. A., Bao, S. M., & Wilson, M. L. (2005). Neighborhood racial composition, neighborhood poverty, and the spatial accessibility of supermarkets in metropolitan. Detroit, MI. *American Journal of Public Health*, *95*(4), 660–667. doi:10.2105/AJPH.2004.042150 PMID:15798127

KEY TERMS AND DEFINITIONS

Built Environment: Provides the setting for human action and activity, including parks, buildings, green spaces, communities, and cities; also a determinant of public health outcomes, health status, access to health care, or the provision of care.

Healthy Parks: Acts as nontraditional continuing education structures to support and benefit from the diverse attributes of public health, social leisure, and lifelong learning.

Learning Cities: Represents the geographical space for implementing lifelong learning among individuals, institutions, communities, state and municipal governments.

Leisure: Describes resulted actions relating to time, activity, state-of-mind; values expressing enjoyment, happiness, satisfaction; or engagements demonstrating physical, mental, social development, group interaction, and collective participation.

Lifelong Learning: Situates the continuance of education during every state of living; an action of social participation for the continued benefit of a society.

Chapter 9
The Role of Self-Efficacy and Aging in Managing Disease

Debra Weiss-Randall
Florida Atlantic University, USA

ABSTRACT

In 1900, life expectancy in the U.S. was 47 years and infectious diseases were the leading cause of mortality; today, life expectancy in the U.S. is almost 80 years and chronic diseases are the leading causes of mortality. Eighty percent of adults 65 and older have multiple chronic health conditions, which are costly to treat. Offering older adults an evidence-based self-management program can reduce medical costs and improve patient outcomes and quality of life. Research has shown that self-efficacy is a key factor in effective self-management programs. The Chronic Disease Self-Management Program (CDSMP) is an evidence-based program that helps patients to boost their self-efficacy and improve their disease self-management, under the supervision of a physician. In addition, the use of evidence-based complementary modalities is recommended as part of an integrative approach to self-management to help patients manage the daily anger, fear, and depression that frequently accompany living with an incurable disease.

INTRODUCTION

Gone are the days when the doctor (usually a male) told the patient what to do and the patient accepted it without reservation. Today patients are consumers, and they select healthcare providers from a roster of names accepted by their health plan. Thanks to the Internet, which has widely disseminated health information through websites such as WebMD, patients are much better informed today than they were 25 years ago. They are also prey to "infomercials" and a host of advertisers selling products that will "cure" them of obesity, cancer, depression, and more, if they pay a monthly fee to receive certain supplements, potions, and balms. *Caveat emptor*—buyer beware.

In the U.S., chronic diseases cause 7 of 10 deaths each year, and treating chronic diseases accounts for 86% of the nation's healthcare costs (Centers for Disease Control and Prevention, 2013). In 2012, about half of all U.S. adults—117 million people—had at least one chronic health condition; 25% of adults

DOI: 10.4018/978-1-5225-0640-9.ch009

had two or more chronic health conditions (Ward et al., 2014). The healthcare provider's aim in dealing with patients who have chronic diseases such as diabetes and asthma is adequate self-management in order to maintain good quality of life. Control over risk factors such as diet, exercise, and smoking make an enormous difference in outcome.

Today patients are partners in their own healthcare. This chapters posits that, for patients to be able to achieve adequate self-management of chronic diseases, they need a chronic disease self-management program that provides education about disease management and helps patients to apply what they have learned at home. Furthermore, in order to feel empowered to act, patients need to develop self-efficacy, i.e., belief in their capacity to exercise control over their lives and effect behavior change. A diagnosis of a serious illness such as cancer can lead to fear, depression, and feelings of powerlessness, which must be treated in order for the patient to be an effective partner in his or her care. Evidence-based non-pharmacologic complementary therapies can be a great help in this regard, providing emotional and psychological support.

This chapter describes the contributions of self-efficacy theory and positive psychology to disease self-management. Next, the chapter provides a review of the literature on chronic disease self-management programs, with a discussion of the Chronic Disease Self-Management Program (CDSMP), an evidence-based program developed in the mid-1990s that has been found to boost patients' self-efficacy and improve outcome measures. The chapter also examines the effectiveness of individual components of chronic disease self-management programs. The chapter then provides a detailed discussion of evidence-based non-pharmacologic complementary therapies, which are a useful adjunctive treatment that should be used under the supervision of a physician. These complementary therapies provide symptom relief, reduce stress, improve patients' ability to perform daily tasks, and facilitate adoption of healthy lifestyle habits.

Next, the chapter looks at the U.S. statistics on aging and disease, and the implications for healthy aging. Aging places an additional burden on patients. Seniors with chronic diseases may feel hopeless about recovery and need supportive services aimed at their age group to encourage self-efficacy and to keep them motivated to participate in rehabilitation. Elderly patients may need adaptive physical activities to accommodate age-related physical limitations. Access to appropriate facilities, and transportation to get there, are two additional challenges seniors face.

The chapter concludes by summing up the recommendations for chronic disease self-management, including the use of an evidence-based self-management plan such as CDSMP, and the use of complementary therapies to provide symptom relief and promote adoption of healthy behaviors. Treatment should be tailored to the patient's specific age cohort and be culturally sensitive as well, respecting the patient's ethnic, racial, and religious background.

SELF-EFFICACY THEORY

Albert Bandura's groundbreaking work in self-efficacy posited that "expectations of personal efficacy determine whether coping behavior will be initiated, how much effort will be expended, and how long it will be sustained in the face of obstacles and aversive experiences" (Bandura, 1977, p. 191).

An outcome expectancy is a person's belief that a particular course of action will produce certain outcomes. Bandura (1977) differentiates it from self-efficacy, which is a person's belief that he or she can successfully execute the behavior required to produce the outcomes. Bandura notes that individuals can believe that a particular course of action will produce certain outcomes, but if they entertain serious doubts about whether they can perform the necessary activities such information does not influence their behavior (Bandura, 1977, p. 193).

Perceived self-efficacy is based on four principal sources of information (Bandura, 1982):

- Performance attainments
- Vicarious experiences observing others
- Verbal persuasion and social influence, and
- Physiological states.

Performance attainments refer to success the person has experienced; these successes build confidence in the person's ability to succeed again in the future. Observing someone who is perceived to be of similar competence succeed can give the observer confidence that she, too, can succeed. Conversely, watching a peer fail can put a damper on one's enthusiasm for tackling a similar task. Pep talks (verbal persuasion) have the greatest effect on those who believe they can produce effects through their actions. Experiencing negative physiological states such as high arousal with tension and agitation (e.g., nerves before a speech), or fatigue with aches and pains (e.g., aching back before a race) may deter a person from continuing toward his goal (Bandura, 1982). The higher the perceived self-efficacy, the more likely the person is to persevere and overcome obstacles to attain the desired goal. Bandura (1982) emphasizes the centrality of the self-efficacy mechanism in human agency. Perceived self-efficacy influences a person's thought patterns, actions, and emotional arousal. The higher the level of self-efficacy, the higher the performance accomplishments will be.

There is an inverse relationship between level of self-efficacy and emotional arousal; the higher the former, the lower the latter. Why is this the case? Emotional arousal is debilitating and, hence, reduces a person's confidence that he or she can complete the desired task. Confidence, in turn, is influenced by one's outlook in life. An optimistic outlook promotes confidence in one's ability to overcome obstacles and achieve a desired outcome. Self-efficacy theory is closely related to positive psychology, which promotes an optimistic outlook on life.

POSITIVE PSYCHOLOGY

Martin Seligman, founder of the positive psychology movement, defines it as "the scientific study of the strengths that enable individuals and communities to thrive" (Seligman, 2015). In contrast to the traditional disease model, which focuses on weaknesses and dysfunction, the positive psychology model focuses on authentic happiness and flourishing (Seligman, 2011). Seligman's PERMA model of well-being has five components:

- Positive Emotions
- Engagement
- Relationships
- Meaning
- Accomplishment

When life is frustrating and a person's efforts to attain desired goals are thwarted, is the glass half full or half empty? From a positive pschology point of view, it is always half full.

Given challenging circumstances, the optimist feels that he or she can persevere and attain a desired goal. The pessimist, on the other hand, doesn't even want to try because it seems like a hopeless cause. Can a person's outlook on life be changed? Positive psychologists believe the answer is "Yes!" Positive psychology posits that a person's thoughts profoundly affect his or her actions. Therefore, thinking positive thoughts will engender positive actions. If you believe in your ability to attain a goal, you are likely to do it!

Positive psychology builds on strength and resilience, with the patient no longer viewed as "a passive vessel," but rather as a decision maker (Bandura, 1989; Seligman, 2011). Rather than emphasizing disease and dysfunction, positive psychology focuses on well-being, optimal experience, happiness, and self-determination. It posits that a positive personality can be *developed* because human beings are adaptive entities. Furthermore, because people and experiences are embedded in a social context, it is vital to take positive communities and institutions into account (Seligman & Csikszentmihalyi, 2000).

How can people change their mindset to a more positive one? In Seligman's view, people can become more optimistic by cultivating kindness, developing friendships, exercising, using their strengths, finding their flow, finding meaning through spirituality, and by expressing gratitude, mindfulness, and hope (Seligman, 2015). Mroczek (2014) argues for the plasticity of the personality, for the possibility that personality traits such as conscientiousness—an important element of self-management—can be cultivated. Some authors (Chapman et al., 2014; Magidson et al., 2014) advocate interventions that cultivate the trait of conscientiousness, which, in turn, leads to improved health behaviors.

When people have a life-threatening chronic disease (such as heart disease or cancer), the coping mechanisms they use, in part, determine their emotional well-being (Carver et al., 1993; Hart et al., 1987; Stanton et al., 2007). When problems are controllable, the most effective strategy, and the one most closely related to emotional well-being, is active coping (problem-solving and seeking information and social support). When problems are uncontrollable, the most effective coping strategies are acceptance of the problem, positive reappraisal of the situation (e.g., considering it an opportunity to adopt a healthier lifestyle, to appreciate the truly important things in life), and the use of a sense of humor (Angeles Ruiz, 2011). A positive attitude toward the illness has a beneficial effect on recovery. Research has found that positive expectations predicted patients' recovery from a myocardial infarction (Agarwal et al., 1995). Dispositional optimism is also an important predictor of recovery from a cardiovascular episode or surgery (Scheier et al., 1989).

REVIEW OF THE LITERATURE

Forty years ago, most patients went to their primary doctor and took whatever medication was prescribed; doctors were in charge of disease management, and patients followed their advice. With the founding of the World Wide Web in 1989, the flow of information on medical diseases and conditions increased exponentially. Patients became health consumers who searched medical websites for information about their health conditions. Today, patients can optimize their quality of life by taking an active role in self-management of their chronic diseases and conditions, under the supervision of a healthcare provider.

Overview of Chronic Disease Self-Management

Lorig and Holman (2003) give an overview of the history of disease self-management. The term "self-management" as applied to chronic disease indicates that the patient is an active participant in treatment. One of its early proponents was Thomas Creer, who used it in his work with chronically ill children at the Children's Asthma Research Institute and Hospital (Creer et al., 1976). For someone with a chronic disease, self-management is generally a lifelong task. The burden of day-to-day disease management falls largely on the patient.

Self-management of chronic disease comprises three tasks—medical management, role management, and emotional management (Lorig & Holman, 2003). The medical management of the disease or condition includes taking medications and monitoring vital signs such as blood pressure and heart rate; it also may necessitate adhering to a special diet and/or using medical devices such as an inhaler for asthma. The role management of the chronic disease or condition involves maintaining, changing, and creating new behaviors or life roles to accommodate the limitations imposed by the disease. For example, people with chronic back pain may need to modify how they participate in a sport (Lorig & Holman, 2003). Emotional management involves dealing with the anger, fear, frustration, and depression that are often experienced by an individual with a chronic, incurable disease; dealing with the disease requires daily management of symptoms and adaptation to the limitations imposed by the disease (Lorig & Holman, 2003). Corbin and Strauss's (1988) research on individuals with chronic diseases and conditions yielded the finding that self-management programs must be problem based, i.e., they need to solve the underlying problem that is perceived by the patient to be the core issue. They cite the example of arthritis: traditional arthritis programs focused on preventing or limiting disability; however, for the patients, pain management was the underlying problem. Therefore, disability prevention should be taught in the context of pain management (Corbin & Strauss, 1988). The first step in self-management program should be a detailed needs assessment to ascertain what the most important issues are for the patient.

In order to execute these tasks successfully, one must master five core self-management skills—1) problem solving, 2) decision making, 3) resource utilization, 4) forming a patient-provider partnership, and 5) taking action (Lorig & Holman, 2003). In solving a problem, one must first define it, then generate ideas for possible solutions, implement a plan to resolve the problem, and then evaluate the results. The Americans with Disabilities Act (ADA), passed by Congress in 1990, prohibited discrimination in employment, public services, public accommodations, and telecommunications. It led to the requirement that public buildings have access ramps for wheelchairs that buses accommodate wheelchairs, and that public services and facilities (including theatres and museums) offer accommodations for individuals with disabilities. Therefore, when a person with a chronic condition or disease has a problem regarding transportation (a frequent concern), it is now easier than it was before ADA to problem solve and get them where they need to go using public transportation. Decision making might revolve around being able to understand when a symptom is serious enough to require a visit to the doctor or hospital, to know how much exercise is "enough," or to know how to read food labels to make sure the item does not contain anything not on the individual's special diet.

The third skill, resource utilization, requires getting the consumer to the resource. It may involve acquiring new skills, such as learning to surf the Web to locate a desired resource. In addition, Lorig and Holman (2003) suggest casting a wide net by contacting several sources of information at once rather than calling only one and waiting for someone to get back to you. The fourth skill, forming a partnership with the physician or other healthcare provider, requires re-thinking the traditional approach to the patient-provider relationship, which was predicated on diagnosing and treating acute, infectious diseases. In the U.S. today, chronic diseases such as heart disease, cancer, and stroke are the major killers, and people live with chronic diseases for decades. When dealing with chronic diseases, the provider-patient relationship has to be a partnership, with the physician supervising and teaching the patient about self-management.

Finally, taking action involves skill mastery and confidence in one's ability to carry out an action plan in the next week or two. The objective should be quite specific and measurable; for example, "This week I will walk to the corner store and back (2 blocks in all) before dinner on Monday, Wednesday, and Saturday." (Lorig & Holman, 2003). In addition, the plan should be realistic and "doable," and the person should be confident that he or she can achieve the objective. On a scale of 1 (totally unconfident) to 10 (totally confident), the person planning to take action should have a confidence score of 7 or above. If it is below 7, more problem solving may be needed (Lorig & Holman, 2003). To improve compliance with an action plan and to make sure that it is appropriate, self-tailoring is needed; this requires that the individual has learned the principles behind behavior change, decision making, and problem solving. In addition, the individual must believe in his or her capacity to effect behavior change, as self-efficacy (Bandura, 1977, 1982, 1989, 1991) is the mechanism driving the success of self-management interventions (Lorig & Holman, 2003). (For a discussion of self-efficacy, see Theoretical Framework.)

Chronic Disease Self-Management Program (CDSMP)

CDSMP is a self-management education program for individuals with chronic illnesses or health conditions. Lorig and colleagues (Lorig et al., 1999) developed it in a longitudinal study at the School of Medicine at Stanford University. The aim of CDSMP is to improve self-management of chronic disease by improving self-efficacy through the use of goal setting, performance mastery, modeling, and social persuasion techniques (Melchior et al., 2014). The Centers for Disease Control and Prevention (CDC) recommends CDSMP as an effective evidence-based tool for chronic disease self-management (CDC, 2016).

The CDSMP randomized controlled trial (RCT) at Stanford University had more than 1,000 participants with heart disease, lung disease, stroke, or arthritis. The outcome measures the researchers studied were changes in the participants' health status (self-rated general health, disability, social limitations, pain/physical discomfort, energy level, shortness of breath, psychological well-being, depression), health care usage (visits to physicians and emergency department, hospitalizations), self-efficacy (to perform self-management behaviors, manage disease in general, achieve outcomes), and self-management behaviors (exercise, manage cognitive symptoms and stress, use community resources, and communicate with physician).

Lorig et al. (1996) state that four factors motivated them to undertake the CDSMP study, namely, 1) an aging population, 2) increases in both chronic disease and comorbidity, 3) new concepts about healthy aging, and 4) a lack of health education programs for those with multiple chronic diseases or conditions (Lorig et al., 1996). The aims of developing such a self-management program were to improve quality of life for an aging population suffering from chronic diseases, and to reduce healthcare costs (Lorig et al., 1996).

The researchers had previous experience with an Arthritis Self-Management Program (ASMP), and developed their theoretical framework for CDSMP based on the results of ASMP Lorig et al., 1989).. They found that participants in ASMP who experienced positive changes in pain reported an increased sense of control over their symptoms, whereas those who did not were more likely to report that nothing could be done for their symptoms. Feelings of control were operationalized as perceived self-efficacy to feel confident that they could manage arthritis symptoms (Lenker et al., 1984). This hypothesis that ASMP increased self-efficacy and that this increase was associated with improvements in pain was tested and demonstrated in subsequent research (Lorig et al., 1999).

The CDSMP RCT offered weekly workshops that taught skills useful for managing chronic diseases and conditions. The workshops were held in community settings such as senior centers, churches, libraries, and hospitals; participants met 2 1/2 hours per week for 6 weeks. The workshops were facilitated by two trained leaders, one or both of whom were non-health professionals with a chronic disease (Lorig et al., 1999). The topics covered in the workshops included: 1) techniques to deal with problems such as frustration, fatigue, pain and isolation, 2) appropriate exercises for strength, flexibility, and endurance, 3) appropriate use of medications, 4) communicating effectively with family, friends, and health professionals, 5) nutrition, 6) decision making, and, 7) how to evaluate new treatments (Lorig et al., 1999).

The Stanford study (Lorig et al., 1999) found that participants who took CDSMP, when compared to those who did not, demonstrated significant improvements in exercise, ability to do social and household activities, communication with physicians, self-reported general health, health distress, fatigue, and disabilities. They also spent fewer days in the hospital. There was a cost to savings ration of approximately 1:4 (Lorig et al., 1999).

From 2008 to 2010, the Healthy Aging Regional Collaborative in South Florida (Melchior et al., 2014) evaluated the effectiveness of CDSMP in a study at multiple agencies in community settings over a six-week period. Seven agencies delivered 108 CDSMP workshops at 81 sites in Broward, Miami-Dade, and Palm Beach Counties. Each weekly 2½-hour workshop was led by two trained instructors; there were a total of 94 instructors. The study comprised a total of 811 participants, who filled out surveys at baseline and at the end of the six-week intervention (Melchior et al., 2014). Topics covered during the 6-week CDSMP intervention included managing fear, anger, and depression; problem solving and decision making; exercise techniques; communication skills; and nutrition. At the end of each workshop, participants created an action plan with a specific weekly goal to be accomplished before the next workshop. Outcome measures included health behavior outcomes (exercise frequency and perceived level of interference in social and daily activities by chronic disease symptoms) and self-efficacy outcomes (self-confidence in ability to manage chronic disease adequately). The outcomes that showed statistically significant improvement included self-efficacy to manage disease ($p = .001$), self-efficacy to manage emotions ($p = .026$), time spent walking ($p = .008$), and perceived social/role activities limitations ($p = .001$). In sum, the intervention found that CDSMP was effective at improving self-efficacy, increasing physical activity, and decreasing perceived limitations in social and daily activities (Melchior et al., 2014).

In addition to improving health outcomes and lifestyle behaviors, CDSMP also has been shown to reduce medical costs (Anh et al., 2013; Ory et al., 2013). In a study of 1,170 community-dwelling CDSMP patients in 17 states, participants showed significant reductions in ER visits (5%) at the 6-month and 12-month follow up assessments, and in hospitalizations (3%) at 6 months (Anh et al., 2013). The researchers calculated that the potential net savings would be $364 per CDSMP participant (Anh et al., 2013). That equates to a national savings of $3.3 billion if 5% of adults with chronic conditions were offered the intervention (Anh et al., 2013). The median age of the study participants was 65.4 years, a geriatric population (Ory et al., 2013). CDSMP has been replicated across the United States and is considered a state-of-the-art intervention for disease self-management (CDC, 2016).

The CDSMP model of chronic disease self-management has been adapted for use with consumers who suffer from chronic mental illnesses and disorders. The Health and Recovery Program (HARP) is a six-session intervention delivered by mental health peer leaders; its aim is to help participant become more effective managers of their chronic illnesses (Druss et al., 2010). The use of peer leaders is growing rapidly in the U.S. as an avenue to address concerns about elevated morbidity and premature mortality among those with chronic mental illnesses (Parks & Svedsen, 2006). Individuals with serious mental illness are at risk of developing a number of chronic medical conditions (Sokal, 2004; Carney et al., 2006; Carney & Jones, 2006).

Effectiveness of Specific Components of Disease Management Programs

Rather than advocating a specific disease management program, Pimouguet et al. (2011) sought to identify the effective components of disease management programs. Their rationale was as follows: "Because disease-management programs are heterogeneous, the effective components need to be identified to improve program implementation" (Pimouguet et al., 2011, E115). They further noted that there was no "consensual definition" of disease management. Pimouguet et al. (2011, p. E116) defined disease management as follows:

the ongoing and proactive follow-up of patients that includes at least two of the following five components: patient education (dietary and exercise counselling, self-monitoring, and knowledge of disease and medication); coaching (the disease manager encourages the patient to overcome psychological or social barriers that impede autonomy or improvement in medication compliance); treatment adjustment (the disease manager is able to start or modify treatment with or without prior approval from the primary care physician); monitoring (the disease manager gets medical data from the patient); and care coordination (the disease manager reminds the patient about upcoming appointments or important aspects of self-care and informs the primary care physician about complications, treatment adjustment or therapeutic recommendations).

Pimouguet et al.'s meta-analysis (2011) focused on disease management in patients with Type 1 and 2 diabetes mellitus. Only RCTs were included in the meta-analysis. The outcome measure evaluated was the impact of specific components of disease management programs on hemoglobin (A.sub.1C) levels. Forty-four studies met the inclusion criteria, but three had missing data on hemoglobin (A.sub.1C) at baseline and so were excluded, leaving a total of 41 RCTs in the meta-analysis. The trials were conducted between 1990 and 2009 and enrolled a total of 7013 participants. The RCTs were international; 26 trials were conducted in the U.S., five in Canada, three in Europe, and seven in Asia. The results showed that diabetes management programs had a clinically moderate but significant impact on hemoglobin (A.sub.1C) levels; effective components of the programs were a high frequency of patient contact and the ability for disease managers to adjust treatment with or without prior physician approval (Pimouguet et al., 2011). Further study might be useful in determining the effectiveness of specific disease management components with different diseases and for various subpopulations, in order to provide self-tailoring of CDSMP and other evidence-based self-management programs.

The following section discusses adjunctive non-pharmacologic therapies that can be used as part of an integrative approach to treatment. All of the modalities described below are evidence-based; it should be noted that they are not alternative, but rather, complementary treatments to be used under a physician's supervision.

Evidence-Based Non-Pharmacologic Complementary Therapies

Evidence-based integrative medicine includes non-pharmacologic complementary therapies that provide symptom relief. Memorial Sloan Kettering Cancer Center, a pioneer in complementary treatments, recommends the following safe, effective, evidence-based complementary modalities: 1) mind-body techniques (yoga, meditation, qi gong, tai chi, and relaxation techniques), 2) music therapy, 3) acupuncture, 4) diet and nutrition, including herbs, 5) physical activity, and 6) massage therapy (Bao, 2014). The six complementary modalities are displayed in Figure 1.

Complementary modalities can be used with older adults, but they need to be tailored to their specific needs; for example, the Integrative Medicine Institute of Memorial Sloan Kettering Cancer Center has a program, *65+*, for older adults with cancer. It is staffed by experts in geriatric medicine, rehab, nutrition, social work, pain, and palliative care. Five mind-body techniques are discussed in the following section.

Complementary modalities should not be confused with alternative therapies, which eschew traditional medical practices. Complementary, or integrative, therapies are rational and noninvasive and have demonstrated safety, value, and benefits (Deng & Cassileth, 2014).

Figure 1. Six evidence-based complementary modalities
Recommended by Memorial Sloan Kettering Cancer Center for disease management (Bao, 2014).

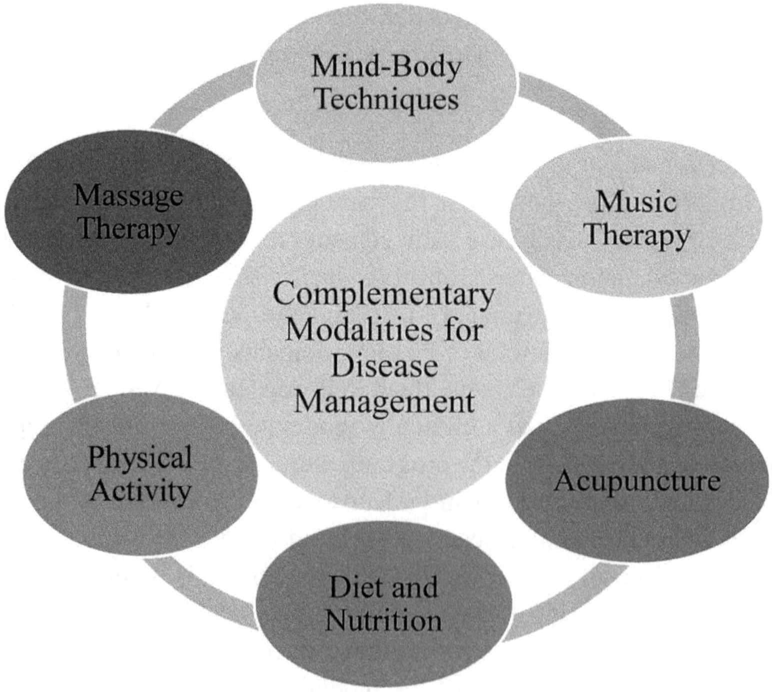

A discussion of the six recommended complementary non-pharmacologic therapies follows. Increasingly, major medical centers are offering these therapies under the umbrella of an Integrative Institute, with all care supervised by a physician, who is part of a healthcare team.

Mind-Body Techniques

Mind-body techniques reflect an integrative approach to health; the body influences the mind, and the mind, in turn, affects the functioning of the body. The evidence-based mind-body techniques used as complementary therapies in the treatment of chronic diseases such as cancer and heart disease are depicted in Figure 2.

Yoga

At Albert Einstein College of Medicine, a longitudinal research study on the effects of mind-body studies on cancer has focused on yoga. This randomized wait-list controlled study began in 2001. The yoga intervention in the Einstein study was developed for use with breast, lung and colorectal cancer patients by Dr. Chirag Shah, a U.S.-board certified oncologist and certified yoga instructor, in consultation with Integral Yoga expert Richard Sisco. The Yoga-based Cancer Rehabilitation Program served 240 patients between 2001 and 2009 (Moadel et. al., 2009). It comprised four components—warm up, yoga asanas (poses), pranayama (yogic breathing), and meditation. To avoid falls, all components were done either seated or laying down, with rests between each pose, and modifications added as needed for lymphedema, abdominal pain, fatigue, and anxiety. Props (mats, blankets, and blocks) were used for support and to minimize pain (Moadel et al., 2009). Improved mood and decreased distress were found in the intervention group compared to the wait group; the intervention helped them to cope better (Moadel, 2010).

Figure 2. Evidence-based mind-body techniques used in disease management

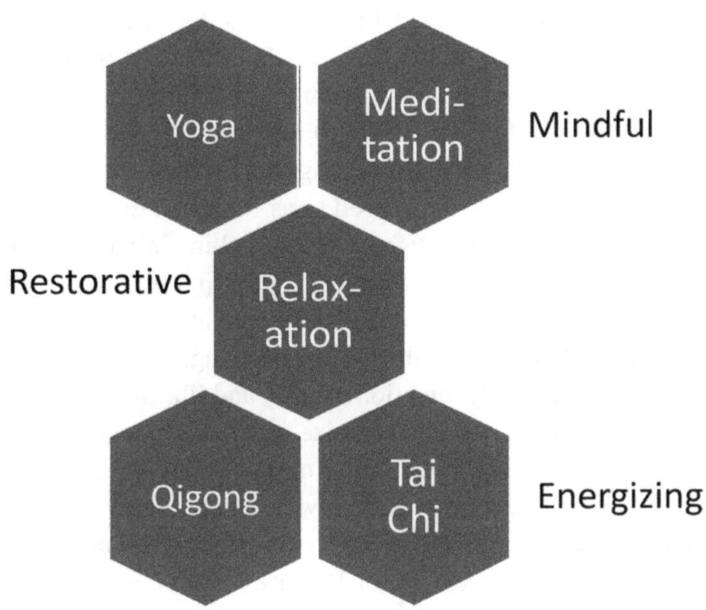

Lin et al. (2011) conducted a meta-analysis of RCTs evaluating the effects of yoga on psychological health, quality of life, and physical health of patients with cancer. Compared to the waitlist control groups, the yoga groups showed significantly greater improvements in psychological health: anxiety ($P = .009$), depression ($P = .002$), distress ($P = .003$), and stress ($P = .006$). However, due to the quality and small number of studies conducted, the findings have to be considered preliminary. More high-quality research using RCTs is needed.

Meditation

Mindfulness meditation is one of the most studied body-mind therapies. Mindfulness is defined as "a state of being attentive to and aware of what is taking place in the present" (Brown & Ryan 2003, p. 822). Mindfulness-based techniques enable an individual to be a detached observer of his or her thoughts, perceptions, and emotions; this detachment allows the person to respond to stressful events in an accepting, nonjudgmental manner (Michel et al., 2014). Mindfulness meditation is frequently offered as part of Mindfulness-Based Stress Reduction (MBSR), an eight-week program that includes mindfulness meditation, body scan, and yoga. Mindfulness-Based Stress Reduction has been found to reduce anxiety and stress, and improve sleep and overall quality of life (Shennen et al., 2011; Ledesma & Kumano, 2009; Cramer et al., 2012b; Zainal et al., 2013; Piet et al., 2012).

Meditation that uses visualization is another complementary technique that is closely tied to the self-efficacy theory of Bandura and positive psychology. A cancer patient may visualize macrophages--cells that attack cancer cells--as blue elephants stomping on cancer cells, sucking them up into their trunks, and squirting them out and eliminating them from the body. Patients may spend up to two hours a day affirming that they can recover, visualizing the cancer being eliminated, and meditating to control the emotional arousal of the mind and create a state of calm equanimity (Barasch, 1994).

Qigong and Tai Chi

Qigong (also spelled ch'i kung) comprises two Chinese words: Qi, which means "life force" or "vital energy," and Gong, which means "accomplishment or skill cultivated through steady practice." The intention of qigong practice is "to restore, circulate, balance and/or enhance personal life energy" (Dunbar, 2015). When qigong is practiced by individuals to improve their own health and well-being, it is referred to as "internal qigong." When a certified qigong practitioner uses the principles of Traditional Chinese Medicine (TCM) to heal others, it is referred to as "external qigong" (Dunbar, 2015). Qigong is considered a form of moving meditation. Qigong developed in China about 5,000 years ago. It enhances healing of the body by improving the flow of energy, or qi (ch'i), along energy pathways known as meridians throughout the body. Acupuncture and acupressure also work on the meridians. In Chinese medicine, good health is believed to be the result of a free-flowing, well-balanced energy system; when vital energy flow is blocked, a systemic dysfunction occurs, and illnesses and disorders result. T'ai-chi ch'üan is a Chinese internal style martial art and exercise for relaxation, energy, and overall well-being. Tai chi, which is a flowing series of poses, grew out of qigong more recently—about 200 years ago.

Kelley and Kelley (2015) completed a systematic review of meta-analyses on meditative movement therapy (MMT) (yoga, tai chi, and qigong) and its effects on Health-Related Quality of Life (HRQOL) in adults. (For more about HRQOL, see Centers for Disease Control & Prevention, 2000). The Kelley and Kelley (2015) review included only randomized controlled trials for adults age 18 and over, and those in which the difference in HRQOL between the intervention group and control group was a primary outcome reported as the standardized mean difference (SMD) effect size. The studies that met the inclusion criteria included the following diseases and conditions: cancer, schizophrenia, low back pain, heart failure, and diabetes. The percentile improvement in HRQOL between the intervention group and the control group by type of modality ranged from 9.9 to 48.9 for yoga (Buffart et al., 2012; Cramer et al., 2012a; Cramer et al., 2013a; Cramer et al., 2013b, Shneerson et al., 2013; Zhang et al., 2012), 25.8 to 42.1 for tai chi only (Pan et al., 2013), 21.9 and 46.3 for qigong only (Wang et al., 2013; Zeng et al., 2014), and 47.4 for tai chi and qigong combined (Zeng et al., 2014). The researchers believe this is the first such study examining the effects of MMT on HRQOL for RCTs. The researchers recommend that, based on their review findings, "it would appear both prudent and safe at this time to suggest that HRQOL may be improved by participating in MMT at least 3 times per week for about 71 minutes per session" (Kelley & Kelley, 2015). They recommend that further research be conducted, and that future studies include cost-effectiveness of the interventions as well as dose-response of the MMT and description of the specific type of MMT (e.g., specify form of yoga used).

Relaxation Techniques

One of the most commonly used complementary modalities for patients with chronic disease and disorders is relaxation techniques. They are used to improve well-being, relieve stress, and elevate mood. The term "relaxation response" was coined by Herbert Benson (Benson & Klipper, 1975/2001), a cardiologist at Harvard Medical School, to describe a physiological and psychological state that was evoked through meditative practices and that was the opposite of the fight or flight response elicited by a stressor. The relaxation response is characterized by

- Decreased metabolism, heart rate, blood pressure, and rate of breathing
- A "calming" in brain activity
- An increase in attention and decision-making functions of the brain
- Changes in gene activity that are the opposite of those associated with stress (Benson & Proctor, 2010)

The relaxation response may be elicited by sitting quietly, focusing on slow, deep breathing, and saying a calming word or sound associated with the person's belief system on each exhale. The mind should focus only on the breath and on relaxing. Research has shown the relaxation response to be effective with hypertension (Benson et al., 1974, Peters et al., 1977) and irregular heartbeat (Benson & Proctor, 2010). It does not require the agility of yoga practice or even the muscular control of progressive muscle relaxation, and so is suitable for frail seniors.

Reig-Ferrer et al.'s (2014) randomized controlled study of seniors in a nursing home was a trial of the effectiveness of Benson's relaxation response with an elderly population. Previous research (Kiecolt-Glaser et al., 2010) had shown that a Jacobson-type muscle relaxation technique improved cellular immune competence in the elderly. Reig-Ferrer et al. (2014) wanted to achieve a similar effect without muscular effort, to accommodate elderly individuals who have muscle and joint disorders. They selected

Benson's relaxation response, which has been shown to decrease stress (Esch et al., 2003) and anxiety, and to enhance cognitive performance in healthy aging (Galvin, 2006). Reig-Ferrer et al. (2014) evaluated the effects of this relaxation technique on psychological well-being and quality of life, biomedical variables, and immune changes of participants compared to a waitlist control group.

The intervention was two weeks, with a 3-month follow up. Reig-Ferrer et al. (2014) hypothesized that the relaxation technique would elevate psychological well-being, which would enhance immune functioning and enhance quality of life. Reig-Ferrer et al.'s (2014) RCT excluded anyone with health problems directly related to immune function or on drugs with significant effects on endocrine or immune function. The following biomedical measures were taken at the beginning of the intervention, 15 days after the intervention concluded, and three months after the intervention concluded: 1) clinical history, 2) functional assessment, using Katz Index of Activities of Daily Living, 3) weight, height, BMI, blood pressure and heart rate, 4) red and white blood cell counts, CBC, hemoglobin hematocryte, MCV, platelets, ESR, and 5) glucose, creatinine, urea, uric acid, lipids, AST, ALT, GGT, total proteins, and serum albumin. Psychological well-being was measured with the Satisfaction with Life Scale (SWLS) and Bradburn's Affect Balance Scale (ABS); Health-Related Quality of Life was measured using the Nottingham Health Profile (NHP) (Reig-Ferrer et al., 2014).

The Reig-Ferrer et al. (2014) trial was the first time a relaxation technique had been used in a nursing home in Spain and in which the psychological, biomedical and immunological measures were obtained. The aim was to test the Benson relaxation method as a psycho-gerontological intervention for enhancing well-being and immune parameters. The results showed a decrease in negative affect, psychological discomfort, and symptom perception in the treatment group, and improved quality of life. There were significant differences in immune parameters after the trial between the intervention group and waitlist group in CD19, CD71, CD97, CD134, and CD137 lymphocyte subpopulations. However, the sample size was very small and further research is needed with larger samples (Reig-Ferrer et al., 2014).

Prasad et al. (2010) administered a cross-sectional, point-of-care survey to patients attending the Cardiology Outpatient Clinic at Mayo Clinic in Rochester, Minnesota to document the use of complementary and alternative (CAM) therapies among patients with cardiovascular disease; the top four modalities used for heart-related symptoms were relaxation techniques, stress management, meditation, and guided imagery. A total of 23.9% of those surveyed reported using mind-body therapies for heart-related symptoms. Improvement in heart-related symptoms after using these therapies was reported by 22.2% for palpitations, 21.8% for sleep disturbance, 20.0% for chest pain, and 19.4% for leg swelling (Prasad et al., 2010).

COPD is a progressive disease associated with an abnormal inflammatory response of the lungs to noxious particles or gases (Volpato et al., 2015). Due to continuous exposure to risk factors and increases in life expectancy, COPD is expected to move from sixth to fourth cause of mortality and morbidity worldwide (Pauwels et al., 2001; Lopez et al., 2006; Murray & Lopez, 1997). Interventions aimed at COPD patients tend to focus on the physical aspects of the disease and to ignore the considerable anxiety, depression, and feelings of helplessness and powerlessness that often accompany the disease as it progresses (Karadag et al., 2008). Volpato et al. (2015) did a systematic review of the literature on the effect of relaxation techniques on anxiety, depression, quality of life, and percentage of Forced Expiratory Volume (FEV_1) in patients with COPD. FEV_1 is the maximal amount of air a person can forcefully exhale in one second. Volpato et al.'s (2015) review included only RCTs, and they had to focus on anxiety, depression, quality of life, and/or percentage of FEV_1. Volpato et al. (2015) found that relaxation techniques can have a moderate positive impact on psychological well-being and respiratory function; they believed that the results sustain the importance of relaxation techniques as a tool for managing COPD. Various relaxation techniques were used in the RCTs, including several different breathing techniques, singing, yoga, and tai chi. Volpati et al. (2015) noted the need for more high-quality research.

Music Therapy

The power of music to improve mood and emotions has been extolled by poets for centuries. Shakespeare put it this way: "If music be the food of love, play on" (Shakespeare, 1602/1623). Music therapy is the clinical and evidence-based use of music interventions by a credentialed professional to address the physical, emotional, cognitive, and social needs of patients (American Music Therapy Association, 2015). Music therapy may be used as part of a complementary medicine program in the context of an integrative approach to disease management. It is important to note that music therapy does NOT replace medical treatment; rather, it is an adjunctive therapy that supports patients by facilitating their coping with pain, anxiety, fear, and depression (Stanczyk, 2011). It is used to promote wellness, manage stress, alleviate pain, express feelings, enhance memory, improve communication, and promote physical rehabilitation (American Music Therapy Association, 2015). With oncology patients, music therapy focuses on the physiological and psychological needs of the patient, including anxiety about the future, fear of pain, and side effects from treatments (Stanczyk, 2011). Controlled trials have found that music therapy reduces anxiety (Salamon et al., 2003), stress, (Allen et al., 2001) depression, and pain (Good et al., 2002). Music therapy was also effective in reducing pain in oncology patients (Zimmerman et al., 1989).

Some cancer treatment centers have implemented drum circles for cancer survivors. At Albert Einstein College of Medicine, the Bronx Oncology Living Daily (BOLD) program offers free mind-body workshops to those in the local community affected by cancer as part of the Psychosocial Oncology program (Moadel, 2010). The BOLD drum circle helps patients to connect, get support, and feel empowered (Bongo therapy, 2011). The BOLD Program followed the model of integrative medicine at Memorial Sloan Kettering Cancer (MSKCC). At MSKCC, music therapy is used to calm agitation and distress, to lower blood pressure, and to help patients relax during difficult tests or procedures (Bao, 2014). Music therapy may be provided pre-treatment, during treatment, and after treatment. Researchers found that providing music therapy to patients prior to receiving radiation treatment decreased State-Trait anxiety and systolic blood pressure in cancer patients (Chen et al., 2013).

Acupuncture

Acupuncture was developed in China more than 3,000 years ago. Insertion of the needles into specific pressure points on the body stimulates the parasympathetic system and calms down the sympathetic nervous system. Acupuncture needles are regulated as a medical device in the United States; they are sterile, single-use, filiform, 32 gauge to 36 gauge, and 30 mm to 40 mm in length. The needle is inserted a few millimeters to a few centimeters into the skin. A typical treatment session lasts for 20 minutes to 40 minutes (Deng & Cassileth, 2014). Acupuncture has been shown to reduce pain (Vickers et al., 2012). Meta-analyses of acupuncture trials for four chronic pain conditions-- back and neck pain, osteoarthritis, chronic headache, and shoulder pain—have found significant effect sizes; acupuncture was superior to no acupuncture control and sham acupuncture, offering greater pain relief in all comparisons ($p<0.001$) (Vickers et al., 2012; Vickers & Linde, 2014). Acupuncture has also has been found to be effective in controlling chemotherapy-induced vomiting (Ezzo et al., 2005). In the hands of a licensed acupuncturist, acupuncture is very safe. Sterile needles are used, and they are disposed of after a single use. For those who cannot tolerate needles, acupressure is a needle-less alternative to acupuncture that uses the same pressure points but without needles (Bao, 2014).

Diet and Nutrition

There is an old saying, "You are what you eat." Making healthy food choices is free and should be easy to implement. However, Americans live in an obesogenic environment where fast food franchises such as McDonalds reign supreme, and where fatty fried foods and soda are the norm. Filmmaker Morgan Spurlock raised public consciousness about the dangers of consuming sugary soda and junk food with his 2004 film, *Supersize Me.* In the film, he ate nothing but McDonalds food for one month to document the adverse health consequences of such a diet. Spurlock pointed out that those marketing healthy food choices, such as the 5 A Day Fruit and Vegetable Campaign of the American Cancer Society, spent a mere $2 million a year on promotion, while McDonald's spent $1.4 billion on direct advertising and Hershey's spent $200 million (*Supersize Me*, 2004). Nevertheless, Spurlock's film did cause McDonald's to stop making Supersize fries; it also stopped frying potatoes in saturated fat after consumers sued McDonald's.

Heart disease is the number one killer in the United States today for both men and women; approximately 610,000 people die of heart disease in the United States every year–that's 1 in every 4 deaths (Centers for Disease Control and Prevention, 2015). More than half of older adults have hyperlipidemia and more than half have hypertension (Racine et al., 2011). Hyperlipidemia is a term that means there are elevated lipids (fats) in the blood; it refers primarily to cholesterol and triglycerides. Cholesterol is found primarily in saturated fat, which comes from animal products (meat, poultry, dairy). The American Heart Association (2015) recommends that adults reduce their consumption of saturated fat to no more than 5 to 6 percent of total calories. For a person who eats 2,000 calories a day, that's about 11 to 13 grams of saturated fat. Trans fat is another source of cholesterol that should be reduced; trans fat causes double trouble, as it raises LDL (low density lipoproteins, the "bad" cholesterol, and lowers HDL (high density lipoproteins, the "good" cholesterol). A person with hyperlipidemia should consult a doctor for medical treatment of the condition. However, medication alone is not sufficient; lifestyle factors are very important. Making healthy diet choices and getting an adequate amount of exercise are important steps in lowering high cholesterol, even if a person is on a statin (American Heart Association, 2015).

Hypertension refers to high blood pressure, defined as a diastolic blood pressure of 90 or above and a systolic blood pressure of 140 or above. High systolic blood pressure is a major risk factor for cardiovascular disease for people 50+ years old. Systolic blood pressure tends to rise with age due to increasing stiffness of large arteries, long-term build-up of plaque, and increased incidence of cardiac and vascular disease (American Heart Association, 2015). The American Heart Association recommends eating a healthy diet low in sodium, exercising regularly, maintaining a healthy weight, managing stress, and avoiding tobacco smoke to prevent hypertension. Regular consumption of green tea also may reduce the risk of hypertension (Yang et al., 2004, Cassileth, 2011).

Once diagnosed with hypertension, your physician may prescribe medication; however, the recommended lifestyle factors should still be followed (American Heart Association, 2015). The National Heart, Lung, and Blood Institute (2015) recommends that adults with risk factors for heart disease, including age 50+, elevated lipids, hypertension, smoking, and a family history, follow the Dietary Approach to Stop Hypertension (DASH) diet. The Dash diet reduces intake of saturated fat, total fat, sodium, and cholesterol, increases intake of fruits and vegetables, and increases consumption of potassium, calcium, magnesium, fiber, and protein. The DASH diet has been found to be effective in reducing blood pressure in adults (Appel et al., 1997; Blumenthal et al., 2010; Dickinson et al., 2006; Elmer et al., 2006). The DASH eating plan goals for a 2,000-calorie-a-day diet are shown in Table 1.

A high-fat, low-fiber diet is a key factor in the current epidemic of Type 2 diabetes mellitus (T2DM) in the U.S. and other countries. It is estimated that 23.6 million people have diabetes (about 20% of those are undiagnosed) in the United States; T2DM represents about 90 to 95 percent of cases of diagnosed diabetes. One-quarter of American adults 65 and over have diabetes (American Diabetes Association, 2015). In other countries, the highest prevalence rates of T2DM are in indigenous peoples who have experienced rapid change in their lifestyle (Venn & Mann, 2004). In the next 20 years, the greatest number of cases of T2DM are predicted to occur in China and India. Diabetes is a chronic disease; its effective management is "a constant juggling act" that requires careful attention to medication dosing, eating, activity, and other variables (DiMeglio, 2013). Unlike Type 1 diabetes, which appears in childhood, T2DM has an onset in adulthood.

Diabetes mellitus is a metabolic disorder characterized by hyperglycemia, insulin resistance and insulin insufficiency; living with diabetes elevates the risk of heart disease and can lead to long-term complications such as neuropathy, retinopathy, and nephropathy. A common sight in America today is middle-aged and older adults in wheelchairs missing one or both legs from amputations due to complications from diabetes. All of the health problems attendant to diabetes decrease quality of life and increase risk of mortality (American Diabetes Association, 2015; Constantino et al., 2013; Santaguida et al, 2005).

Dietary management of a case of presumed diabetes was first documented in 1500 B.C., with the recommendation that the patient consume wheat grains, grapes, honey, and berries (Leeds, 1979). Many other dietary prescriptions were tried between then and 1921, when insulin was discovered. The Food and Agriculture Organization (FAO) of the World Health Organization (WHO) recommends a diabetes-prevention diet in which the bulk of carbohydrates consumed are rich in nonstarch polysaccharides and have a low glycemic index (GI), with liberal intake of cereals, vegetables, legumes, and fruits (FAO/

Table 1. Daily and weekly DASH eating plan goals for a 2,000-calorie-a-day diet

Food Group	Daily Servings
Grains	6–8
Meats, poultry, and fish	6 or less
Vegetables	4–5
Fruit	4–5
Low-fat or fat-free dairy products	2–3
Fats and oils	2–3
Sodium	2,300 mg*
	Weekly Servings
Nuts, seeds, dry beans, and peas	4–5
Sweets	5 or less

*1,500 milligrams (mg) sodium lowers blood pressure even further than 2,300 mg sodium daily.
Source: National Heart, Lung, and Blood Institute. National Institutes of Health, U.S. Department of Health & Human Services.

WHO, 1998). Diabetes organizations in many countries, including Australia, the United Kingdom, the United States, and continental Europe, have endorsed the dietary recommendations of the FAO/WHO for prevention of T2DM as well as for treatment of both types I and II diabetes mellitus (Venn & Mann, 2004).

The development of T2DM is associated with a number of risk factors (Venn & Mann, 2004):

- Excess energy intake, leading to obesity
- High intakes of saturated and trans fats
- High intakes of fiber-depleted refined grain foods
- Lack of physical exercise

Medical nutrition therapy (MNT) is an important component of management of diabetes management. A registered dietician can help set up a menu for diabetic patients. People with diabetes are advised to avoid fried and fatty foods, and processed, refined carbohydrates, which have high advanced glycation end products (AGEs); foods with high AGEs can increase chronic inflammation and contribute to heart disease and other complications from diabetes (Weisenberger, 2014). A review of the literature on nutrition management of type II diabetes mellitus (T2DM) found strong support for the high intake of whole grain foods being a protective factor against the development of type II diabetes mellitus (T2DM). Adults who consumed approximately three servings per day of whole grain foods were less likely to develop T2DM than were low consumers (<3 servings per week), with a risk reduction of 20%-30% (Venn & Mann, 2004). Mirmiran et al. (2014) recommend consuming a whole-grain diet of functional foods to manage T2DM. They note that previous studies have shown that dietary carbohydrate modification in patients with metabolic syndrome has had favorable results, including increased insulin sensitivity and decreased adipocyte cell size (Laaksonen et al., 2005; Kallio et al., 2007). Mirmiran et al. (2014) propose a novel approach to NMI, one that makes functional foods-- especially whole grains, phytochemical-rich fruits and vegetables, legumes, nuts, dairy products, green tea and some spices--a required component of a health-promoting diet for diabetic patients. Bioactive compounds in whole grain foods (e.g., rye, oatmeal, barley, brown rice) have shown promise in regulating glycemic response, increasing insulin sensitivity, improving pancreatic β-cell functions, and increasing insulin secretion (Rosén et al., 2009; Shen et al., 2011). The American Diabetes Association recommends the Mediterranean diet, which is rich in whole grains, vegetables, legumes, nuts and seeds, and fruits; it uses heart-healthy monounsaturated olive oil and polyunsaturated oil (from nuts and seeds) rather than saturated fat Neithercott, 2014).

Herb and dietary supplements are a commonly used complementary modality in the self-management of many chronic diseases and conditions. The Memorial Sloan Kettering Cancer Center (MSKCC) Integrative Medicine website provides an extensive listing of herbs, botanicals, and other supplements used as adjunctive therapy for cancer treatment (MSKCC Integrative Medicine, 2015). In addition, MSKCC's Bendheim Integrative Medicine Center offers Nutritional and Dietary-Supplement Counseling for its on patients and for those in the community (MSKCC Bendheim Integrative Medicine Center, 2015).

Caution should be used in taking herbs and other dietary supplements as an adjunctive treatment for disease management; since they are not regulated substances, their quality and strength may vary. In addition, they may interact with medications and other medical treatments. An integrative approach to treatment is recommended, with the healthcare provider supervising all dietary supplements to make sure that there are no harmful side effects or drug interactions.

Physical Activity

Physical activity is a leading health indicator for our nation (*Healthy People 2020*). Getting regular physical activity that meets the federal guidelines (*Healthy People 2020*) is critical to maintaining a healthy weight. In 2012, half of adults age 18 and over met the guidelines for aerobic physical activity (at least 150 minutes per week of moderate physical activity, or 75 minutes per week of vigorous physical activity, or an equivalent combination). The levels of aerobic physical activity varied by gender: more adult males (53.8%) than females (46.5%) met the federal guidelines. The levels also varied by race; the number of non-Hispanic white adults who met the federal guidelines for aerobic physical activity was nearly one and a half times that of both Hispanic/Latino adults and non-Hispanic black adults. For adults with activity limitations, only 30.5% met the federal guidelines for aerobic physical activity, versus 53.9% of adults without activity limitations. All of the percentages are age-adjusted. (*Healthy People, 2020*).

Encouraging Americans to get regular exercise is a key factor in the fight against obesity. We live in an obesogenic environment that has produced an epidemic of obesity: more than one-third of American adults and 17% of youth are obese, with a Body Mass Index (BMI) of 30 or greater (Ogden et al., 2014). Among non-Hispanic Blacks and Hispanics, the age-adjusted prevalence rates of obesity are 47.8% and 42.5%, respectively. Obesity rates vary with age; prevalence is 39.5% among adults aged 40-59 years old. Obesity is a risk factor for heart disease, diabetes, stroke, and cancer. The fight against obesity comprises two main components: 1) changing eating habits to include high-fiber, low-fat items; and 2) increasing the level of physical activity.

Increasing one's level of physical activity aids in weight management. In addition, meeting the federal guidelines for aerobic physical activity reduces the risk of cardiovascular disease, (Wannamethee & Shaper, 2001; Sesso et al., 2000), ischemic stroke (Hu et al., 2000; Gorelick et al., 1999; Wannamethee & Shaper, 1999), T2DM (Hu et al., 2001; Pfohl & Schatz, 2001; Fulton-Kehoe et al., 2001), colon cancer (Brownson et al., 1991; Giovannucci et al., 1995), osteoporosis (Kohrt et al., 1995), depression (Fox, 1999; Camacho et al., 1991; Weyerer, 1992), and fall-related injuries (Meyer et al., 1993; Jaglal, 1993).

The first step in physical activity participation among adults is being knowledgeable about the benefits of physical activity. Once adults are aware that getting adequate physical activity is likely to lengthen their life and to reduce their risk for heart disease, ischemic stroke, diabetes, cancer, osteoporosis, depression, and fall-related injuries, they should be motivated to exercise, right? Unfortunately, knowledge alone may not be sufficient to facilitate physical activity. In the Dallas Heart Study, a 7-year longitudinal study of cardiovascular health in a multi-ethnic adult population, participants were asked about their physical activity and health beliefs (Mathieu et al., 2012). A whopping 94% of participants felt that physical activity was effective in preventing a heart attack; yet only 46% of Hispanics, 59% of African-Americans, and 78% of Whites participated in physical activity. Whites had higher rates of participation in physical activity than did African-Americans or Hispanics. Lack of physical activity was associated with higher cardiovascular mortality overall and among African Americans in particular. The researchers concluded that there were other ethnic-specific factors that required further study (Mathieu et al., 2012).

The second step in physical activity participation among adults is health promotion, including counselling, to encourage physical activity. In the Netherlands, chronically ill patients pay regular visits to their family practitioner to monitor their disease; during the visit the practice nurse provides lifestyle counseling. The most common type of promotion is verbal advice, followed by print and computer-based interventions. It is not clear which type of exercise promotion works best in the long term (Foster et al., 2005). One method that shows great promise is computer-based patient self-management programs such as mHealth (mobile phone Apps) and other E-health applications, which facilitate patient self-management (McDermott & While, 2013).

Verwey et al. (2014a) developed a smartphone physical activity App, called *It's Life*, embedded in a Self-management Support Program (SSP). They are testing the tool and the SSP in a randomized controlled trial of participants who have been diagnosed with either COPD or T2DM. The trial has three arms: the use of a monitoring and feedback tool embedded in the SSP (group 1), the SSP without the tool (group 2), and usual care (group 3). The participants are 40-70 years old, in primary care, and do not comply with national standards of physical activity (Verwey et al., 2014a). The primary outcome measure is physical activity in daily life, and the hypothesis is that the intervention group will increase their physical activity compared to the control group. The secondary outcome measures are self-efficacy (measured by General Self-Efficacy Scale and Exercise Self-Efficacy Scale (Everett et al., 2009)), quality of life (measured by SF-36), and health status (measured by Diabetes Symptom checklist-revised for T2DM participants and Chronic Respiratory Questionnaire for COPD participants). The trial began with a pre-measurement period during which time participants got used to wearing and entering comments on their accelerometer (part of the tool). They received two sessions about barriers, facilitators, and activity planning, with the aim of modifying factors known to influence physical activity, such as social support and self-efficacy (Verwey et al., 2014a). After two weeks, patient and nurse set a goal of physical activity per day; then the patient received feedback in the form of tips, encouragement, rewards, suggestions—all written in a positive tone.

***In the pilot study, a positive trend was seen for use of the tool; the mean level of physical activity increased by more than 10 minutes per day and patients reported a higher quality of life (Verwey et al., 2014b). The results of the longitudinal RCT, when completed, should yield valuable data on how to increase physical activity for patients suffering from serious chronic illnesses.*

Massage Therapy

In the Who's rock opera, *Tommy*, the protagonist sings "See me, feel me, touch me, heal me!" Touch is healing; it may be vital to survival at an early stage in life. In the 1940s, psychoanalyst Rene A. Spitz studied child development. He observed that infants in foundling homes who were well fed and warm but not held or touched, tended to wither and die. Of 91 babies he observed, 27 died in infancy, followed by seven more in their second year of life; in some foundling homes, up to 90 percent of the babies died in early infancy (Cassileth & Vickers, 2004). Human touch was needed for proper development. Therapeutic massage relaxes muscular tension. When licensed massage therapists work with chronically ill patients, special training is recommended to enable them to work on patients safely and effectively (Miner, 2007). Therapeutic massage with oncology patients reduces pain and anxiety, and improves quality of life; it also has been shown to reduce chemo-induced nausea and vomiting (Calenda, 2006; Bao, 2014). The use of therapeutic massage in cancer centers and hospitals in increasing. Massage has a positive effect on the body's biochemistry, increasing the neurotransmitter dopamine, the lymphocytes, and the natural killer cells (Calenda, 2006).

Healing Touch is another complementary therapeutic modality used by many nurses and health providers today. It is a form of massage that involves only light touching or stroking. The Healing Touch practitioner works on the patient's energy field surrounding his or her body, rather than directly on the muscles themselves. Healing Touch is a good choice of modality for frail patients, as it is gentle but penetrating. It was first offered as a continuing education program for nurses in the 1980s. The principle behind Healing Touch is promoting well-being through work with the energy system of the body (Mentgen, 2002). It is used in the U.S. and around the world at outpatient pain centers, in private practices, and in operating rooms.

Wardell and Weymouth (2004) did a systematic review of studies using Healing Touch with chronically ill patients. In their review of the literature on Healing Touch, Wardell and Weymouth (2004) categorized studies by disease or disorder. Nine of the studies of Healing Touch used the modality for chronic pain relief; three studies used Healing Touch with cancer patients for functional status, well-being, mood, fatigue, blood pressure, and pain; four studies used Healing Touch to improve immune system functioning; three used the modality on patients who had had cardiovascular procedures or were critical ill with CV disease; five studies were with elderly dementia patients; four studies were with mentally ill patients (depression, PTSD, anxiety, chronically stressed); two were in theoretical areas, and one was in pediatrics (Wardell & Weymouth, 2004). Seven of the nine pain studies showed decreased pain with Healing Touch, and an eighth showed a decrease when reflexology and Healing Touch were used together. The cancer studies showed that both massage therapy and Healing Touch were more effective in reducing pain, fatigue, and blood pressure in chemotherapy patients than was Caring Presence or standard care alone. Among the elderly who received Healing Touch, compared to the control group, the intervention group improved significantly on all ten behavioral items (appetite, sleep, freedom from pain, orientation, compliance with daily routine, socialization, emotional stability, nonverbal responses, conversational communication, and freedom from jargon). Elderly dementia patients who were given Healing Touch three times a week for four weeks showed significant decreases in agitation. Outcomes from the studies with elderly adults were positive; the intervention groups showed enhanced appetite, improved sleep, and reduced pain; worry and outbursts were decreased. Functional ability and compliance with daily routines increased. The other areas studied had limited or inconclusive results.

In sum, Healing Touch is supported for use with older adults. Further study with larger sample sizes and rigorous methods is needed to replicate these finding, which show great promise for use of Healing Touch for pain relief, as an adjunctive therapy with cancer treatment, and with elderly patients suffering from dementia (Wardell & Weymouth, 2004).

SUMMARY: USE OF NON-PHARMACOLOGIC COMPLEMENTARY MODALITIES

In conclusion, the use of non-pharmacologic complementary modalities as an adjunctive treatment in chronic disease self-management can significantly enhance patients' quality of life, reduce symptoms, relieve stress, and give much-needed support. The main complementary modalities that have been shown to be effective with cancer and other chronic diseases are 1) mind-body techniques (yoga, meditation, relaxation techniques, qigong, and tai chi), 2) music therapy, 3) acupuncture, 4) diet and nutrition, 5) physical activity, and 6) massage therapy. Participation in complementary modalities must be done under the supervision of a physician. All complementary practitioners must have undergone special training to deal safely and effectively with a frail, sick, and aging patient population. Increasingly, complementary therapies are being offered by major medical centers through their own Integrative Medicine Institutes, which facilitates smooth coordination of care.

AGING AND CHRONIC DISEASE

In 2010, there were 40 million adults age 65 or over in the United States, accounting for 13% of the population (U.S. Census Bureau, 2010). By 2030, the adult population 65 and over is expected to grow to 72 million, or almost 20% of the total population (Federal Interagency Forum on Aging-Related Statistics, 2012). In *Older Americans 2012: Key Indicators of Well-Being,* the Federal Interagency Forum (Forum) on Aging-Related Statistics (2012) describes the condition of U.S. adults aged 65 and over using 37 indicators in the following five broad areas:

- Population
- Economics
- Health status
- Health risks and behaviors
- Health care

Three of the five areas involve health, which reflects the national concern over the skyrocketing costs of healthcare for an aging elderly population.

The report compiles data from more than a dozen federal agencies to construct broad indicators of well-being for adults 65 and over. The report forecasts increasing numbers of older women in the workforce, declining poverty rates, increasing housing problems, increasing obesity, and increasing use of hospice. A natural consequence of aging is a decline in the immune response, which renders a person more susceptible to disease (Panda et al., 2009). Almost half of all Americans have at least one chronic disease; 31.5% of Americans suffer from multiple chronic conditions (MCC) (Gerteis et al., 2014. Prevalence of MCC increases with age; 80% of adults 65 and over suffer from MCC. The healthcare costs of MCC are staggering; 71% of all healthcare spending in the U.S. goes towards treating people with MCC (Gerteis et al., 2014). Chronic diseases/health conditions for adults 65 and over in the United States are listed in Table 2.

The leading causes of death for Americans 65 and over in 2009 were heart disease, cancer, and chronic respiratory diseases, followed by stroke and Alzheimers Disease. From 1998 until 2006, stroke was the third leading cause of death, but it was surpassed in 2008 by chronic respiratory diseases and fell to fourth place. Deaths from Alzheimers disease climbed from 1998 to 2009, surpassing deaths from influenza/pneumonia and diabetes in 2003 to become the fifth leading cause of mortality for adults 65 and over (Federal Interagency Forum on Age-Related Statistics, 2012). Almost a quarter of adults 65 and over reported being in fair or poor health, and 13.7% reported suffering from clinical depression.

Dietary adequacy was assessed using 12 components from the total Healthy Eating Index-2005 score. The total score was 67 out of 100, or poor. The lowest ratings were for dark green and orange vegetables and legumes (36), whole grains (34), and sodium (33). Given the dietary recommendations for a Mediterranean diet low in sodium and high in vegetables, legumes, and whole grains, the diet was far from adequate (Federal Interagency Forum on Age-Related Statistics, 2012). Diet quality for adults aged 65 and over is shown in Table 3.

Although physical activity level for adults 65 and over increased from 1998 to 2010, it still was very low; only 5.5% of senior adults met the federal guidelines for physical activity (Federal Interagency Forum on Age-Related Statistics, 2012). Physical activity levels for adults 65 and over are shown in Table 4.

Table 2. Chronic health conditions: Percentage of people age 65 and over who reported having selected chronic health conditions, by sex and race and Hispanic origin, 2009–2010

	Heart Disease	Hyperten-sion	Stroke	Asthma	Chronic Bronchitis or Emphysema	Any Cancer	Diabetes	Arthritis
Total	30.4	55.9	8.6	11.3	10.3	24.0	20.5	51.2
Men	36.9	54.1	9.1	9.7	9.6	27.6	23.5	44.8
Women	25.5	57.2	8.2	12.5	10.8	21.2	18.2	56.1
Non-Hispanic White	32.1	54.2	8.5	11.3	10.9	26.9	18.0	52.6
Non-Hispanic Black	25.1	69.2	11.7	11.5	8.4	13.9	31.6	51.0
Hispanic	22.2	57.2	7.2	11.1	7.1	10.4	32.5	43.8

Note: Data are based on a 2-year average from 2009-2010. See data sources for the definition of race and Hispanic origin in the National Health Interview Survey.

Source: Federal Interagency Forum on Age-Related Statistics (compiled from CDC, National Center for Health Statistics, National Health Interview Survey).

Table 3. Diet quality: Average diet scores, population age 65 and over, by age group, 2007–2008

	Age		
	65 and Under	65-74	75 and Over
Total Healthy Eating Index-2005 Score	67	66	67
Adequacy components			
Total fruit	90	86	94
Whole fruit	100	100	100
Total vegetables	84	86	82
Dark green and orange vegetables and legumes	36	36	35
Total grains	100	100	100
Whole grains	34	32	37
Milk	60	58	63
Meat and beans	100	100	100
Oils	75	77	73
Moderation components			
Saturated fat	60	59	63
Sodium	33	32	35
Solid fats, alcoholic beverages, added sugar	59	59	59

Note: The Healthy Eating Index-2005 (HEI-2005) has 12 components, and a higher score indicates a higher quality diet. The moderation components (e.g., sodium) are scored in reverse; i.e., excessively high intakes get 0 percent and as intakes decrease towards the standard, scores increase up to 100 percent.

Reference population: These data refer to the resident noninstitutionalized population.

Source: Federal Interagency Forum for Age-Related Statistics (compiled from multiple agencies).

Table 4. Percentage of people age 45 and over who reported participating in leisure-time aerobic and muscle-strengthening activities that meet the 2008 Federal physical activity guidelines, by age group, 1998–2010.

Year	45-64	65	65-74	75-84	85 and Over
1998	11.4	5.5	7.0	3.9	2.0
1999	11.9	5.9	7.7	4.5	0.9
2000	12.8	6.9	8.4	5.7	1.9
2001	13.1	6.7	7.7	6.1	3.1
2002	14.2	7.1	8.8	5.8	2.1
2003	14.6	7.6	9.2	6.7	2.9
2004	14.0	7.8	9.7	6.4	3.5
2005	14.4	7.9	10.5	5.7	3.0
2006	13.8	7.5	9.1	6.5	3.0
2007	15.0	7.9	9.5	6.6	4.1
2008	16.3	9.5	11.3	9.3	2.3
2009	16.9	10.0	12.8	7.9	2.8
2010	17.8	10.5	13.6	7.3	4.0

Note: The measure reflects the 2008 Federal Physical Activity Guidelines for Americans to perform 1) at least 150 minutes a week of moderate-intensity or 75 minutes a week of vigorous-intensity aerobic physical activity, and 2) moderate- to high-intensity muscle-strengthening activities for major muscle groups at least two days a week. The measure shows the percentage who met both guidelines.

Reference population: These data refer to the resident noninstitutionalized population.

Source: Federal Interagency Forum on Age-Related Statistics (compiled from CDC, National Center for Health Statistics, National Health Interview Survey).

IMPLICATIONS FOR HEALTHY AGING

The population in the United States is aging. People are living longer, and many—especially women—are working longer. With most infectious diseases under control in the U.S. (STDs are an exception), disease management is largely about chronic conditions. People's expectations have changed, too. Television commercials advertise sexual aids for seniors, along with a host of products to make older adults feel, look, and act younger. Healthy Aging isn't about cosmetic surgery and botox, however; it is about adopting healthy lifestyle habits, especially making healthy dietary choices, exercising regularly, avoiding tobacco, and practicing stress management. Depression, anxiety, fear, and feelings of helplessness often follow a diagnosis of a chronic disease such as cancer or COPD. Complementary therapies such as yoga, meditation, qigong, tai chi, and relaxation techniques can be helpful in reducing negative affect and distress, and in enhancing feelings of well-being. Massage therapy (including Healing Hands), acupuncture, and qigong can provide effective non-pharmacologic pain relief.

It is estimated that one-third of Americans—about 100 million people—experience chronic pain, and 5 to 8 million of them treat it with opioid drugs (National Institute on Drug Abuse, 2015). Opioids are highly addictive, and opioid abuse is rampant. In 2012, more than 259 million prescriptions were written in the U.S. for opioid painkillers such as Vicodin and OxyContin. That amounts to one bottle of pain pills for every U.S. adult. In 2011, 17,000 people died from prescription painkiller overdoses (National Institute on Drug Abuse, 2015). There is a safe, healthy alternative to opioids for pain. Research has shown that use of complementary modalities such as acupuncture, massage therapy, qigong, and music therapy aid in pain relief and should be incorporated into disease management plans for patients who experience chronic pain. Even medically fragile seniors can benefit from music therapy and Healing Hands, or learn MBSR or Benson's relaxation technique; none of these modalities requires physical strength or agility.

When assessing an older patient for a disease management plan, the CDSMP model is useful; it has been effective with both physical and mental health conditions. An integrative approach that incorporates evidence-based non-pharmacologic complementary modalities has been found to improve health outcomes. In our high-tech age, with new drugs coming out every few months, it is tempting to rely on medication as the first and primary defense against chronic disease. Even the most effective medications have some side effects, especially after long-term use. It is wise to keep in mind the old medical dictum, "To do no harm." It might take a little longer to train a patient to learn MBSR or a Benson relaxation technique than it does to pop a pill, but in the end, it is worth the effort. It saves money and reduces potential harm to the patient.

CONCLUSION

Disease is a function of interaction among three entities—host, agent, and environment. Self-management of chronic diseases deals primarily with the host and the environment. For example, to manage the host (mind-body), a patient with T2DM follows a healthy low-fat, low-sodium, non-AGE diet, exercises moderately, avoids tobacco and alcohol, and monitors blood sugar and insulin therapy, all under physician supervision. To manage the environment, a person suffering from asthma or COPD avoid triggers such as pet dander or industrial pollutants that might provoke an exacerbation. Self-management of chronic diseases is a growing concern for both patients and healthcare providers. The CDSMP model reminds us that "one size does not fit all." A detailed needs assessment of each group and topic is recommended to help the supervising physician tailor the CDSMP for each patient. The problem-solving model of CDSMP is useful in identifying the underlying issue that is bothering the patient. After identifying the issue, the provider can help the patient to make decisions about daily activities, such as how much exercise is enough for a given session, or whether a pain in the lumbar spine is a severe enough to call the doctor. The patient and doctor form a partnership, or management team. The doctor provides the patient with knowledge about his or her conditions and steers the patient toward resources to support self-management.

To persevere at self-management, patients need to believe in themselves and their ability to take care of the multi-faceted job of management, including following dietary and exercise recommendations, avoiding tobacco, and practicing some form of relaxation, meditation, or stress-reduction technique to deal with the emotional toll of living with a chronic disease. This self-efficacy should be coupled with a positive psychology outlook that sees things from an optimistic point of view.

There are many medical and complementary therapy websites that offer patients free information on their specific conditions. *Caveat emptor* (buyer beware) of infomercials that are selling supplements, not health promotion. Major medical centers and research studies recommend sticking to safe, evidence-based complementary modalities. Before using any complementary modality, patients should ask their supervising doctor about it to make sure that it is safe and appropriate. Alternative treatments may be harmful, interacting with medical treatments.

The last century saw enormous medical advances, with the life expectancy increasing 60%, the development of antibiotics, organ transplants, and artificial limbs. Who knows what the next century will bring? We may see paralyzed patients walk, artificial skin on burn victims, and a life expectancy of 120 years. Health-related quality of life should to continue to improve in the U.S. thanks to the information revolution on the Internet and social media, advances in medical technology and electronic record-keeping, and proactive patient self-management of health conditions.

REFERENCES

Agarwal, M., Dalal, A., Agarwal, D., & Agarwal, R. (1995). Positive life orientation and recovery from myocardial infarction. *Social Science & Medicine*, *40*(1), 125–130. doi:10.1016/0277-9536(94)E0058-Z PMID:7899916

Allen, K., Golden, L. H., Izzo, J. L. Jr, Ching, M. I., Forrest, A., Niles, C. R., & Barlow, J. C. et al. (2001). Normalization of hypertensive responses during ambulatory surgical stress by perioperative music. *Psychosomatic Medicine*, *63*(3), 487–492. doi:10.1097/00006842-200105000-00019 PMID:11382277

American Diabetes Association. (2015). Making healthy food choices. Retrieved from: http://www.diabetes.org/food-and-fitness/food/what-can-i-eat/making-healthy-food-choices/?loc=ff-slabnav

American Heart Association. (2015). Prevention and treatment of high blood pressure. Retrieved from: www.heart.org/HEARTORG/Conditions/HighBloodPressure/PreventionTreatmentofHighBloodPressure

American Music Therapy Association (AMTA). (2015). About Music Therapy & AMTA. Silver Spring, MD: AMTA. Retrieved from http://www.musictherapy.org/about/musictherapy/

Americans with Disabilities Act (ADA). (1990). Washington, D.C.: U.S. Department of Justice.

Ángeles Ruiz, M.; Sanjuan, P.; Pérez-García, A.M.; Rueda, B.& (2011). Relations between life satisfaction, adjustment to illness, and emotional distress in a sample of men with ischemic cardiopathy. *Spanish Journal of Psychology*, 14(1), 356.

Anh, S., Basu, R., Smith, M. L., Jiang, L., Lorig, K., Whitelaw, N., & Ory, M. G. (2013). The impact of chronic disease self-management programs: Healthcare savings through a community-based intervention. *BMC Public Health*, *13*(1), 1141. doi:10.1186/1471-2458-13-1141 PMID:24314032

Appel, L.J., Moore, T.J., Obarzanek, E., Vollmer, W.M., Svetkey, L.P., Sacks, F.M., Bray, G.A., Vogt, T.M., Cutler, J.A., & Windhauser, M.M., Lin-P-H, & Karanja, N. (1997). A clinical trial of the effects of dietary patterns on blood pressure. *N ENlg. Journal of Medicine*, *336*, 1117–1124.

Bandura, A. (1977). Self-efficacy: Toward a unifying theory of behavioral change. *Psychological Review*, *84*(2), 191–215. doi:10.1037/0033-295X.84.2.191 PMID:847061

Bandura, A. (1982). Self-efficacy mechanism in human agency. *The American Psychologist*, *37*(2), 122–147. doi:10.1037/0003-066X.37.2.122

Bandura, A. (1989). Human agency in social cognitive theory. *The American Psychologist*, *44*(9), 1175–1184. doi:10.1037/0003-066X.44.9.1175 PMID:2782727

Bandura, A. (1991). Social-cognitive theory of self-regulation. *Organizational Behavior and Human Decision Processes*, *50*(2), 179–211. doi:10.1016/0749-5978(91)90022-L

Bao, T. (2014). Integrative oncology: 65+ workshop. Treating symptoms & improving well- being. Memorial Sloan Kettering Cancer Center. Retrieved from: https://www.mskcc.org/cancer-care/treatments/symptom-management/integrative- medicine.

Barasch, M. I. (1994). The amazing power of visualization. *Natural Health*, *24*(4), 64.

Benson, H., & Klipper, M. (1975/2001). *The relaxation response*. New York: HarperCollins.

Benson, H., & Proctor, W. (2010). *Relaxation revolution: Enhancing your personal health through the science and genetics of mind body healing*. New York: Scribner.

Benson, H., Rosner, B. A., Marzetta, B. R., & Klemchuk, H. M. (1974). Decreased blood pressure in pharmacologically treated hypertensive patients who regularly elicited the relaxation response. *Lancet*, *303*(7852), 289–291. doi:10.1016/S0140-6736(74)92596-3 PMID:4130474

Blumenthal, J. A., Babyak, M. A., Hinderliter, A., Watkins, L. L., Craighead, L., Lin, P.-H., & Sherwood, A. et al. (2010). Effects of the DASH diet alone and in combination with exercise and weight loss on blood pressure and cardiovascular biomarkers in men and women with high blood pressure: The ENCORE study. *Archives of Internal Medicine*, *170*(2), 126–135. doi:10.1001/archinternmed.2009.470 PMID:20101007

Bongo therapy. (2011). *Einstein: The Magazine for Alumni and Friends of Albert Einstein College of Medicine.* Summer/fall, 9. Retrieved from https://www.einstein.yu.edu/docs/publications/einstein-magazine/einstein-magazine-summer-fall-2011.pdf

Brown, K. W., & Ryan, R. M. (2003). The benefits of being present: Mindfulness and its role in psychological well-being. *Journal of Personality and Social Psychology*, *84*(4), 822–848. doi:10.1037/0022-3514.84.4.822 PMID:12703651

Brownson, R. C., Chang, J. C., Davis, J. R., & Smith, C. A. (1991). Physical activity on the job and cancer in Missouri. *American Journal of Public Health*, *81*(5), 639–642. doi:10.2105/AJPH.81.5.639 PMID:2014869

Buffart, L. M., van Uffelen, J. G., Riphagen, B. J., & Brown, W. J. (2012). Physical and psychosocial benefits of yoga in cancer patients and survivors, a systematic review and meta-analysis of randomized controlled trials. *BMC Cancer*, *12*(1), 559. doi:10.1186/1471-2407-12-559 PMID:23181734

Calenda, E. (2006). Massage therapy for cancer pain. *Current Pain and Headache Reports*, *10*(4), 270–274. doi:10.1007/s11916-006-0031-1 PMID:16834941

Camacho, T. C., Roberts, R. E., Lazarus, N. B., Kaplan, G. A., & Cohen, R. D. (1991). Physical activity and depression: Evidence from the Alameda County Study. *American Journal of Epidemiology*, *134*, 220–231. PMID:1862805

Carney, C. P., & Jones, L. E. (2006). Medical comorbidity in women and men with bipolar disorders: A population-based controlled study. *Psychosomatic Medicine*, *68*(5), 684–691. doi:10.1097/01.psy.0000237316.09601.88 PMID:17012521

Carney, C. P., Jones, L. E., & Woolson, R. F. (2006). Medical comorbidity in women and men with schizophrenia: A population-based controlled study. *Journal of General Internal Medicine*, *21*(11), 1133–1137. doi:10.1111/j.1525-1497.2006.00563.x PMID:17026726

Carver, C., Pozo, C., Harris, S., Noriega, V., Scheier, M., Robinson, D., & Clark, K. et al. (1993). How coping mediates the effect of optimism on distress: A study of women with early stage breast cancer. *Journal of Personality and Social Psychology*, *65*(2), 375–390. doi:10.1037/0022-3514.65.2.375 PMID:8366426

Cassileth, B. R. (2011). Green Tea (Camellia sinensis). *Oncology (Williston Park)*, *14*, 1432–1433. PMID:22329195

Cassileth, B. R., & Vickers, A. J. (2004). Massage therapy for symptom control: Outcome study at a major cancer center. *Journal of Pain and Symptom Management*, *28*(3), 244–249.

Centers for Disease Control and Prevention. (2000). *Measuring healthy days: Population assessment of health-related quality of life*. Atlanta, GA: Centers for Disease Control and Prevention.

Centers for Disease Control and Prevention. (2013). Death and Mortality. NCHS FastStats Web Site. Retrieved from: http://www.cdc.gov/nchs/fastats/deaths.htm

Centers for Disease Control and Prevention, National Center for Health Statistics. (2015). Underlying Cause of Death 1999-2013.

Chapman, B. P., Hampson, S., & Clarkin, J. (2014). Personality-informed interventions for healthy aging: Conclusions from a National Institute on Aging work group. *Developmental Psychology*, *50*(5), 1426–1441. doi:10.1037/a0034135 PMID:23978300

Chen, L.-C., Wang, T.-F., Shih, Y.-N., & Wu, L.-J. (2013). Fifteen-minute music intervention reduces pre-radiotherapy anxiety in oncology patients. *European Journal of Oncology Nursing*, *17*(4), 436–441. doi:10.1016/j.ejon.2012.11.002 PMID:23218591

Constantino, M. I., Molyneaux, L., Limacher-Gisler, F., Al-Saeed, A., Luo, C., Wu, T., & Wong, J. et al. (2013). Long-term complications and mortality in young-onset diabetes: Type 2 diabetes is more hazardous and lethal than type 1 diabetes. *Diabetes Care*, *36*(12), 3863–3869. doi:10.2337/dc12-2455 PMID:23846814

Cooperative Program Centers for Disease Control and Prevention. (2016). *Self-management education. CDC- recommended programs. Chronic Disease Self-Management Program (CDSMP).* Atlanta, GA: Centers for Disease Control and Prevention.

Corbin, J., & Strauss, A. (1988). *Unending work and care: Managing chronic illness at home.* San Francisco: Jossey-Bass.

Cramer, H., Lange, S., Klose, P., Paul, A., & Dobos, G. (2012a). Yoga for breast cancer patients and survivors: A systematic review and meta-analysis. *BMC Cancer, 12*(1), 412. doi:10.1186/1471-2407-12-412 PMID:22988934

Cramer, H., Lauche, R., Haller, H., & Dobos, G. (2013a). A Systematic review and meta- analysis of yoga for low back pain. *The Clinical Journal of Pain, 29*(5), 450–460. doi:10.1097/AJP.0b013e31825e1492 PMID:23246998

Cramer, H., Lauche, R., Klose, P., Langhorst, J., & Dobos, G. (2013b). Yoga for schizophrenia: A systematic review and meta-analysis. *BMC Psychiatry, 13*(1), 32. doi:10.1186/1471-244X-13-32 PMID:23327116

Cramer, H., Lauche, R., Paul, A., & Dobos, G. (2012b). Mindfulness-based stress reduction for breast cancer-a systematic review and meta-analysis. *Current Oncology (Toronto, Ont.), 19*(5), e343–e352. doi:10.3747/co.19.1016 PMID:23144582

Creer, T., Renne, C., & Christian, W. (1976). Behavioral contributions to rehabilitation and childhood asthma. *Rehabilitation Literature, 37*, 226–232, 247. PMID:959645

Deng, G., & Cassileth, B. R. (2014). *Integrative oncology: An overview. American Society of Clinical Oncology Education Book* (pp. 233–242). New York: Integrative Medicine Service, Memorial Sloan Kettering Cancer Center.

Dickinson, H. O., Mason, J. M., Nicolson, D. J., Campbell, F., Beyer, F. R., Cook, J. V., & Ford, G. A. et al. (2006). Lifestyle interventions to reduced raised blood pressure: A systematic review of randomized control trials. *Journal of Hypertension, 24*(2), 215–233. doi:10.1097/01.hjh.0000199800.72563.26 PMID:16508562

DiMeglio, L. (2013). Help yourself form healthy habits. Alexndria, VA: American Diabetes Association. Retrieved from http://www.diabetesforecast.org/2013/jul/help-yourself-form-healthy-habits.html

Druss, B. G., Zhao, L., von Esenwein, S. A., Bona, J. R., Fricks, L., Jenkins-Tucker, S., & Lorig, K. et al. (2010). The health and recovery peer (HARP) program: A peer-led intervention to improve medical self-management for persons with serious mental illness. *Schizophrenia Research, 118*(1-2), 264–270. doi:10.1016/j.schres.2010.01.026 PMID:20185272

Dunbar, J. (2015). Qigong Therapy. Magic Tortoise Taichiquan School. Retrieved from: http://www.magictortoise.com/qigong_therapy.htm

Elmer, P. J., Obarzanek, E., Vollmer, W. M., Simons-Morton, D., Stevens, V. J., Young, D. R., & Svetkey, L. P. et al. (2006). Effects of Comprehensive lifestyle modification on diet, weight, physical fitness, and blood pressure control: 18-month results of a randomized trial. *Annals of Internal Medicine, 144*(7), 485–495. doi:10.7326/0003-4819-144-7-200604040-00007 PMID:16585662

Esch, T., Fricchione, G. L., & Stefano, G. B. (2003). The therapeutic use of the relaxation response in stress-related diseases. *Medical Science Monitor, 9*, RA23–RA34. PMID:12601303

Everett, B., Salamonson, Y., & Davidson, P.M. (2009). Bandura's exercise self-efficacy scale: Validation in an Austrian cardiac rehabilitation setting. *Int. J. Nurs. Stud., 46*(6), 824-829.

Ezzo, J., Vickers, A., & Richardson, M. A. (2005). Acupuncture-point stimulation for chemotherapy-induced nausea and vomiting. *Journal of Clinical Oncology, 23*(28), 7188–7198. doi:10.1200/JCO.2005.06.028 PMID:16192603

FAO/WHO. (1998). Carbohydrates in human nutrition. *FAO Food and Nutrition Paper*, 1998, 66.

Federal Interagency Forum on Aging-Related Statistics. (2012). *Older Americans 2012: Key indicators of well-being*. Washington, D.C.: U.S. Government Printing Office.

Foster, C., Hillsdon, M., Thorogood, M., Kaur, A., & Wedatilake, T. (2005). Interventions for promoting physical activity. *Cochrane Database of Systematic Reviews*, (1): CD003180. PMID:15674903

Fox, K. R. (1999). The influence of physical activity on mental well-being. *Public Health Nutrition, 2*(3a3A), 411–418. doi:10.1017/S1368980099000567 PMID:10610081

Fulton-Kehoe, D., Hamman, R. F., Baxter, J., & Marshall, J. (2001). A case-control study of physical activity and non-insulin dependent diabetes mellitus (NIDDM). The San Luis Valley Diabetes Study. *Annals of Epidemiology, 11*(5), 320–327. doi:10.1016/S1047-2797(01)00218-6 PMID:11399446

Galvin, J. A., Benson, H., Deckro, G. R., Fricchione, G. L., & Dusek, J. A. (2006). The relaxation response: Reducing stress and improving cognition in healthy aging adults. *Complementary Therapies in Clinical Practice, 12*(3), 186–191. doi:10.1016/j.ctcp.2006.02.004 PMID:16835029

Gerteis, J., Izrael, D., Deitz, D., LeRoy, L., Ricciardi, R., Miller, T., & Basu, J. (2014). *Multiple chronic condition chartbook: 2010 medical expenditure panel survey data*. Rockville, MD: Agency for Healthcare Research and Quality.

Giovannucci, E., Ascherio, A., Rimm, E. B., Colditz, G. A., Stampfer, M. J., & Willett, W. C. (1995). Physical activity, obesity, and risk for colon cancer and adenoma in men. *Annals of Internal Medicine, 122*(5), 327–334. doi:10.7326/0003-4819-122-5-199503010-00002 PMID:7847643

Good, M., Anderson, G. C., Stanton-Hicks, M., Grass, J. A., & Makii, M. (2002). Relaxation and music reduce pain after gynecologic surgery. *Pain Management Nursing, 3*(2), 61–70. doi:10.1053/jpmn.2002.123846 PMID:12050837

Gorelick, P. B., Sacco, R. L., Smith, D. B., Alberts, M., Mustone-Alexander, L., Rader, D., & Rhew, D. C. et al. (1999). Prevention of a first stroke: A review of guidelines and a multidisciplinary consensus statement from the National Stroke Association. *Journal of the American Medical Association*, *281*(12), 1112–1120. doi:10.1001/jama.281.12.1112 PMID:10188663

Hart, K. E., Turner, S. H., & Cardozo, S. R. (1987). Ongoing research. Stress, personality, coping and well-being: A four-wave longitudinal process study. *Personality and Individual Differences*, *8*(4), 591–593. doi:10.1016/0191-8869(87)90226-1

Healthy People 2020. (n. d.). Physical activity. Washington, D.C.: U.S. Department of Health & Human Services.

Hu, F. B., Manson, J. E., Stampfer, M. J., Colditz, G., Liu, S., Solomon, C. G., & Willett, W. C. (2001). Diet, lifestyle, and the risk of type 2 diabetes mellitus in women. *The New England Journal of Medicine*, *345*(11), 790–797. doi:10.1056/NEJMoa010492 PMID:11556298

Hu, F. B., Stampfer, M. J., Colditz, G. A., Ascherio, A., Rexrode, K. M., Willett, W. C., & Manson, J. E. (2000). Physical activity and risk of stroke in women. *Journal of the American Medical Association*, *283*(22), 2961–2967. doi:10.1001/jama.283.22.2961 PMID:10865274

Jaglal, S. B., Kreiger, N., & Darlington, G. (1993). Past and recent physical activity and risk of hip fracture. *American Journal of Epidemiology*, *138*, 107–118. PMID:8342529

Kallio, P., Kolehmainen, M., Laaksonen, D. E., Kekäläinen, J., Salopuro, T., Sivenius, K., & Uusitupa, M. et al. (2007). Dietary carbohydrate modification induces alterations in gene expression in abdominal subcutaneous adipose tissue in persons with the metabolic syndrome: The FUNGENUT Study. *The American Journal of Clinical Nutrition*, *85*, 1417–1427. PMID:17490981

Karadag, F., Ozcan, H., Eskin, M., Karul, A. B., Ceylan, E., Tufek, Y., & Cildag, O. (2008). Psychological distress in chronic obstructive pulmonary disease patients. *Stress and Health*, *24*(2), 115–122. doi:10.1002/smi.1178

Kelley, G. A., & Kelley, K. S. (2015). Meditative movement therapies and health-related quality- of-life in adults: A systematic review of meta-analyses. *PLoS ONE*, *10*(6), e129181. doi:10.1371/journal.pone.0129181 PMID:26053053

Kiecolt-Glaser, J. K., Christian, L., Preston, H., Houts, C. R., Malarkey, W. B., Emery, C. F., & Glaser, R. (2010). Stress, inflammation, and yoga practice. *Psychosomatic Medicine*, *72*(2), 113–121. doi:10.1097/PSY.0b013e3181cb9377 PMID:20064902

Kohrt, W. M., Snead, D. B., Slatopolsky, E., & Birge, S. J. Jr. (1995). Additive effects of weight- bearing exercise and estrogen on bone mineral density in older women. *Journal of Bone and Mineral Research*, *10*(9), 1303–1311. doi:10.1002/jbmr.5650100906 PMID:7502701

Laaksonen, D. E., Toppinen, L. K., Juntunen, K. S., Autio, K., Liukkonen, K. H., Poutanen, K. S., & Mykkänen, H. M. et al. (2005). Dietary carbohydrate modification enhances insulin secretion in persons with the metabolic syndrome. *The American Journal of Clinical Nutrition*, *82*, 1218–1227. PMID:16332654

Ledesma, D., & Kumano, H. (2009). Mindfulness-based stress reduction and cancer: A meta- analysis. *Psychooncology, 18,* 571-579. Leeds, A.R. (1979). The dietary management of diabetes in adults. *The Proceedings of the Nutrition Society*, *98*, 365–371.

Lenker, S. L., Lorig, K., & Gallagher, G. (1984). Reasons for the lack of association between changes in health behavior and improved health status: An exploratory study. *Patient Education and Counseling*, *6*(2), 69–72. doi:10.1016/0738-3991(84)90036-3 PMID:10268098

Lin, K. Y., Hu, Y. T., Chang, K. J., Lin, H. F., & Tsauo, J. Y. (2011). Effects of yoga on psychological health, quality of life, and physical health of patients with cancer: A meta- analysis. *Evidence-Based Complementary and Alternative Medicine*. PMID:21437197

Lopez, A. D., Shibuya, K., & Rao, C. (2006). Chronic obstructive pulmonary disease: Current burden and future projections. *The European Respiratory Journal*, *27*(2), 397–412. doi:10.1183/09031936.06.00025805 PMID:16452599

Lorig, K. R., Chastain, R. L., Ung, E., Shoor, E., & Holtman, H. R. (1989). Development and evaluation of a scale to measure perceived self-efficacy in people with arthritis. *Arthritis and Rheumatism*, *32*(1), 37–44. doi:10.1002/anr.1780320107 PMID:2912463

Lorig, K. R., & Holman, R. H. (2003). Self-management education: History, definition, outcomes, and mechanisms. *Annals of Behavioral Medicine*, *26*(1), 1–7. doi:10.1207/S15324796ABM2601_01 PMID:12867348

Lorig, K. R., Sobel, D. S., Stewart, A. L., Brown, B. W. Jr, Ritter, P. L., González, V. M., & Holman, H. R. et al. (1999). Evidence suggesting that a chronic disease self- management program can improve health status while reducing utilization and costs: A randomized trial. *Medical Care*, *37*(1), 5–14. doi:10.1097/00005650-199901000-00003 PMID:10413387

Lorig, K. R., Stewart, A. L., Gonzalez, V. M., Laurent, D. D., & Lynch, J. (1996). *Outcome Measures for Health Education and Other Health Care Interventions*. Thousand Oaks, CA: Sage Publications.

Magidson, J. F., Roberts, B. W., Collado-Rodriguez, A., & Lejuez, C. W. (2014). Theory driven intervention for changing personality: Expectancy value theory, behavioral activation, and conscientiousness. *Developmental Psychology*, *50*(5), 1442–1450. doi:10.1037/a0030583 PMID:23106844

Mathieu, R.A., Powell-Wiley, T.M., Ayers, C., McGuire, D.K., Khera, A., & Das, S.R., & Lakoski, S. G. (2012). Physical activity participation, health perceptions, and cardiovascular disease mortality in a multiethnic population: The Dallas Heart Study. *American Heart Journal*, *163*(6), 1037–1040. doi:10.1016/j.ahj.2012.03.005 PMID:22709758

McDermott, M. S., & While, A. E. (2013). Maximizing the healthcare environment: A systematic review exploring the potential of computer technology to promote self-management of chronic illness in healthcare settings. *Patient Education and Counseling*, *92*(1), 13–22. doi:10.1016/j.pec.2013.02.014 PMID:23566427

Melchior, M. A., Seff, L. R., Albatineh, A. N., McCoy, H. V., Page, T. F., & Palmer, R. C. (2014). Intermediate outcomes of chronic disease self-management program offered by members of the Healthy Aging Regional Collaborative in South Florida. *Research on Aging*, *36*(4), 431–449. doi:10.1177/0164027513500054 PMID:25651315

Memorial Sloan Kettering Cancer Center (MSKCC) Bendheim Integrative Medicine Center. (2015). Nutritional and dietary-supplement counseling. Retrieved from: https://www.mskcc.org/locations/bendheim-integrative-medicine

Memorial Sloan Kettering Cancer Center (MSKCC) Integrative Medicine. (2015). About herbs, botanicals, and other products. Retrieved from https://www.mskcc.org/cancer-care/treatments/symptom-management/integrative-medicine/expertise

Mentgen, J. (2002). Healing touch. *The Nursing Clinics of North America*, *36*(1), 143–157.

Meyer, H.E., Tverdal, A., & Falch, J.A. (1993). Risk factors for hip fracture in middle-aged Norwegian women and men. *American Journal of Epidemiology*, *137*, 1203–1211.

Michel, A., Bosch, C., & Rexroth, M. (2014). Mindfulness as a cognitive-emotional segmentation strategy: An intervention promoting work-life balance. *Journal of Occupational and Organizational Psychology*, *87*(4), 733–754. doi:10.1111/joop.12072

Miner, W. (2007). Training massage therapists to work in oncology. *Journal of the Society for Integrative Oncology*, *5*(4), 163–166. doi:10.2310/7200.2007.015 PMID:19087760

Mirmiran, P., Bahadoran, Z., & Azizi, F. (2014). Functional foods-based diet as a novel dietary approach for management of type 2 diabetes and its complications: A review. *World J. Diabetes*, *5*(3), 267–281. doi:10.4239/wjd.v5.i3.267 PMID:24936248

Moadel, A. (2010). Einstein on Cancer: Dr. Alyson Moadel. Psychosocial oncology: Coping with cancer. Bronx, NY: Albert Einstein College of Medicine. Retrieved from http://www.einstein.yu.edu/video/?VID=259#top

Moadel, A. B., Shah, C., & Sisco, R. (2009). Description of the Yoga-based Cancer Rehabilitation Program of the Montefiore-Einstein Cancer Center. Retrieved from: https://www.einstein.yu.edu/docs/faculty/profiles/479-alyson-moadel/integral-hatha-yoga-protocol-description-MECC-rehab-ca-pgm.pdf

Mroczek, D. (2014). Personality plasticity, healthy aging, and interventions. *Developmental Psychology*, *50*(5), 1470–1474. doi:10.1037/a0036028 PMID:24773109

Murray, C. J. L., & Lopez, A. D. (1997). Alternative projections of mortality and disability by cause 1990-2020; Global Burden of Disease Study. *Lancet*, *349*(9064), 1498–1504. doi:10.1016/S0140-6736(96)07492-2 PMID:9167458

National Heart, Lung, and Blood Institute. (2015). Description of the DASH eating plan. National Institutes of Health. U.S. Department of Health & Human Services. Retrieved from http://www.nhlbi.nih.gov/health/health-topics/topics/dash/

National Institute on Drug Abuse (NIDA). (2015). *DrugFacts: Prescription and over-the-counter medications*. Washington, D.C.: National Institute of Health.

Neithercott, T. (2014). A Mediterranean food plan can protect health. Diabetes Forecast: The Healthy Living Magazine. Alexandria, VA: American Diabetes Association. Retrieved from http://www.diabetesforecast.org/2014/08-aug/a-mediterranean-food-plan-can.html?loc=ymal

Ogden, C. L., Carroll, M. D., Kit, B. K., & Flegal, K. M. (2014). Prevalence of Childhood and Adult Obesity in the United States, 2011-2012. *Journal of the American Medical Association*, *311*(8), 806–814. doi:10.1001/jama.2014.732 PMID:24570244

Ory, M. G., Anh, S. N., Jiang, L., Lorig, K., Ritter, P., Laurent, D. D., & Smith, M. L. et al. (2013). National Study of Chronic Disease Self-Management: Six-Month Outcome Findings. *Journal of Aging and Health*, *25*(7), 1258–1274. doi:10.1177/0898264313502531 PMID:24029414

Pan, L., Yan, J., Guo, Y., & Yan, J. (2013). Effects of Tai Chi training on exercise capacity an quality of life in patients with chronic heart failure: A meta-analysis. *European Journal of Heart Failure*, *15*(3), 316–323. PMID:23099355

Panda, A., Arjona, A., Sapey, E., Bai, F., Fikrig, E., Montgomery, R. R., & Shaw, A. C. et al. (2009). Human innate immunosenescence: Causes and consequences for immunity in old age. *Trends in Immunology*, *30*(7), 325–333. doi:10.1016/j.it.2009.05.004 PMID:19541535

Parks, J., & Svedsen, D. (2006). *Morbidity and mortality in people with serious mental illness*. Alexandria, VA: National Association of State Mental Health Program Directors.

Pauwels, R. A., Buist, A. S., Calverley, P. M. A., Jenkins, C. R., & Hurd, S. S. (2001). Global strategy for the diagnosis, management, and prevention of chronic obstructive pulmonary disease: National Heart Lung and Blood Institute and World Health Organization Global Initiative for Chronic Obstructive Lung Disease (GOLD): executive summary. *Respiratory Care*, *46*(8), 798–825. PMID:11463370

Peters, R. K., Benson, H., & Peters, J. M. (1977). Daily relaxation response breaks in a working population: 2. Blood pressure. *American Journal of Public Health*, *67*(10), 954–959. doi:10.2105/AJPH.67.10.954 PMID:333958

Pfohl, M., & Schatz, H. (2001). Strategies for the prevention of type 2 diabetes. *Experimental and Clinical Endocrinology & Diabetes*, *109*(Suppl. 2), S240–S249. doi:10.1055/s-2001-18585 PMID:11460574

Piet, J., Wurtzen, H., & Zachariae, R. (2012). The effect of mindfulness-based therapy on symptoms of anxiety and depression in adult cancer patients and survivors: A systematic review and meta-analysis. *Journal of Consulting and Clinical Psychology*, *80*(6), 1007–1020. doi:10.1037/a0028329 PMID:22563637

Pimouguet, C., LeGoff, M., Thiebaut, R., Dartigues, J.F., & Helmer, C. (2011). Effectiveness of disease-management programs for improving diabetes care: A meta-analysis. *Canadian Medical Association Journal, 183(2)*, E115.

Prasad, K., Sharma, V., Lackore, K., Sarah, M., Jenkins, S. M., Prasad, A., & Sood, A. (2010). Use of complementary therapies in cardiovascular disease. *The American Journal of Cardiology*, *111*(3), 339–345. doi:10.1016/j.amjcard.2012.10.010 PMID:23186602

Racine, E., Troyer, J. L., Warren-Findlow, J., & McCauley, W. J. (2011). The effect of medical nutrition therapy on changes in dietary knowledge and DASH diet adherence in older adults with cardiovascular disease. *The Journal of Nutrition, Health & Aging*, *15*(10), 868–876. doi:10.1007/s12603-011-0102-9 PMID:22159775

Reig-Ferrer, A., Ferrer-Cascales, R., Santos-Ruiz, A., Campos-Ferrer, A., Prieto-Seva, A., Velasco-Ruiz, I., & Albaladejo-Blazquez, N. et al. (2014). A relaxation techniques enhances psychological well-being and immune parameters in elderly people from a nursing home: A randomized controlled study. *BMC Complementary and Alternative Medicine*, *14*(1), 311. doi:10.1186/1472-6882-14-311 PMID:25151398

Rosén, L. A., Silva, L. O., Andersson, U. K., Holm, C., Ostman, E. M., & Björck, I. M. (2009). Endosperm and whole grain rye breads are characterized by low post-prandial insulin response and a beneficial blood glucose profile. *Nutrition Journal*, *8*(1), 42. doi:10.1186/1475-2891-8-42 PMID:19781071

Salamon, E., Bernstein, S. R., Kim, S. A., Kim, M., & Stefano, G. B. (2003). The effects of auditory perception and musical preference on anxiety in naïve human subjects. *Medical Science Monitor*, *9*, R396–CR399. PMID:12960929

Santaguida, P. L., Balion, C., Hunt, D., Morrison, K., Gerstein, H., Raina, P., & Yazdi, H. et al. (2005). Diagnosis, prognosis, and treatment of impaired glucose tolerance and impaired fasting glucose. *Evidence Report/Technology Assessment (Summary)*, 128,1–11. PMID:16194123

Scheier, M., Matthews, J., Owens, J., Magovern, G., Lefebvre, R., Abbott, R., & Carver, C. (1989). Dispositional optimism and recovery from coronary artery bypass surgery: The beneficial effects on physical and psychological well-being. *Journal of Personality and Social Psychology*, *57*(6), 1024–1040. doi:10.1037/0022-3514.57.6.1024 PMID:2614656

Seligman, M. E. P. (2011). *Flourish: A visionary new understanding of happiness and well- being*. New York: Simon and Schuster.

Seligman, M. E. P. (2015). Authentic happiness. University of Pennsylvania Positive Psychology Center. Retrieved from https://www.authentichappiness.sas.upenn.edu/content/about-us

Seligman, M. E. P., & Csikszentmihalyi, M. (2000). Positive psychology: An introduction. *The American Psychologist*, *55*(1), 5–14. doi:10.1037/0003-066X.55.1.5 PMID:11392865

Sesso, H. D., Paffenbarger, R. S. Jr, & Lee, I. M. (2000). Physical activity and coronary heart disease in men: The Harvard Alumni Health Study. *Circulation*, *102*(9), 975–980. doi:10.1161/01.CIR.102.9.975 PMID:10961960

Shakespeare, W. (1602/1623). Twelfth Night, Act 1, scene 1, 1-3. First Folio. British Library.

Shen, R. L., Cai, F. L., Dong, J. L., & Hu, X. Z. (2011). Hypoglycemic effects and biochemical mechanisms of oat products on streptozotocin-induced diabetic mice. *Journal of Agricultural and Food Chemistry*, *59*(16), 8895–8900. doi:10.1021/jf200678q PMID:21749041

Shennan, C., Payne, S., & Fenlon, D. (2011). What is the evidence for the use of mindfulness- based interventions in cancer care? A review. *Psycho-Oncology*, *20*(7), 681–697. doi:10.1002/pon.1819 PMID:20690112

Shneerson, C., Taskila, T., Gale, N., Greenfield, S., & Chen, Y. F. (2013). The effect of complementary and alternative medicine on the quality of life of cancer survivors: A systematic review and meta-analyses. *Complementary Therapies in Medicine*, *21*(4), 417–429. doi:10.1016/j.ctim.2013.05.003 PMID:23876573

Sokal, J., Dickerson, F. B., Kreyenbuhl, J., Brown, C. H., Goldberg, R. W., & Dixon, L. B. (2004). Comorbidity of medical illnesses among adults with serious mental illness who are receiving community psychiatric services. *The Journal of Nervous and Mental Disease*, *192*(6), 421–427. doi:10.1097/01.nmd.0000130135.78017.96 PMID:15167405

Spurlock, M. (Writer & Dir.). (2004). *Supersize Me*.

Stanczyk, M. M. (2011). Music therapy in supportive cancer care. *Reports of Practical Oncology and Radiotherapy*, *16*(5), 170–172. doi:10.1016/j.rpor.2011.04.005 PMID:24376975

Stanton, A., Revenson, T., & Tennen, H. (2007). Health psychology: Psychological adjustment to chronic disease. *Annual Review of Psychology*, *58*(1), 565–592. doi:10.1146/annurev.psych.58.110405.085615 PMID:16930096

U.S. Census Bureau. (2010). Facts for features: Older Americans month. May 2010. Retrieved from http://www.census.gov/newsroom/releases/pdf/cb10-ff06.pdf

Venn, B. J., & Mann, J. I. (2004). Review: Cereal grains, legumes, and diabetes. *European Journal of Clinical Nutrition*, *58*(11), 1443–1451. doi:10.1038/sj.ejcn.1601995 PMID:15162131

Verwey, R., van der Weegen, S., Spreeuwenberg, M., Tange, H., van der Weijden, T., & de Witte, L. (2014a). A monitoring and feedback tool embedded in a counseling protocol to increase physical activity of patients with COPD or type 2 diabetes in primary care: Study protocol of a three-arm cluster randomized controlled trial. *BMC Family Practice*, *15*(1), 93. doi:10.1186/1471-2296-15-93 PMID:24885096

Verwey, R., van der Weegen, S., Tange, H., Spreeuwenberg, M., van der Weijden, T., & de Witte, L. (2014b). A pilot study of a tool to stimulate physical activity in patients with COPD or type 2 diabetes in primary care. *Journal of Telemedicine and Telecare*, *20*(1), 29–34. doi:10.1177/1357633X13519057 PMID:24414397

Vickers, A. J., Cronin, A. M., Maschino, A. C., Lewith, G., MacPherson, H., Foster, N. E., & Linde, K. et al. (2012). Acupuncture for chronic pain: Individual patient data meta-analysis. *Archives of Internal Medicine*, *172*(19), 1444–1453. doi:10.1001/archinternmed.2012.3654 PMID:22965186

Vickers, A. J., & Linde, K. (2014). Acupuncture for chronic pain. *Journal of the American Medical Association*, *311*(9), 955–956. doi:10.1001/jama.2013.285478 PMID:24595780

Volpato, E., Banfi, P., Rogers, S. M., & Pagnini, F. (2015). Relaxation techniques for people with chronic obstructive pulmonary disease: A systematic review and a meta-analysis. *Evidence-Based Complementary and Alternative Medicine*, *2015*, 1–22. doi:10.1155/2015/628365 PMID:26339268

Wang, F., Man, J. K., Lee, E. K., Wu, T., Benson, H., & Fricchione, G. L. (2013). The effects of qigong on anxiety, depression, and psychological well-being: A systematic review and meta-analysis. *Evidence-Based Complementary and Alternative Medicine*. PMID:23401706

Wannamethee, S. G., & Shaper, A. G. (1999). Physical activity and the prevention of stroke. *Journal of Cardiovascular Risk*, *6*(4), 213–216. doi:10.1177/204748739900600404 PMID:10501271

Wannamethee, S. G., & Shaper, A. G. (2001). Physical activity in the prevention of cardiovascular disease: An epidemiological perspective. *Sports Medicine (Auckland, N.Z.)*, *31*(2), 101–114. doi:10.2165/00007256-200131020-00003 PMID:11227978

Ward, B. W., Schiller, J. S., & Goodman, R. A. (2014). Multiple chronic conditions among US adults: A 2012 update. *Preventing Chronic Disease*, 2014, 11. PMID:24742395

Wardell, D. W., & Weymouth, K. F. (2004). Review of studies of Healing Touch. *Journal of Nursing Scholarship*, *36*(2), 147–154. doi:10.1111/j.1547-5069.2004.04012.x PMID:15227762

Weisenberger, J. (2014). Foods high in AGEs. Diabetes Forecast: The Healthy Living Magazine. Alexandria, VA: American Diabetes Association. Retrieved from http://www.diabetesforecast.org/2014/11-nov/foods-high-in-ages.html?loc=ymal

Weyerer, S. (1992). Physical inactivity and depression in the community. Evidence from the Upper Bavarian Field Study. *International Journal of Sports Medicine*, *13*(06), 492–496. doi:10.1055/s-2007-1021304 PMID:1428382

Yang, Y. C., Lu, F.-H., Wu, J.-S., Wu, C.-H., & Chang, C.-J. (2004). The protective effect of habitual tea consumption on hypertension. *Archives of Internal Medicine*, *164*(14), 1534–1540. doi:10.1001/archinte.164.14.1534 PMID:15277285

Zainal, N. Z., Booth, S., & Huppert, F. A. (2013). The efficacy of mindfulness-based stress reduction on mental health of breast cancer patients: A meta-analysis. *Psycho-Oncology*, *22*(7), 1457–1465. doi:10.1002/pon.3171 PMID:22961994

Zeng, Y., Luo, T., Xie, H., Huang, M., & Cheng, A. S. (2014). Health benefits of qigong or tai chi for cancer patients: A systematic review and meta-analyses. *Complementary Therapies in Medicine*, *22*(1), 173–186. doi:10.1016/j.ctim.2013.11.010 PMID:24559833

Zhang, J., Yang, K. H., Tian, J. H., & Wang, C. M. (2012). Effects of yoga on psychologic function and quality of life in women with breast cancer: A meta-analysis of randomized controlled trials. *Journal of Alternative and Complementary Medicine*, *18*(11), 994–1002. doi:10.1089/acm.2011.0514 PMID:22909345

Zimmerman, L., Pozehl, B., Duncan, K., & Schmitz, R. (1989). Effects of music in patients who had chronic cancer pain. *Western Journal of Nursing Research*, *11*(3), 298–309. doi:10.1177/019394598901100304 PMID:2750142

KEY TERMS AND DEFINITIONS

Alternative Medicine: If a non-mainstream healing or therapeutic practice is used in place of conventional medicine, it's considered "alternative."

Complementary Medicine: When a non-mainstream healing or therapeutic practice is used together with conventional medicine, it's considered "complementary."

DASH Diet: Dietary Approach to Stop Hypertension (DASH) diet. The Dash diet reduces intake of saturated fat, total fat, sodium, and cholesterol, increases intake of fruits and vegetables, and increases consumption of potassium, calcium, magnesium, fiber, and protein.

Integrative Medicine: Healing-oriented medicine that takes account of the whole person (body, mind, and spirit), including all aspects of lifestyle. It emphasizes the therapeutic relationship and makes use of all appropriate therapies, both conventional and complementary.

Positive Psychology: The scientific study of the strengths that enable individuals and communities to thrive, a branch of psychology whose aim is authentic happiness and flourishing.

Self-Efficacy: A person's belief that he or she can successfully execute a particular behavior to achieve a certain outcome.

Chapter 10
Stress and Its Relationship to Leadership and a Healthy Workplace Culture

David B. Ross
Nova Southeastern University, USA

Julie A. Exposito
Broward College, USA

Tom Kennedy
Nova Southeastern University, USA

ABSTRACT

Every organization needs to be driven by effective leaders. In higher education, many leadership courses are designed to transfer knowledge and critical thinking. Other professional development workshops, seminars, and conferences in leadership also offer leadership training and development to assist individuals to understand human capital, and create an organization free from toxicity. A toxic working environment can lead to low morale, disruption in productivity and motivation, high rate of absenteeism, individuals using sick days when they are not sick, cause emotional and physical health issues, and even submitting derailed projects beyond deadlines. When there is an upsurge of stress in the workplace within employees and administrators, the organization will struggle. Negative information dynamics affect health and contribute to stress. Stress management capacity is the ability to manage stress and is vital in the prevention of a negative impact of stress. Stress management can be improved for leaders and organizations.

INTRODUCTION

Stress impacts all levels of employees within an organization. Organizational stress is situational, based upon diverse perspectives of the employees and individuals who hold titled positions. Leaders in modern global organizations sustain increased levels of stress (Campbell, Baltes, Martin, & Meddings, 2007). Campbell, Baltes, Martin, and Meddings (2007) reported 88% of leaders indicated work is the main

DOI: 10.4018/978-1-5225-0640-9.ch010

cause of stress. High amount of stress can impact the ability to make good decisions and formulate sound judgments. When the stress response is triggered, cortisol is released into the blood, this elevated cortisol level is associated with impairments in a host of cognitive processes including decision making, memory, and attention (Dickerson & Kemeny, 2004). Decision making involves emotional intelligence (EI) since leading others involves human interaction (Doty & Fenlason, 2013); this interaction may lead to stressful conditions and affect productivity and morale levels.

Leadership is a broad term that more recently encompasses both intelligence quotient (IQ) and EI (Hendrickson, Lane, Harris, & Dorman, 2013). Emotional intelligence is the ability to read the emotions of others, adjust to situations, understand different perspectives, and build relationships with people (Doty & Fenlason, 2013). It is the responsibility of the organizational leadership to help others adjust to stressful situations by encouraging others to think creatively and preparing for the future by guiding towards personal and organizational change (Goffee & Jones, 2006; Goleman, 2004). The leaders who use a combination of analysis and intuition are better decision makers, therefore helping others to cope with organizational stress (Huang, 2012). Awareness of IQ and EI are important for leaders (Thompson, 2007, 2010; Yadav, 2014). Yadav (2014) claimed by EI, people within organizations can learn how to manage emotions to improve productivity. Counseling sessions and psychological development programs can help employees to better understand work-related behaviors (Yadav, 2014). In addition, courses that teach leadership and decision making through simulations can provide another avenue to help employees manage relevant working conditions within the organization, such as teamwork, productivity, and understanding the behavior of others (Thompson, 2010).

The plasticity of human brain and cognition continues through life; the human brain influences the way people process information (Zhou & Fischer, 2013). According to Thompson (2007), if a leader experiences stress, neurotransmitters and hormones are released and the leader may experience a short period of increased focus and reaction time. But if the stress exists for a long enough period of time, there will be negative consequences. Characteristics of these negative behaviors include (a) lack of listening, (b) over analysis, (c) failure to make decisions, and (d) erratic, fearful or angry emotional decisions. Thompson contended that the release of neurotransmitters and hormones affect the prefrontal cortex (PFC) and the amygdala. Successful leadership necessitates both the PFC and the amygdala. The PFC is associated with cognitive functions that control logic, analysis, and decision making. The amygdala is considered the emotional response to stimuli. High amounts of stress impair the function of the PFC, which results in decreased cognitive ability while the amygdala increases, resulting in a heightened emotional state. Leaders can experience temporary paralysis in their decision making and the inability to function as a leader (Thompson, 2007). Thompson measured a group of leaders under normal conditions and then under simulated stressful situations, and found a decrease in EI.

The two types of decision-making processes (i.e., emotional, cognitive) are impacted by different factors. Emotion-based decisions are affected by egocentric factors, but cognitive-based decisions are impacted by allocentric factors (Haas, Anderson, & Filkowski, 2015). The success of social relationships and survival is based on the ability to see the cause of another person's emotional reaction (Haas et al., 2015). Haas et al. (2015) conducted a study to investigate the behavioral and brain functions involved in emotion attribution decisions. Sixteen adults were given an Interpersonal Reactivity Index to note differences in making emotional and cognitive decisions. Then participants had a magnetic resonance imaging while making the emotion attribution decisions. The neuroimages indicated a dual process model during decision making. Higher scores of stress were associated with faster emotional decisions and increased anterior insula activity. On the other hand, lower scores of distress were associated with delayed emotion decision making and increased prefrontal cortex and premotor activity.

Research on socialcognitive neuroscience has extinguished outdated explanations of decision making in leadership. The current combination of intuitive and analytical approaches to decision making means a reassessment, development, and manangement of inituition at the workplace (Hodgkinson, Sadler-Smith, Burke, Claxton, & Sparrow, 2009). Changing work environments from technological advances and information processing capacities requires leaders to sort, interpret, and act in short amounts of time; this strategic competence uses dual-process theories of judgment and decision making. Intuitive judgment has been associated with quality and timeliness of decision making. Hodgkinson, Sadler-Smith, Burke, Claxton, and Sparrow (2009) admonished the dual-process theory should be a framework for management development and education programs. The conceptual knowledge stems from experience and expertise as much as insight, vision, and intuition. Hodgkinson et al. proposed a blend of conceptual and analytical knowledge with experiential knowledge. Formal leadership education should be aligned with professional development and practice accompanied with constructive feedback. Leaders should (a) acquire intuitive expertise, (b) develop self-awareness, (c) manage strategic decision making, and (d) create creative situations (Hodgkinson et al., 2009).

Riaz, Riaz, and Batool (2014) utilized a cross-sectional survey of 300 respondents to examine rational, intuitive, avoidant, dependent, and spontaneous style of decision making and the effects on individuals and organizations. Decision-making styles vary in efficacy and outcome on an individual and organizational level. Training of rational and intuitive decisions can achieve optimal individual and organizational results, and stress among employees can be utilized to promote innovative ideas. However, stress must be managed effectively (Edwards, Franco-Watkins, Cullen, Howell, & Acuff; 2014; Riaz, Riaz, & Batool, 2014; Thompson, 2010).

According to Edwards et al. (2014), it is unrealistic to remove stressors for improved decision making, job satisfaction, and job performance; stress is commonplace. Performance could be influenced by the perception of stress more than the actual stress; therefore, managing the perception of stress is more realistic than changing the situation. Stress management should include training people to view hindrances as challenges and adaptive strategies for controlling emotional reactions, focusing of tasks, and dealing with stressors. Also, providing resources and support can help employee morale.

WORKPLACE STRESS

A natural additive to stress in any environment is people. An increase of people involves more interactions and a greater potential for challenges that may increase levels of stress. People who are unclear on their roles and responsibilities while holding positions of importance could add stress to the organizational culture. These individuals are responsible for others to adhere to institutional policies and procedures. If they fail to follow these institutional guidelines, it can lead to occupational stress among others, low levels of motivation and performance, self-esteem, conflict among individuals, and low level of dedication (Shambrook, 2007; Welch, 2006), especially if not making enough money while working an increase of hours and trying to meet demands; these demands can be from clients, owners, students, supervisors, and other stakeholders. People bring stress from home and when they enter a stressful situation, everything is aspirated. Home environments, daily commutes with traffic delays, and organizational stress fuels a perfect storm. "People are not capable of separating work stress and their personal lives and that one's life was a filter through which work stress was strained" (Cameron, 2012, p. 15).

There are many aspects that will lead to an employee's stress level while employed at any organization. Cameron (2012) felt there are many aspects to occupational stress and stated "occupational stress is the negative physical and/or emotional responses that occur as a result of discrepancy between the expectations of the position and the capabilities of the worker resulting in diminishing health, illness, or injury" (p. 14). Administrators who create a hostile, abusive work environment can add an increase of stress by placing unrealistic goals on people. When administration creates a hostile environment, non-stop nagging, bullying and mobbing, this abusive behavior leads to emotional break down and mind games played on others. In addition, an administrator may hold grudges towards employees that stem from personal dislike, other unrelated personal reasons, or low self-esteem. Whether the employee is the right person for the position or any task performed by the employee; administration has been known to give false scores on the evaluation process of others (Davenport, Schwartz, & Elliott, 2005; Duffy & Sperry, 2014; Namie & Namie, 2003).

From an administrative point of view, employees are looked upon as individuals who can either add stress to the job or to add less stress by adding input and solutions to the organizational day-to-day issues (Katsapis, 2008). If employees are not performing properly it can also impact the supervisor's position; performance is key. This can be found in professional sports when a team does not perform well or win games, the coach's position is on the chopping block. This can align with a teacher who does not have increased students' scores. In addition, a principal and/or superintendent may suffer job security if in public scrutiny, especially with a superintendent who is mostly in an elected political position.

The concept of equal rank from employee to employee is another area that may add stress within the organization. Cameron (2012) commented that job characteristics can have a direct impact on satisfaction within the workplace. Personal factors and attitudes of others, although not consistent with one another, can cause job stress and a different belief in working conditions. Other employees can be jealous toward another person based on pay scales and/or having more responsibility than another person; favoritism and nepotism plays a big part in this area of creating a stressful and toxic culture.

Work place stress is generally defined as the physiological and psychological changes that occur in response to workplace environments that pose an appraised threat or challenge to the employee (Colligan & Higgins, 2005). It is important to have a general understanding of how stress influences one's physical and mental states in order to appreciate the profound impact stress has on an employee and on the overall workplace environment. A well-established model of stress that was first articulated by Lazarus in 1966 was more recently expanded by Magnusson (1996) and others to include biological factors. This model of stress incorporates how an individual appraises the complex, dynamic interplay between environmental demands (like those experienced in the workplace), and the individual and social resources an individual has to cope with these demands (Lazarus, 1966). The key to this biopsychosocial model of stress, is that an individual's interpretation of a threat is more important than the stressful event itself.

When a workplace event occurs that an individual's perceives (through perceptual, cognitive and emotional processes) as challenging or threatening a cascade of biological and physiological processes occur simultaneously as the amygdala communicates with the hypothalamus which stimulates adrenaline from the adrenal medulla (see Figure 1).

In the biopsychosocial model, the mind and body are conceptualized as interconnected and this connection is bidirectional. Factors that affect psychological, cognitive, emotional, social, and behavioral well-being affect physiological well-being and vice versa. For example, in response to a stressful situ-

Figure 1. Mind-body interaction. Environmental, psychological, behavioral, and social contextual factors, and the functioning of an individual in a specific situation
Magnusson (1996).

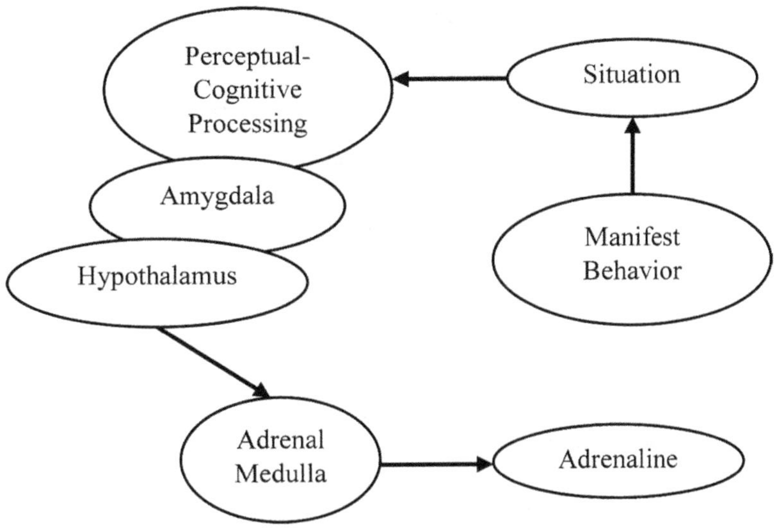

ation in the work place, an individual's heart rate and blood pressure may rise leading to anxiety, this anxiety may exacerbate the physical symptoms leading to angina. Thus, stress creates these negative feedback loops, with physical symptoms making psychological symptoms worse, in an unremitting cycle. Thoughts, feelings, attitudes, beliefs, behaviors and biology are interconnected in ways that can either (a) contribute to illness and job strain, or (b) potentiate health, productivity and well-being. All of these physical and emotional byproducts of stress have a profound influence on the individual and on the organization as a whole. Stress events in the workplace impact employees (physically and emotionally) and creates a more toxic environment, which in turn may lead to even more perceived threats by employees. This unrelenting cycle can be extremely damaging to an organization.

Stress theory provides a framework for investigating the psychological and physiological interactions inherent in the biopsychosocial model. An individual may experience what is considered good or bad stress in the workplace. Selye developed this idea of stress as a continuous variable from eustress (good stress) to distress (bad stress). Although good stress is important for employees to meet goals and work place productivity, distress can lead to poor performance, burnout, and general frustration (Buselli, 1999). Distress (the focus of this chapter) affects three major pathways in the body: (a) the physiological pathway, (b) the psychological pathway, and (c) the social-behavioral pathway. Distress occurs when an individual has a stress response to something in the workplace that they appraise as negative.

The stress response is triggered in the workplace when an employee perceives a situation to be a threat to the physical or emotional well-being and believes one's coping abilities are inadequate to deal effectively with the demand. The perception of threat to one's physical or psychological well-being in the workplace may generate a cascade of biochemical events originating in the central nervous system and affecting the entire body, specifically the muscular skeletal system (MSS), the autonomic nervous system (ANS), and the pituitary-neuroendocrine system (PNE) system (see Figure 2).

Figure 2. The stress response
Buselli (1999).

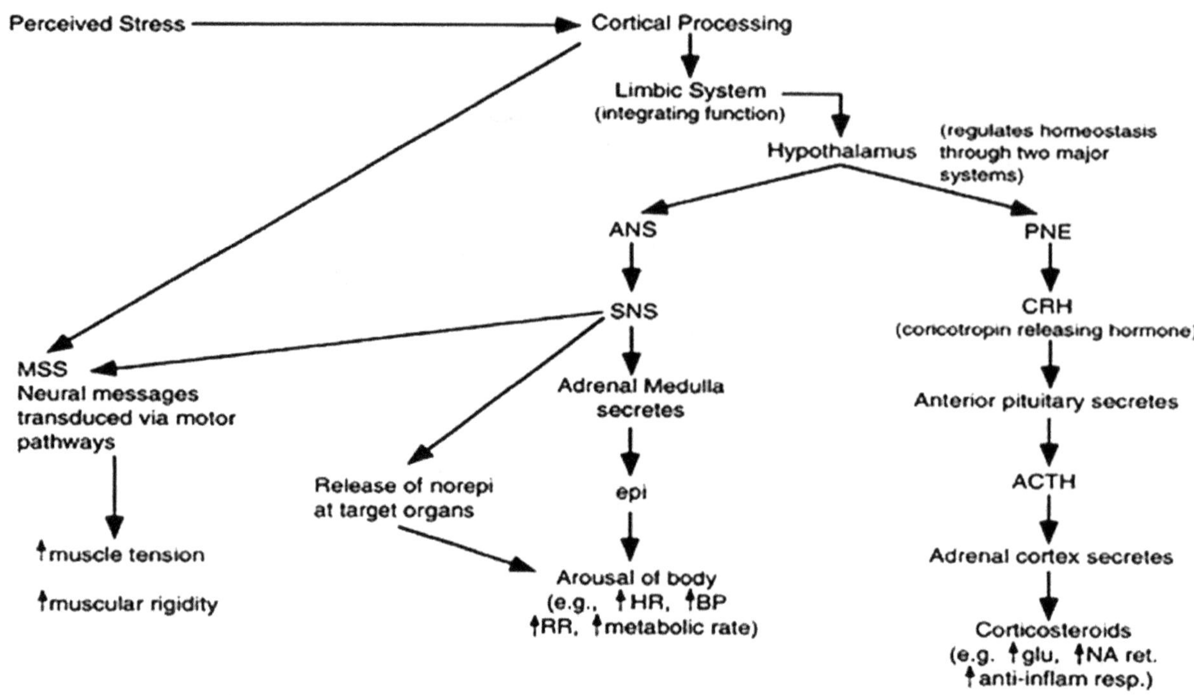

The limbic portion of the central nervous system assimilates thoughts, feelings, and emotions, whereas the hypothalamic portion of the limbic system specifically controls homeostasis and provides constant feedback between mind and body. In response to stress, the MSS is activated. The cerebral cortex processes the perception of threat triggering an increase in muscle tension and rigidity.

The ANS is also activated in response to stress. Once the perception of a threat is processed in the cerebral cortex, it is then communicated through the limbic system, the hypothalamus, and, subsequently, the sympathetic branch of the ANS. Neural messages are passed along through the ANS by two hormones (epinephrine and norepinephrine). These hormones, called neurotransmitters, act on specific organs to produce the generalized arousal state known as the fight-or-flight response (increased heart rate, blood pressure, and respiratory rate).

In response to stress, the PNE system (hypothalamic-pituitary-adrenal) is also affected. These physiological reactions to stress directly impact mood states, social functioning, health behaviors, work productivity and life-meaning. Lazarus (2000) suggested that this cascade of physiological events occur at three levels, acute stress (triggered by new challenges or threats), episodic stress (similar to acute stress but occurs more frequently and consistently) and chronic stress (characterized by persistent and long term stressors). Each of these three levels of stress have a different impact on the individual in the workplace. The byproduct of these levels of stress range from worry and anxiety to aggressiveness, job strain and long term illness respectively (Lazarus, 2000).

Effective Management of Stress in Decision Making

Due to the aforementioned deleterious impact of stress, it is important to explore various ways of stress management in the workplace. Stress management capacity is the ability to manage stress and is vital in the prevention of a negative impact of stress (Thompson, 2010). Stress management can be improved for leaders and organizations. Stretching one's comfort zone can provide an effective method for managing stress. Training, learning, and practicing in high stress environments help manage stress to produce effective decision making. An example is placing employees in a simulation-based platform that mimics a real-world experience. A flight simulator is a good case; however, there are many other platforms to include experiences in medicine, sports, driving, and other related job functions. This places the employees in a certain environment with a specific issue to make decisions either individually or as a group. Either way, employees will need to collaborate and strategize on issues and challenges, and then finalize an optimal solution.

Fractal organizations (i.e., organizations that imitate systems in nature and grow relationships) promote relationship development and have shared purpose and participation of shared ideas. In organizations that practice the fractal theory, relationships can develop at all levels and create cohesive groups (Raye, 2014). However, Raye (2014) contended that when there is an increase of stress in high ranks of employees, the organization will flounder. Internal competition, employee turnover, and unhealthy workers are common in organizations that are micromanaged and decision making is restricted. In one study, excessive work, lack of work and personal life balance, and job loss were the highest sources of stress affecting employees. People who mistrust one another will make faulty decisions, and little change will occur if is driven from the top. Lencioni (2002) illustrated multiple dysfunctions of a team; one of particular importance is the absence of trust. With this dysfunction, when members of a team fail to understand one another and lose trust in each other, results cannot be achieved. Leaders need a more conscious shared vision with collaboration, creativity, and innovation to promote sustainable teams. Developing sound judgment is important for an individual, but there will be great benefits when teams formulate decisions. Sometimes, poor decisions are based on lack of experience or insufficient information, but other times it may be due to stress. There are two types of stressors: acute stressors and chronic stressors. Acute stressors occur and disappear, and chronic stressors exist for longer periods of time. Campbell et al. (2007) admonished individuals suffer from information overload and information anxiety due to excessive amounts of mental stimulus: technological overload, multitasking, and general cognitive overload. Stress will continue to challenge leaders and organizations. There is an uncertainty about the future, and if there is a high level of stress for an extended time, short-term and long-term memory and the awareness of surroundings will diminish (Thompson, 2007).

Leadership within the organization should be vigilant of stressful situations. Experts function well in an ambiguous environment with high quality information; beginners can function as well as experts in the same environment with low quality information, as long as there is access to a lot of information (Huang, 2012). In order to avoid catastrophic leadership failure, Thompson (2007) recommended hiring people with high EI, train employees in EI, and reduce both individual and organizational stress. Additional techniques include (a) assessing IQ, EI, and stress; (b) educating employees on EI and stress; (c) utilizing EI coaching, providing individual and organizational stress coping strategies; (d) making changes to reduce and/or remove stressors; (e) enforcing stress management; (f) monitoring both individual and organizational stress levels; (g) using stress coaches; and (h) building strong teams. Interventions could include therapy, coaching, feed-back systems, or other strategies (McCleskey, 2013).

An effective employee or leader of an organization must continually reward and influence their colleagues-employees based more on intrinsic values than extrinsic values. Pink (2009) illustrated the difference between what he labels Type I and Type X behaviors regarding motivation of people. Type I behavior is when an individual is more concerned with an activity needing no external incentive, compared to Type X behavior when a person cares more about the external rewards of an activity. Pink opined that individuals who are Type I are better coworkers, and stated "if you want to work with more Type I's, the best strategy is to become one yourself" (2009, p. 105). The term leader can be an employee who has a titled or non-titled position; this person shows expertise in their specific area, not always the administrator. Most non-titled employees have situational power to influence others based on their expertise and experiences for specific circumstances. Employees want to be rewarded based on influence and develop that sense of belonging. Otherwise, the willingness to participate, learn, and be part of the organizational structure will weaken. Whether an employee or an individual with a titled position of an organization, power can be used to either influence or control people. These philosophies have different levels of influencing or manipulating others. The influence point of view is based on shared power and a servant leadership approach. The power of control is an entirely different approach with an opposing position of narcissistic characteristics. Using power through exploiting others by virtue of one's entitlement, authority, arrogance, and self-absorption can destroy any organization and the mission of its existence; this narcissism is toxic to any organization.

Executives must know what it takes to lead. Throughout history, leadership theories have evolved to reflect events occurring within the societies of the current time. According to Goffee and Jones (2002), there are three dominant qualities that seem to be fundamental to all successful leaders and have also been an historical continuum in leadership theories. Successful leaders are inspirational leaders and they must know how to engage people and encourage their commitment to the goals of the company. Goffee and Jones listed the four common characteristics found in inspirational leaders: (a) approachability and humanity and the ability to reveal weaknesses, (b) reliance on intuition and soft data to make certain decisions data, (c) demonstration of empathy with their employees, and (d) courage to be different and express their uniqueness.

Leadership is not only about the personal development of one person, but rather the formation of a learning organization. In the 1900s, learning organizations dramatically improved firms like General Electric, Honda, Johnsonville Foods, Pacific Bell, Nokia, Quad Graphics, Samsung, and Sheerness Steel. Some examples that made these corporations improve are focusing on (a) customer value and meeting customer needs; (b) operational excellence and continuous development; (c) innovative processes to improve equipment, facilities, and technology; (d) becoming more accessible to others and especially to customers with disabilities; (e) allowing workers to lead and make decisions; and (f) gaining support from customers and the community. Companies noted Senge's emphasis of learning organizations where people learn and employees become knowledge workers. This process led to institutionalized subsystems. Senge (2006) proposed five basic disciplines of organizational learning: (a) personal mastery, (b) mental models building, (c) a shared vision, (d) team learning, and (e) systems thinking. Thinking in systems will sustain a learning organization, and learning can take place at the individual, group, and organizational level via adaptive, action, and anticipatory methods. A successful organization: (a) adapts, (b) develops new products and processes, (c) learns from competition, (d) transfers knowledge, (e) learns from mistakes, (f) utilizes company talent, (g) seeks improvement, (h) attracts top talent, and (j) increases commitment and innovation (Marquardt, 2011).

Marquardt (2011) examined over three hundred of the top learning organizations worldwide and concluded that in order to be a true learning organization, there are five subsystems that must exist: (a) learning, (b) organization, (c) people, (d) knowledge, and (e) technology. These five incorporated subsystems interface and complement each other. This core system of a learning organization requires all five subsystems for efficacy. Companies that have used this form of institutionalized innovation have benefited, profited, and improved. Case studies describe how established companies that are learning organizations have created a new growth focus (Anthony, Johnson, & Sinfield, 2008). In order to survive, people must recognize, restructure, and reengineer for success (Marquardt, 2011). Successful survival requires remaining, obtaining and sustaining continual transformational learning.

Leadership becomes an organizational and societal issue. A characteristic of a successful leader is encouraging people and supporting the accomplishments of tasks without being directed or micromanaged. The visionary leader who pursues creative approaches to leadership will find success in positive and measurable ways. This has been amply demonstrated by Harvard University (e.g., giving control to alumni, autonomy), Starbucks Coffee (e.g., company-owned system, employee service to customers), and Southwest Airlines (e.g., employee-focused, enthusiasm of management and staff) representing a few examples of flagship organizations among a growing number of leaders who have embraced the demand for accountable and goal focused servant leadership. These examples illustrate how employees care more about the organizational accomplishments by possessing a Type I behavior of intrinsic motivation (Pink, 2009). Today more than ever, leaders in any setting must encourage people to become critical and intrinsic thinkers in order to focus upon new and creative ideas.

Individual learning has been found to have multiple effects on organizations. Ruiz-Mercader, Merono-Cerdan, and Sabater-Sanchez (2006) found that when individual learning occurs at high levels, the learning at this level positively and significantly affects the overall learning at the organization system and infrastructure level. Additionally, organizational leaders can ensure training opportunities are provided to individuals in areas where knowledge or development of skills is needed or required (Bollinger & Smith, 2001). In addition to an organizations' need to be efficient and increase productivity, it is equally as significant for organizational leaders to produce innovative ideas from within themselves and to promote it through employee learning. Knowledge management is the tools, techniques, and strategies used to retain, analyze, organize, improve, and share business expertise (Goffee & Jones, 2012).

Employees in an organization or students in a classroom have limited resources, but still must be led to perform at an optimum level and beyond. For an organization to be effective, real and valued input is encouraged from its people. Leadership decisions may not appease everyone when implementing change. Drucker's research on positive humanistic leadership and organizational management is one of the many pioneers responsible for the paradigm shift away from the outdated autocratic style of leadership. According to Drucker (1998), "one does not manage people as previously assumed. One leads them" (p. 166). Servant leadership is not about oppressing or rejecting the ideas and values of others because of personal conflict, differing opinions, or insecurities. To step aside from the power-control image of a leader, the servant leader actually reframes the partnership with coworkers and promotes others to rise above their current status. A servant leader values coworkers by selecting the right people for tasks. A servant leader utilizes positive reinforcement to facilitate personal growth in the organization.

Deming (1986) observed that leaders must become empowering by tapping the potential of an organization's most important resource: The people who are dedicated and committed to the organizational mission, vision, and core values. "The greatest waste in America is failure to use the abilities of people" (Deming, 1986, p. 53). Among the many components that make up an organization are people and teams of people. They are not only important; they are unique, emotional beings who are subject to cultural conditioning. To understand people, a leader needs to know and be aware of their interactions with each other, the system in which they work and learn, and their motivations (Deming, 1986; Marquardt, 2011).

In order to retain a foothold in the market, executives need to seek continuous improvement by identifying, quantifying, and eliminating waste and by seeking innovative strategies for survival and success. Weldy and Gillis (2010) noted one strategy for organizational improvement, survival, and success is regarding people and their knowledge as an asset. Action learning groups that include the members in the problem-solving process have decreased stress, increased work commitment, responsibility, knowledge of results, and feelings of empowerment (Krishna & Marquardt, 2007). Developing skills and experiential learning involves (a) receiving feedback, (b) acquiring data, (c) finding new solutions to problems, and (d) questioning (Marquardt, 2011). Continuous learning nurtures an environment where all members learn at the individual, team, and organizational levels. The dimensions of a learning organization include but are not limited to (a) continuous learning, (b) dialogue, (c) team learning, (d) systems, (e) empowerment, and (f) leadership (Weldy & Gillis, 2010).

Team member skills can impact organizational development. Hall and Hord (2015) defined organizational development as the "interactive process of people doing their work rather than on the technical substance of the work" (p. 255). Understanding the group and individual skill processes is helpful when implementing change, and individuals, teams and organizations can more effectively solve work problems when using developed generalized process skills (Hall & Hord, 2015). Furthermore, Hall and Hord admonished there is a greater flexibility for change after identifying the process skills and training of work teams where teams make decisions and work is completed within teams. Core skills of effective teams include ideal teams, team decision making, developing consensus, data and feedback, brainstorming, force-field analysis, meeting skills, and team process strategies (Hall & Hord, 2015). An individual rarely has all the necessary knowledge or experience for the problem. The exchange of ideas leads to innovative ideas that would not have been created without collaboration. Involvement in decision making strengthens organizational commitment. A work team or a *community of practice* is comprised of a group of people who have a common objective, a desire to achieve that objective, the necessary skills to get the job done, mutual accountability for results, and ways of measuring performance. Community of practice is comprised of "people who share a concern or a passion for something they do and learn how to do it better as they interact regularly" (Smith, 2009, para. 5). Mutual accountability is accountability for individual tasks and the team being accountable for its results. In other words, it is team responsible for the success or failure of the change, not the leader.

According to UCSF Human Resources (n.d.), team building helps turn a work group into a cohesive unit that shares objectives, supports one another, manages diversity, and respects individual differences. Team building can lead to increased (a) communication, (b) productivity for organizational success, (c) motivation, (d) cooperation and collaborative problem-solving, (e) commitment, (f) support, and (g) diverse and successful work groups. In fact, intercultural relationships built during teamwork enhance intercultural understanding and improve team functioning and operations. Building team commitment through involvement is an important component of a work team. There are different types of teams, such as natural work groups, project teams of all kinds, standing teams, informal teams (social committees), and special situation teams (emergency response teams). High performance teams excel in direction, execution, and results. Teams need to identify the mission (the team's purpose), the issue (the problem to be solved), goals (performance measures and targets), the roles within the team, rules and process checks, and skill sets of team members.

It is important to have effective communication between management and the team to describe what to work on and the expected outcome. The team members, the project, the objective (including how much improvement and by when), the scope of the project, performance measures, and expected results should be clearly stated. Included in the project plan are the milestone dates and responsibilities. Effective decision making should also include communication with all stakeholders. When the team is disbanded, the improvements may slowly vanish and be replaced by the status quo, but by establishing a *process owner* who has ongoing responsibility to the project, the improvement can be maintained. Finally, the team needs to get meaningful recognition in a timely way, so that its members are encouraged to be involved in additional projects. Skills, commitment, accountability make teams happen, with ensuing performance results. In order for teams to meet management, organizational and member expectations, key people involved in the team need to understand and fulfill their roles and responsibilities.

Even with significant leadership and organizational barriers, teams can succeed. The members are people who have first-hand knowledge of the work and represent a variety of perspectives. The team member's role adds value to the team by active participation in any activities that will further accomplish the team's mission. Teams work best when each key member has specific guidelines and a specific role (e.g., leader, scribe, timekeeper, team sponsor, the facilitator, resource specialist). A leader is responsible for managing the team that is fixing the problem or making the improvement. He or she can be at any level in the company and must have a vested interest in the result. The team leader's role is to manage the team toward accomplishing its task and to be the binding force between the sponsor and the team. The leaders also coordinate the team's resources and activities to ensure that the mission is accomplished, remains impartial, and focuses on the process rather than the content of the discussion. A leader may provide training and coaching in continuous improvement tools, problem solving, process improvement methodology, and team process skills. A leader also works through problem behavior. A scribe and timekeeper could also be roles within a team. The scribe can provide accurate, complete documentation of team activities by keeping notes and uses flip charts or a computer with a large display, so everyone sees what is being recorded. The timekeeper can help the team stay on schedule during the meeting. These roles could also be rotated among the team members.

The team sponsor, the facilitator, and any resource specialists are partners rather than members. The facilitator is a coach who provides tools and guidance. He or she helps the team with relational and process issues, but is not there to provide expert knowledge on solving the problem. The facilitator's role is to assist the team leader by acting as a training and coaching resource to the team, team leader, and team members by transferring process skills to the team. A facilitator provides best thinking, retrieves input for the team from co-workers, and communicates team results to co-workers. The sponsor can provide direction and resources to the team and to whom the team can turn for help if there are a lack of resources or if the problem is not what it seemed to be. The team sponsor decides what the team needs, provides resources, and is a partner in the team's success. With input from the facilitator, a team sponsor selects and develops the team leader and ensures that the team has a project plan, assesses progress, and redirects the team if necessary. The team sponsor ensures that the results are quantified. The sponsor attends team meetings if invited. The resource specialist is not a team member, but can provide expert advice.

Changes in organizational structure require communication, problem-solving, and interpersonal skills that allow members to function as part of a team. Team building provides an opportunity for authentic communication and flexibility between disciplines, setting a core purpose and secondary purposes, as well as establishing behavior standards and objectives for effective functioning. The team building process involves establishing team charters, describing team functions and instituting team improvement plans through training, education, and development (Southard, 1993). The foundation of a team work group is developing a workable team charter, which is an essential document used to clarify and agree on expectations. When finalized, it is the contract between the team and is helpful for keeping the team focused on its mission. In the team charter, the problem is identified, which can be an unwanted effect or a result that deviates from the norm. A good problem statement should be an unbiased and objective description of an undesirable effect; how the problem is described will affect the data collection and analysis of the problem. There should be observable results that show something is wrong. Within the description of the problem, *what*, *where*, *when*, and *how much* should be probed; for example, questioning the problems with a current inventory control system or identifying what a wellness program will remedy (i.e., absenteeism, turnover, accidents).

There are complexities of organizational learning, and each member of the team differs in their understanding, willingness, and ability to implement a particular change. Furthermore, some will change quickly, others will take longer, and some may never change (Hall & Hord, 2015). Hall and Hord (2015) provided indicators of a context for change: (a) reducing isolation, (b) increasing staff capacity, (c) providing a caring and productive environment, and (d) promoting increased quality. Weldy and Gillis (2010) found a need for increased communication, participation, access to information, empowerment, and decision making at all levels of the organization. Weldy and Gillis concluded that managers are more likely to believe that employees are being empowered, share the vision, and are motived by decision making. However, employees do not share the same beliefs. Learning organizational models stress the importance of teamwork and empowerment; consequently, more initiatives need to be implemented to empower employees in their knowledge and decision making (Weldy & Gillis 2010). Weldy and Gillis also suggested that not all team members are informed or aware of improvements in knowledge.

Many organizations have difficulty developing high performance teams. Skills, roles, responsibilities, and relationships can be established and developed by clarifying the mission, vision, and plan. Centralized decision making is both hierarchical and authoritarian in the decision-making process, but decentralized decision making is collaborative (Collins & Porras, 1991). Leadership should encourage, excite, and value employees and strengthens the team (Mink, 2012). Organizations would benefit from participative management and work teams where employees at all levels are involved in the problem-solving, communication, and strategic planning (Ross, Matteson, & Exposito, 2014).

There is an increase in work productivity among employees when they are part of self-managed teams involved in the decision-making process and are empowered to offer new ideas (Garvin, Edmondson, & Gino, 2008; Northouse, 2012). Collaboration among team members, team performance, and team learning are characteristics of a learning organization (Bierema, 1999). A successful organization recognizes and values the talent of its members and increases commitment and innovation (Marquardt, 2011). A learning organization can gain a competitive edge by empowering its members and investing in a collective intelligence that has an ability to learn and transform systems by training, adapting, re-skilling, and continuous development of work teams.

Effective companies network and are linked to systems learning. Companies such as Cisco, General Electric, Genzyme, Intel, and Procter & Gamble have attained market leadership through innovation strategies. Some organizations fail to recognize the challenging complexities of organizational learning, and suffer from a decentralized decision making. Centralization is measured by both hierarchy and authority in the decision-making process pushing the decision making out of the hands of many and into the hands of a few (Collins & Porras, 1991). If leaders demonstrated a willingness to listen and entertain alternative points of view, employees would feel emboldened and empowered to offer new ideas (Garvin, Edmondson, & Gino, 2008).

Leaders assume to change an organization to learning involves just the articulation of a clear vision, offering employee incentives, and a great deal of training. However, only a handful of companies have known the importance of vison. Recently, a broader group of organizations have realized the importance and vitality of vision. Vision removes the fuzziness surrounding goals, direction and future (Collins & Porras, 1991). It sets the image of an organization within itself a part of vision in brand leadership. Brand is identity and identity is destiny. Consider Apple, AT&T, FedEx, Ford, CBS, McDonald, and Microsoft; when a brand is *credible*, *compelling*, and *connecting*, people become passionate about the brand. The successful branding of these organizations was based on innovation, create new solutions, speed in communication, new logos, and focusing on inspiring people's dreams and aspirations, trust and value, understanding customer's mindsets and loyalty. This causes employees and consumers to bond with certain brands and images for life (McEwen, 2005). The branding vision becomes nostalgic in the culture of the organization.

Enhancing and establishing organizational culture forms beliefs, customs, practices, and values. This organizational culture influences a firm effectiveness (Gregory, Harris, Armenakis, & Shook, 2009). The rich impact of culture encourages empowerment, self-management, sharing, and team work. These influences tend to lead to firm organizational effectiveness (Gregory et al., 2009). Strong corporate culture is often the result of a well-laid plan. Strategy is referred to as an action plan, goals, steps, methodologies, and tactics. Such contextual factors affect all probabilities as to whether organizational strategy will occur. These elements must be allowed to operate if the organization wishes to accomplish its desired results. This implies that the strategy provides or produces structure.

There are previous models of human resource development that include training, education, and development, but there is a difference between training (a discontinuous process) and development (a continuous process) (Kumpikaitė, 2008). Based on the model presented by Juli (2011), there are action steps for transforming the people subsystem (i.e., build vision, nurture collaboration, promote team performance, cultivate team learning, ensure team delivers results). Kumpikaite (2008) stated human resource is a process, which includes (a) training of new employees, (b) employee adaptation, (c) professional development, (d) re-skilling, (e) career development, (f) personal and teamwork performance, (g) combined organizational and personal objectives, and (h) continuous development. The learning organization uses collective intelligence, ability to learn, and creativity to transform systems (Bierema, 1999). Employees believe their work is important and meaningful, and employers should recognize that employees who care about the organization and their career will be more committed. Juli (2011) proposed greater accountability and commitment to an organization when people feel included and valued. Encouraging collaboration, team performance, and team learning by reflection and correction can ensure results.

The people subsystem of the learning organization needs to be empowered and enabled to learn; it involves learning by the employees, managers/leaders, customers, and business partners (Marquardt, 2011). The values of a post material society are based on self-expression through innovation and creativity and a desire to use mental capacity and emotional intelligence at work. Work is becoming more collaborative and focused on teamwork (Wilenius, 2014). Action learning involves people in the problem-solving process, and according to Marquardt (2011), the groups are effective if they are diverse. Collaboration can (a) broaden environmental scanning, (b) widen an analytical range, (c) overcome routines, (d) improve the learning of members, and (d) evolve new organizational forms.

Krishna and Marquardt (2007) stressed that action learning groups have higher affective organizational commitment, higher level of responsibility and greater organizational commitment, higher knowledge of results, and higher levels of empowerment. Leading companies see business from the organizational perspective (Wilenius, 2014). Employees see their own future as part of the future of the organization. This means an organization must give opportunities for learning. Other factors like developing skills are considered even more important. According to Marquardt (2011), experiential learning involves: (a) seeking feedback; (b) obtaining data from various perspectives, (c) encouraging new actions for both old and new problems; and (d) recognizing the values in questioning ideas, assumptions, attitudes, and actions.

Healthy Leadership

The philosophy of servant leadership is to place the needs of the organization and people first and help others increase their knowledge, skills, and abilities, so they can contribute to the organizational mission and vision. The following characteristics help a servant leader focus on the needs of their people: healing, stewardship, serving others, listening, foreseeing the future, compassion, conceptualization, ability to persuade, knowledge of what is going on around them, sense of group closeness, and desire to help people grow (Barbuto & Wheeler, 2007). When people are pleased with their workplace environment and treated well by their peers and leaders, they are productive and committed to the organization. Servant leadership has a *pay it forward* philosophy as well: If a leader instills a stress-free environment where an employee is happy, the employee could display positive behavior towards others within the organizational environment, potentially limiting psychological, physiological, and emotional stress. The servant leader also benefits from this process by understanding ethics and power along with awareness of the value of organizational trust and its integrity. To become a servant leader, leaders must provide positive reinforcement and influence, so people can perform at an optimal level.

A significant issue for effective leadership in the future is to place the internal customer (the employee) first. This effort builds a confidence level within an organization in several ways. Employees feel part of a group, develop a sense of team within the group, and learn that they possess many talents. Garfield (1992) spoke with leaders of three companies to explore what leaders face and will have to overcome in their future. The leaders' philosophy of giving empowerment to the people helps build trust and respect between the leader and follower. By involving everybody and focusing on the employee, the employee takes pride in his or her work, feels part of a team, and develops a strong commitment to the organization. "Rigid, authoritarian styles of management are being discarded in favor of greater employee participation in decision making" (Garfield, 1992, p. 9).

Leading companies see business from the organizational perspective (Wilenius, 2014). Most organizations utilize various types of work teams for learning and decision making. Other research had admonished that an organization can transform by celebrating learning, team learning, building learning communities, and expanding individual and group knowledge.

Organizations are using collaboration and teamwork and involving people in the decision making (Wilenius, 2014). Collaboration can (a) broaden environmental scanning, (b) widen an analytical range,

(c) overcome routines, (d) improve the learning of members, and (d) evolve new organizational forms (Marquardt, 2011). Work teams have higher levels of responsibility and greater organizational commitment, higher knowledge of results, and higher levels of empowerment, which can lead to increased organizational effectiveness (Gregory, Harris, Armenakis, & Shook, 2009; Krishna & Marquardt, 2007).

It is important to understand the dynamics of work teams as more organizations use multiple work teams. Group decision making can be a frustrating experience if team members have not developed skills to work collaboratively (Hall & Hord, 2015). Hall and Hord (2015) delineated characteristics of effective teams: talk is task-centered and understood by all members, full participation where members actively listen, comfortable environment, criticism is shared and accepted, team leaders are not controlling, and group decisions are made. Establishing work teams involve careful team-processing skills (i.e., establishing ideal teams, encouraging team decision making, developing consensus, and obtaining feedback) (Hall & Hord, 2015). Understanding the dynamics of work teams will increase collective intelligence, ability to learn, collaboration, organizational efficacy, and creativity to transform systems (Bierema, 1999).

Servant leadership models are successful in higher education and any other global organizations. Servant leadership, particularly in higher education, builds collaboration, trust, empathy, ethics, and various conditions (e.g., cultural, demographic, economic, sociological) to meet the needs of all stakeholders. If this leadership model is applied to the context of higher education, it can be a long-term process, not a tactic to deceive employees. Instead, it creates a buy-in approach to fixing past organizational issues of high attrition, mistrust, poor performance, union conflicts, and low morale.

The theory and concepts behind servant leadership are in sharp contrast to the notion that managers and leaders serve as power brokers and standardize discipline. In 1970, Greenleaf coined servant leadership as the idea that places servants first, shifting from the *tough love style* leadership paradigm. Today, the visionary leader recognizes that a lack of business and political acumen, along with a misunderstanding of the organizational culture and demands, can result in placing psychological, physiological, and emotional stress on employees and be closely associated with poor productivity, low morale, dissention among employees, employee absenteeism, and a total breakdown within the organizational structure.

Servant leadership focuses on the leader serving the people under them. Servant leaders are entirely different than traditional leaders, but only because they have observed the value among corporate boardrooms and public sector agencies and have grown to recognize that both sectors are pleading for change. Servant leaders do not hide behind their subordinates but rally among coworkers from the front lines in a similar fashion to one of the original pioneers of servant leadership: General Stonewall Jackson serving during the Civil War.

Private and public institutions have significantly improved their organizational cultures and services through developing and supporting a vertical and horizontal culture of servant leadership. Relationships are important in developing functional organizations or groups of people focused upon common goals. The lack of understanding this organizational restructuring will not promote effective change. Leadership is an art and involves a multitude of variables that require attention.

The importance of relationships is another principle foundation of servant leadership. Interpersonal relationships are critical elements within any organization as they afford a basis for how effectively the organization and its people function, perform tasks, and react to the external environment (Baron, 1996; Flum, 2015). It seems safe to assume that numerous scientific studies undertaken by researchers and supporters of servant leadership, including Stephen Covey, Margaret Wheatley, Kenneth Blanchard, James Collins, Peter Senge, and Max DePree, corroborate the measures of organizational performance outcomes through well designed skills and are more interested in building positive relationships. These types of organizations are full of valued team members much like the employees of the Herman Miller Furniture Company. These employees have not only enjoyed the feeling of empowerment through servant leadership for over 42 years, but the company demonstrates low attrition and high production of quality goods and outstanding customer service that has led it into its premier status as leading the industry standard for goods and services.

By focusing on the needs and wants of a group, the organization can improve relationships. No one feels threatened and retaliation becomes an outdated concept. Individual leaders and managers are not the focus. Relationships can be developed through compassion; this trait is the ability to consider an employee's personal circumstances while performing job tasks. Leaders can be approached with questions and concerns that may not be directly related to job functions, and suffer vicariously through the employees. This compassions leads to greater personal and organizational relationships; a leader understands that personal affairs may impact the employee, yet considers this when delegating job functions. This in turn leads to greater attachment and confidence with the leader, and employees feel more comfortable addressing concerns with their leaders that are external to the work environment. The mutual association that can be created when the group knows its needs come before their leader is astronomical. When the leader reframes the previously held notions of power and authority brokers as being the dominant member of the organization, the organizational relationship will significantly improve as individual needs are met. A persuasive leader influences others to perform; if one follows based on a desire rather than a need, a personal relationship of loyalty and fellowship will be established (Barbuto & Wheeler, 2007).

Toxic Leadership

Leadership which has been researched for decades covers many terminologies such as transformational, transactional, autocratic, participative, laissez-faire, as well as the toxic side of operating an organization with the increase of narcissism permeating the 21st century (Villarreal, 2014). Bolman and Deal (2009) stated that a person can avoid the toxic side of leadership by gaining a sense of self, building on strengths and weaknesses through feedback and reflection, and looking for trust within their organization. Leona Helmsley, known as the *Queen of Mean,* had a type of leadership that was toxic and abusive. Not only was she convicted of tax evasion and mail fraud, she used coercive power to terrorize all levels of the organizations people from staff to the leadership teams. She demanded perfection from employees, and if they did not meet her standards, she insulted them while using profanity (Bolman & Deal, 2006). This behavior occurred at her hotels as well as her residences. A toxic leader causes isolation; this type of leader is unaware of his or her faults. Trust is also a virtue that is lacking in a toxic environment. There is a cost to distrust within an organization, which is a trend occurring in the past decades; particularly within the political arena. Covey (2010) demonstrated the media reports of many scandals of corporate or political leaders that have violated the public trust. The banking system, Wall Street, and other corporate giants have placed disgust in the American people, who consequently demonstrated in the streets and in the nation's capital. Covey stated that "as trust goes down, speed goes down, and costs go up" (2010, p. 10). To rid distrust and toxic leadership within organizations, there needs to be a change in direction. For organizational leaders to be influenced and inspired by their people, building and modeling trust is vital. In addition, transparency is extremely important to build trust and collaboration.

"Toxic leadership is a multidimensional construct that includes elements of abusive supervision along with narcissism, authoritarianism, self-promotion, and unpredictability" (Dobbs, 2014, p. 15). Research has found that toxic leadership impacts various organizations and sectors. These areas include (a) physical and mental health of employees, (b) increased dysfunctional group behaviors, (c) increased absenteeism and tardiness, (d) reduced productivity, and (e) resignation or transfers. In addition, toxic leaders possess the following characteristics: unethical or bad behavior, self-promotion, abusive and tyrannical supervision, downward hostility toward others, engages in destructive and demotivational behaviors, and narcissistic and authoritative tendencies (Dobbs, 2014; Schmidt, 2014).

Schmidt (2014) found certain organizations with rigid hierarchical structures similar to the military had characteristics of subordination and abusive control. Bandura (1973) claimed people who considered leaders to have strong authority also had high rank. In some situations, there necessitates autocratic leadership; however, the term subordinate within other industries can lead to arrogance, hubris, abuse of power, mistrust, and performance issues. "Military experience is a powerful way to test and develop oneself as a warrior" (Bolman & Deal, 2009, p. 16). Bolman and Deal (2009) consider a warrior as a leader who can build a stable organization; they recognize conflict and strive for reaching the goals of the organization. Leadership style(s) become fluid and represent a juxtaposition opportunity for meaningful dialogue among organizational stakeholders in most industries, with the exception of these few autocratic missions like the armed forces.

It is questionable that observations would not produce levels of arrogance, hubris, and bullying within any organization. An argument for the skewed "feel good" human brain neurotransmitter behavior suggests that pleasure is sought and many times obtained from those in titled positions of authority because they lack effective skills as leaders and managers. If a manager-leader lacks confidence in his or her own skill sets, the more prone he or she may be to the use of abusive tactics to control operations and people. This abuse can increase with longevity within the company. It is rare to find authentic leaders who are secure with their own skills and are willing to embrace-promote and encourage more creative thought provoking staff who can take the organization to a more advanced position of critical thinking in a regulatory-driven and competitive business.

It is unlikely a perfect "organizational fit" exists; however, there is an expectation of a humanistic approach to leadership of most organizations, and is more dominant than symbolic, political, and structural approaches (Bolman & Deal, 2003). Given the current issues with unemployment and underemployment conditions in the United States, it would be reasonable to postulate that people want and need jobs to support their families and become employed full time in a job with fair benefits. It would not be uncommon to find employees who are willing to accept and be mistreated by organizational managers-leaders who choose to abuse their own position of authority and power to exploit others they feel are inferior to their organizational fit. This resembles a co-dependent relationship where employees could be so connected to their job but fear the unknown of losing their job, leading to the thought that life is over and they will never be successful. One of the most damaging types of abuse is the marginalization of employees over non-merit factors or feelings of jealousy for those who have developed more advanced levels of critical thinking and are viewed as threats to those in current leadership positions.

In 1943, Maslow developed a theory that individual needs exist in a hierarchical format. The individual needs for survival are those related to physiological, security, and belongingness (lower level of the triangle); and esteem and self-actualization (upper level of the triangle) (Huitt, 2007). These needs affect an employee in the workplace. People must have their lower level needs met to be motivated to do their job well. For example, this could be a safe working environment or pay that is fitting for the responsibilities the person has. If an employee is pleased, then they are likely to be motivated when increased job responsibilities, status, and challenging work assignments are given to them. Although the application of this theory to a work setting may be simple, this theory is little researched and not very useful if put in place.

Drawing from Maslow's Hierarchy of Needs, people want to feel a part of the mission of the organization and not be excluded from improving skills and contributing to the overall goals and outcomes. However, there are ill-prepared and toxic people at all levels who hinder productive outcomes stifling healthy and productive ones. People who remain in this environment perpetuate dysfunction within an organization.

Global leaders must be sensitive to the needs of people in their organizations. An aloof and distant autocratic manager who seeks to impress and gain favor from upper level management has diminished the organizational culture and its human assets. The sycophant approach to leadership and management is a clever con game causing extensive damage that stagnates performance and morale within the organization. This type of approach is used by individuals who pretend to be a *yes-man* or *yes-woman* and *suck-up* to their supervisors to gain advantage over others. If treated correctly, most staff members are willing to engage in any task to advance the mission and goals of the organization. Servant leadership as applied to the workplace suggests employees demand for authentic leadership and loyalty as it can be applied to groups of diverse populations seeking common goals.

The crisis in institutional leadership also impacts productivity, motivation, morale, trust, and confidence. In some workplaces and the organizational structure and environment, there is an inclusion of mobbing, also called workplace bullying (Davenport, Schwartz, & Elliott, 2005; Duffy & Sperry, 2014; Namie & Namie, 2003). If this type of behavior infiltrates the organization, the *so-called leader* with no true leadership qualities would be the main contributor to the crisis. A person who is ineffective as a leader uses the chaos theory to control and bully people. With this type of philosophy, a so-called leader promotes a lack of knowledge of organizational direction so people will rely on this so-called leader for answers and directions. This *control tactic* creates great crisis in the organization.

Leaders set the emotional tone of a workplace environment (Gilbert, Carr-Ruffin, Ivancevich, & Konopaske, 2012). Goleman (2004) found direct correlations between business success and emotional intelligence, but when leaders face great amounts of stress and uncertainty in a fast changing global society, it can negatively impact critical thinking, judgement, and the systemic process of decision making. Increased amounts of stress affect cognitive and emotional intelligences (Thompson, 2010; McVicar, 2015). Stress was named the 20th century disease and is becoming the 21st century disease. Workplace stress costs industries approximately 350 million dollars and is linked to the top six leading causes of death (Thompson, 2007). Baker (2013) claimed failed corporations share two common characteristics: ineffective leadership and faulty decision making. Stress affects decision making at both the conscious and unconscious level (Thompson, 2010). Catastrophic Leadership Failure is when high levels of stress impair a leader's ability to effectively utilize both cognitive ability and EI in making timely and effective decisions (Thompson, 2007). Thompson (2007) concluded a leader can experience enough stress to cause a decrease in IQ and EI, at which point there will be a catastrophic decrease in performance.

ATTRITION IN THE WORKPLACE

Another bi-product of stress that deserves specific attention is attrition in the workplace. Rosenbach, Taylor, and Youndt (2012) noted that there are many definitions of leadership being studied and observed, yet leadership remains little understood except to recognize that leaders are not born; leaders are made. Theories of leadership can be measured by its effectiveness in various sectors. Leadership has many traits, whether they are behavioral theories where leadership is learned or acquired, or based on the trait theory that people are born leaders (Mehta, 2012). There is no specific best-fit style of leadership as many theorists base leadership on decision making, goal structure, structuring of group tasks, power, personality, and situations (Mehta, 2012). "Leadership effectiveness can be achieved by ensuring a fit between the leadership style and the demand of the situation" (Mehta, 2012, p. 24).

Leadership can be further explained as a process of social influence within diverse organizational environments in which there is a set of common traits for every situation. Rosenbach, Taylor, and Youndt (2012) explained that understanding leadership is necessitated by organizational and environmental dynamics and the increasing complexities of the workplace. With the workforce becoming increasingly diverse, leaders have more pressure and responsibility to deal with the challenges presented by employees. The employees of today's workforce need to be influenced by effective leaders who can protect their interests while pursuing the goals of the organization.

Poor leadership may lead to attrition. Considering the competing result of scarce resources to recruit and retain good employees, attrition issues become one of the most sobering matters facing institutional leaders today. Employees can find themselves negatively impacted by the culture of the organization and miserable from being exposed to the degradation that runs rampant within their jobs. There is a high demand for control and expectations from the organizational leaders, and employees are bound to fail. Poor supervisory practices account for a significant number of employees who feel dissatisfaction and hold negative feelings. If a leader lacks certain elements of power, they have found to be tyrants and "on other occasions to be more aggressive or abusive than others" (Lee-Chai & Bargh, 2001, p. 119). Raven and Kruglanski (as cited in Lee-Chai & Bargh, 2001) mentioned that coercive power and tactics are used by people who lack confidence and other levels of power, such as expertise and informational power. Four areas which can be identified as problematic and noteworthy are (a) disruption in the work setting; (b) lack of communication with policies and procedures; (c) abusive, tyrannical, and inept leadership; and (d) organizational failure.

High attrition rates can become fiscally monumental. Large attrition is not unique to most organizations. A considerable amount of turnover occurs in state and federal agencies where costs can easily exceed thousands of dollars and higher to recruit and train individuals for employment, excluding relocation and other costs. It takes several years to adequately train an individual in their field of expertise. There is a drain of qualified people and the loss of productivity, lower morale, and safety issues surrounding high turnover rates. Also, the number of complaints and the potential for civil liability increases the argument for a review of the servant leadership model. To help curtail attrition, servant leadership certainly offers any organization an opportunity to develop into a learning organization, becoming a healthier, comfortable, and empowering place to work, and be recognized for achievement and growth. To create a healthier professional environment for all stakeholders (i.e., employees, supervisory levels), there is a need for equity, equality, respect, core values, open communication, continual training, and other incentives to develop an internal self-confidence. An organizational structure should foster a sense of camaraderie and encourage growth for everyone to pursue a common set of goals, which leads to a strong sense of belonging and personal motivation to remain employed within the institution. Moreover, the personal empowerment of these employees is further supported by working in a learning environment where the culture supports ownership in the organization through active participation of managers and leaders who are open to new ideas and change (Marquardt, 2011).

Aside from ownership within the organization, most employees desire the opportunity to be treated in a fair and balanced manner by the agency leadership. A few of those examples include fair promotions, mutual respect, educational opportunities, and consistent increases in annual pay and benefits. Employee attitudes can range from disempowered to empowered. A disempowered employee places recognition in the hands of the organization; whereas an empowered employee is responsible for his or her own sphere of influence. No matter what an individual's position is in any organization, the recognition process affects an individual's ability to reward and recognize others. "Empowerment implies that employees throughout the organization have the authority to do whatever is necessary to meet requirements and satisfy customers and are trusted to make the best choices without having to wait for approval from management. It is a process of power sharing" (Schultz, 2014, p. 44). This influences employees to develop self-esteem and job satisfaction, thus increasing the organization's productivity and therefore the value of the organization. It is leadership that fosters the growth of new ideas.

MOTIVATIONAL FRAMEWORK

Organizations are grappling to fulfill the needs of their employees, decrease stress, and increase motivation. Motivation plays a major role in urging people to perform at their full potential. Motivation is derived from the word movere, which is Latin for "to move," (i.e., voluntary effort). Effective employees are key components in the success of an organization (Muo, 2013). Motivation may also be affected by four components: situation-the environment and external stimulus, temperament-the state and organism internal state, goal-the purpose of behavior and attitude, and tool-what is needed to reach the target (Graham & Weiner, 1996).

Motivational theories have been studied and applied because of their importance/need in the organizational sciences, especially within the field of organizational behavior. There is not one motivational theory that has been accepted as universal; this reflects its complexity and the different applications that theories may have. One application in particular can be applied to the motivation of employees in stressful working conditions. People react differently to stress; stress can motivate or hinder employee behavior. Employers must understand the relationship between motivation and various psychological, physiological, and emotional stressors. It is a complex task to investigate the relationship between stress and motivation in an organization. Motivation serves as a foundation to understand stressors within an organization. Herzberg designed the motivator-hygiene theory, which resembles Maslow's hierarchy of needs, specifically to how individuals are motivated in their place of work. Herzberg (2003) suggested that meeting the lower-level needs (i.e., hygiene factors) would not motivate individuals to put forth the extra effort, but would only prevent them from being dissatisfied. Higher-level needs (i.e., motivators) have to be met for individuals to be motivated. Motivation of workers takes place because a manager focuses change towards an intrinsic nature and content. This is accomplished by enriching employees' autonomy and their opportunities to take on additional responsibility, gain recognition, and develop their skills and careers (Herzberg, 2003).

Factors That Affect Motivation

Motivating employees is a difficult task that organizations all over the world face (Muo, 2013). Verner, Babar, Cerpa, Hall, and Beecham (2014) examined team motivational factors (e.g., project management, software development, external and practitioner factors) to determine the relationship with team motivation. Team motivation, the impact of culture on motivation, and the impact of project success were examined. A positive association was found between project completion and team motivation in an examination of both successful and failed projects. Participants represented the United States, Australia, Chile, and Vietnam. No difference in motivation existed between the United States, Australia, and Chile, but a difference existed between these three countries and Vietnam. Vietnamese employees have very high levels of motivation. Cultural factors played a role in team motivation (Verner et al., 2014).

McClelland's learned needs theory suggested individuals learn needs from the culture in which they live and are considered to be a member. Three needs in this theory are the need for affiliation, the need for power, and the need for achievement. The need for affiliation is to establish social relationships with others. The need for power is to control both the environment in which they work and the ability to have influence over others. The need for achievement is to take responsibility, set challenging goals, and obtain performance feedback. When one of these areas is strong in a person, it increases the level of satisfaction one can reach. It then should become a manger's goal to understand the employee's needs so that the employee's job can be structured in a way that promotes job satisfaction, increases job security in the workplace, consequently reducing stress. Jaramillo, Locander, Spector, and Harris (2007) claimed that motivation is a psychological state that encourages engagement in particular behavior. In order for management to achieve company objectives effectively and ethically, an understanding of motivation is important (Guillén, Ferrero, & Hoffman, 2015). Guillén et al. (2015) stated culture is important within an organization and proposed finding a greater holistic understanding of the interrelationship between employee diversity. To exemplify this, in higher spiritual cultures there is a higher number of spiritual motives vs. greater material motivation in a more materialistic culture. Cooperative behaviors and cross-cultural interactions create positive interdependence (Robbins, DeCenzo, & Wolter, 2013). There are challenges within a global work environment stemming from cultural variations and legal or regulatory requirements (Metcalf, 2014). Metcalf (2014) noted achievement, recognition, work responsibility, and advancement as motivator factors, whereas company policy, administration, supervision, salary, working conditions, and interpersonal relationships were not motivator factors.

Decision making in individualistic Western cultures happens on an individual basis, whereas decision making in collectivistic Eastern cultures happens as a group (Moberg & Leasher, 2011). Moberg and Leasher (2011) conducted a study investigating the differences of motivation from a cross-cultural context and found attributes related to job performance vary by culture. A motivation analysis profile was utilized to glean motivation consistencies within regions. The Chally Assessment measured traits, temperaments, competencies, and behaviors related to job performance from a sample of 123,791 applicants between 1998 and 2008. Power distance relates to inequalities of wealth, status, and authority. High-power distance cultures have rigid structures, while low-power distance cultures are more decentralized and merit-based. People from lower-power distance cultures may find positions of power more motivating than those from high-power distance cultures. Consequently, those from low-power distance cultures will be more driven and motivated. Culture also plays a role in the dimension of achievement vs. relationship. Task completion motivates achievement-oriented cultures, whereas relationship-focused cultures stress the importance of relationships and networks. It was found that Western cultures had a greater need for achievement, relationships, and power than those from the Eastern culture. Contrary to previous cross-cultural research, Moberg and Leasher found that Western cultures displayed a need for relationships, which could be a result of current business emphasis on the development of relationships. When an organization is recruiting, training, and motivating a team to operate in global markets, cross-cultural differences impact motivation and employee performance.

Corporate social responsibility (CSR) includes sound business practices for a better society. Based upon McClelland's theoretical foundation of three motivational needs (i.e., achievement, affiliation, power), Kim and Scullion (2013) investigated employee motivation in a multi-national setting and the interaction of political, institutional, and cultural dynamics. They found that motivation varies based on culture, societal norms, and political and economic settings. Data from 53 semi-structured interviews was collected from varied cultural and hierarchical structures to answer the effects of motivation on CSR in a comparative context. Employees from Korea were motivated for affiliation needs, but employees from the UK were motivated by individual achievement. The role of power was not evident, perhaps from the belief that CSR is not viewed as a form of control but rather from a humanitarian approach. Kim and Scullion concluded that a relationship exists between employee-centered CSR and employee-work motivation, thus CSR may positively impact employee motivation.

Culture and context play a vital role in the workplace and affect how employees participate and acquire knowledge (Merrifield, 2012). Merrifield (2012) examined the workplace, employees, and unions, as well as the influence of social, economic, and political factors on motivation and learning. Past life experiences (e.g., parental education, prior learning experience), current life situations (e.g., age, gender), and social and historical contexts (e.g., ethnicity, social class, family demands, surrounding community, work environments) create motivators and barriers that affect the workplace. Confidence was a factor in increased engagement, which increased staff morale, involvement in teamwork, communication, and productivity. Cultural and workplace contexts form motivators and de-motivators. Intrinsic motivators relate to learning and self-improvement, while intrinsic de-motivators relate to cultural and attitudinal barriers. Extrinsic motivators relate to rewards like promotions and financial incentives, where extrinsic de-motivators include lack of rewards for learning. Moberg and Leasher (2011) contended that more cross-cultural research on differences of global employee motivation would aid in employee recruitment and development in global markets. Multi-national corporations could achieve greater success by adjusting business strategies to the cultural norms of its employees.

Several studies (Cowherd & Levine, 1992; Cowley & Smith, 2014; Něměčková, 2012; Thomas & Holley, 2012; Wang, Yang, & Wang, 2012) examined motivation in relation to the type of business or organization in which the employee works and the position the employee holds within the business or organization. Wang et al. (2012) compared job satisfaction and job turnover rates within the public and private sector of employees in Taiwan. The control variables for the 500 respondents included age, gender, position, and job tenure. The results indicated that public employees have lower extrinsic and higher intrinsic job satisfaction that employees in the private sector. Cowley and Smith (2014) used the World Values Survey to compare intrinsic motivation among 30,000+ workers in 51 countries working within the public and private sector. The World Values Survey is a self-report instrument that focuses on work-related motivation and general life activity motivation. While data presented in this study supported the indication of higher intrinsic motivation in the public sector in 21 of the 51 countries, it was not found to be universally true around the world. The public sector attracts workers with a mission to serve; however, corruption within public sector organizations was found to impact the ability of the organization to fulfill its mission to the public. Cowherd and Levine (1992) reviewed equity theory and distributive justice theory as they related to issues of employee pay differentials and work production and found "the research suggests pay equity influences three aspects of lower-level employee motivation: commitment to top-management goals, effort, and cooperation" (p. 307). Cowherd and Levine designed a study of 102 business units in 41 corporations in North America and Europe. They found a positive relationship between interclass pay equity for hourly workers and lower-level employees and product quality. Product quality and perceptions of fairness increased when egalitarian interclass reward distributions were put into practice. They further found that high pay for top-level workers did not result in improved product quality unless those on the lower pay scales also received higher wages.

Něměcková (2012) examined the benefit of employee education as it relates to motivation and retention. The research included the responses of 142 bank employees in the Czech Republic, all with secondary or university education levels, as they rated 18 possible company benefits. The findings showed that more middle managers ranked the benefit of continued education more important than did top management. Middle managers and entry-level employees related further educational opportunities with assurance of employability. Top managers indicated (in round table discussions) that their heavy workloads made this benefit less attractive.

Workers in repetitive task jobs, such as assembly line production, may become bored and complacent in their work, leading to a loss of productivity and job dissatisfaction. Thomas and Holley (2012) examined the motivating factors of those in repetitive task jobs by focusing their study on librarians. They found that motivation could be increased in repetitive task jobs through enriching the work experience, offering appropriate incentives, treating employees as individuals, and effectively communication with employees. Thomas and Holley (2012) offered several suggestions for motivating the repetitive task employee. Employee work experiences can be enriched by offering avenues for learning and mind engagement, opportunities to lead or coach others, and assigning strategic tasks to be accomplished in teams or individually. Supervisors should encourage open communication and be open-minded about what they hear. Staff incentives beyond money include praise, thanks, casual Fridays, and special events. Supervisors and managers should pay attention to the individuals they supervise and their motivating factors as they may change over time.

Liao-Troth and Dunn (1999) surveyed volunteer managers and volunteers to ascertain perceptions of motivating factors in the volunteers' work. They found that managers have an accurate perception of what motivates the volunteer worker. In order to reduce volunteer turnover and burnout, job rewards should be closely tailored and aligned to volunteer preferences as this leads to a better volunteer-assignment match. Whether supervising paid or volunteer workers, supervisors must have a true understanding of employee's motivation to work (Liao-Troth & Dunn, 1999). Regardless of the work sector or position within the organization, it is through knowing the employee and their motivating factors, that the supervisor will be able to tailor their approach to employee motivation.

Motivational Methods

Leaders should place more emphasis on how to get high-quality service from each of their employees; but unfortunately, they place much of their time in trying to increase and improve the production of products.

There has been a significant increase in the amount of studies on motivational techniques used to urge better performance from employees. However, it is hard to find one technique suitable for the numerous complex needs of each employee (Vranova, 2012). Employers should not view their workers as service providers, but as an essential resource contributing to the accomplishment of the business (Muscalu & Muntean, 2013). Some of the circumstances that impact motivation is compensation, human resource management, and working conditions (Muo, 2013).

Extrinsic and intrinsic factors are two key components involved in motivation (Vranova, 2012). The extrinsic factors are related to those motivating factors from external sources. Examples include money, working conditions, and leadership style. Money is a common extrinsic motivator (Cosma & Gilceava, 2014). Motivating with cash is an impelling influence that encourages workers to reach an anticipated goal (Muo, 2013). Using cash as a motivator for employees goes as far back as the twentieth century. Many believe it is a good motivating factor because it is known, desired and required across the world (Cosma & Gilceava, 2014). However, there are elements that impact the effects of this factor. One of these factors includes how the process of receiving these funds is applied. Aarabi, Subramaniam, and Akeel (2013) believed money to be the most influential motivating factor.

On the other hand, intrinsic factors are personal and expressive in nature and derive from within a person. Intrinsic factors are often said to be more significant; having a sense of achievement from reaching a goal is an example of intrinsic motivation (Aworemi, 2011). Employers are increasing their knowledge on these motivation factors and the processes needed to implement them to improve their employees' work habits (Aarabi et al., 2013). When an employee is motivated, he or she is more consistent in performance and eager for constant improvement. Building teams and relationships are needed to keep the organizational goals on a positive path. Without motivation, communication, collaboration, and social relations, there could be a disruption in the flow of the organization. The goal-setting theory posits that goals are the most important factors affecting the motivation and behavior of employees. Specific goals often involve quantitative targets for improvement in a behavior of interest. Specific performance goals are much more effective than those in which a person is told to do their best (Locke & Latham, 2005).

Human resource management has a very distinguished role in assisting organizations in meeting their goals of recruiting, choosing, and creating highly qualified employees (Muscalu & Muntean, 2013). Organizations must create an environment that encourages these employees to put forth their best efforts (Muo, 2013). This may include providing professional development, recognizing exemplary work habits, and offering support within the organization. This environment increases the organization's ability to recruit and retain workers, as well as enriches the overall success of the organization.

The aforementioned practices of recruiting and retaining employees are the primary purpose for human resource management (Vranova, 2012). Aarabi et al. (2013) believed that human resource management should take the initiative in providing organizations with more motivational strategies. Employees thrive from having an effective leader and being active members of a prosperous organization (Muo, 2013). Organizations must invest in their employees in an effort to ensure longevity and success (Muscalu & Muntean, 2013). Therefore, human resource management has a duty and responsibility to create and implement motivating techniques within organizations.

The structure of today's working environment has become more unwelcoming (Muscalu & Muntean, 2013). Aarabi et al. (2013) believe there is a strong connection between a risk-free working environment and employees functioning at high levels on the job; these employees typically had good attendance and a strong work ethic. Employees must feel valued, respected, and have a sense of ownership in the organization (Muo, 2013). Vranova (2012) believed the aforementioned features increase job fulfillment;

these individuals have a tendency to have a positive demeanor and are more conscientious on the job. Aarabi et al. found it imperative that leaders put forth even a stronger effort in creating a pleasant working environment. Organizations must develop some type of plan to increase their employees' commitment to work (Aworemi, 2011). Creating an employee friendly environment is a prerequisite for warranting a high achieving organization (Muscalu & Muntean, 2013). This type of working environment is known to improve on the job performances of employees. Therefore, leaders must focus on interacting more with their employees in an effort to know them on a personal yet professional level (Aarabi et al., 2013).

Motivating employees is a very cumbersome but worthwhile process (Muscalu & Muntean, 2013). Therefore, organizations must continue to discover and implement methods to enhance the productivity of their workers. This implementation is more beneficial when it is done in a respected and employee-friendly working environment. Many times these conditions produce intrinsically motivated employees (Gilbert, 2011). There is a strong relationship between effectively motivating employees and the success of an organization (Cosma & Gilceava, 2014). Discovering ways to limit stress and motivate employees is more vital than ever before. Considering the various motivational theories, organizations that implement methods to inspire their employees in working to their full potential will produce a lucrative organization (Aworemi, 2011; Muo, 2013). However, it is wise to remember that no one theory or method may be successful to meet the needs of every employee and organizational structure because each entity is an individual with varying needs (Muscalu & Muntean, 2013). These methods must be individualized to meet the needs of the employees and should be utilized in a consistent manner. The Hawthorne Effect (n.d.) illustrated that employees are more productive when they know their work is being observed or accessed, when they are provided feedback, and when allowed to offer input into the work process. Recognition is sought by employees for assurances that they are doing their job well and reassurance is needed to prove that an employee's opinion matters as well. When all of this happens, motivation to work becomes high for both the employee and the organization.

The equity theory suggests that individuals engage in social comparison by comparing their efforts and rewards with those of others. The perception of individuals about the fairness of their rewards relative to others influences their level of motivation. Equity exists when individuals perceive that the ratio of efforts to rewards is the same for them as it is for others to whom they compare themselves (Burgess & Huston, 2013). Inequity exists when individuals perceive that the ratio of efforts to rewards is different (usually negatively) for them than to others. According to the equity theory, individuals are motivated to reduce what they consider to be their inequity and attempt this in different ways. For example, an employee may change his or her level of effort; an employee who feels under-rewarded is likely to work less. A person may also try to change his or her rewards, for example by asking for time off or for a raise. Another possible option is by changing the behavior of the person. This is done when someone is encouraged to put forth more in their actions. Finally, a person experiencing inequity may change by drawing a comparison to a different person to assess equity. For managers, the equity theory emphasizes the importance of a reward system that is perceived as fair by employees (Barnet, 2015).

RECOMMENDATIONS TO HANDLE STRESS

Implementing change agents is complex and requires skill in changing the behaviors of individuals and the organizations (Forman, 2015). Russell (2014) investigated the relationship between stress, burnout in high-risk jobs, and the influence of leadership. Russell surveyed 379 police officers from southern and southwestern United States agencies and found that workplace stress increases burnout, but transformational leadership diminishes the stress and burnout in moderate stressful conditions. Transformational leadership influences and motivates followers for the benefit of the organization. Organizational and operational factors were the strongest sources of stress, and a lack of participation in decision making and unfair workplace treatment contributed to increased stress levels. Stress affected both the individual and organization. Russell recommended investigating the effects of transformational leadership on performance, behavior, and psychological well-being in high risk occupations.

Edwards, Franco-Watkins, Cullen, Howell, and Acuff (2014) merged the challenge-hindrance and the sociocognitive models of stress to demonstrate the impact of stress in job performance. Edwards et al. conducted two studies to measure the effect on perceived stress, on-task effort, and negative affective thoughts. In the first study, perceived stress and performance was reconciled by on-task effort and negative affective thoughts. In the second study, the stressor strength was manipulated by assigning time pressure or no time pressure. The time pressure reduced performance and increased perceived stress. The seriousness of the stressor affected whether people saw the stressor as a challenge or a hindrance. It also affected work performance. Edwards et al. reported individual differences in perceived stress affected performance more than actual stressors with no time pressure. Edwards et al. emphasized the importance of weighing the type and severity of the environmental stressor as well as the individual differences in perceived stress. A relationship existed between perceived stress and performance; individual differences in positive and negative stress perceptions have the greatest impact when there is not a high stressor. Furthermore, individuals with high EI face less perceived stress than those with lower EI (Goleman, 2004).

Individual perception, character, and duration of stressful situations play a role in decision making. Leaders perceive situations differently; perception is dependent upon resources, urgency, uncertainty, and influence (McVicar, 2015). The decision-making process is both a cognitive and emotional process that is affected by physical and mental comfort, personal stress, time pressures, adequacy of information, and control over the situation. Stress can positively or negatively impact decision making. McVicar (2015) found stress produces a hormonal reaction that increases alertness and sharp cognitive functioning in the initial stages of decision making. However, there may be negative consequences like impaired cognitive reasoning, planning, concentration, and memory recall in prolonged stressful situations. In an article from the Educational Testing Service (2014), it was suggested that both real-world and virtual-world interactive learning environments, games, simulations, intelligent tutors, and organizational teaming can provide leaders with management of stress within the decision-making process. There are techniques for building stress resilient emotional intelligence, but it takes skill and effort to use these techniques: (a) awareness, (b) thinking about emotions, (c) monitoring emotional sensations, and (d) rest and recovery. Training, desensitization of emotions in low-stress environments, and reprogrammig somatic markers will devolp stress resilient emotional intelligence.

REFERENCES

Aarabi, M. S., Subramaniam, I. D., & Akeel, A. B. (2013). Relationship between motivational factors and job performances of employees in Malaysian service industry. *Asian Social Science*, *9*(9), 301–310. doi:10.5539/ass.v9n9p301

Anthony, S. D., Johnson, M. W., & Sinfield, J. V. (2008). Building an engine that produces a steady stream of innovative growth businesses is difficult, but companies that are able to do it differentiate themselves from competitors. Retrieved from sloanreview.mit.edu/article/institutionalizing-innovation

Aworemi, J. R. (2011). An empirical study of the motivational factors of employees in Nigeria. *International Journal of Economics and Finance, 3*(5), 227-233. doi:10.5539 /ijef.v3n5p227

Baker, M. W. (2013). *A multiple case study of the dark side of leadership: An exploration of executives who led their companies to disastrous results versus exemplary CEOs who did not* (Order No. 3570902).

Bandura, A. (1973). *Aggression: A social learning analysis*. Englewood Cliffs, NJ: Prentice Hall.

Barbuto, J., & Wheeler, D. (2007, October). Becoming a servant leader: Do you have what it takes? *NetGuide*. Retrieved from http://www.ianrpubs.unl.edu /epublic/live/g1481/build/g1481.pdf

Barnet, T. (2015). Motivation and motivation theory. Retrieved from http://www.referenceforbusiness.com/management/Mar-No/Motivation-and-Motivation-Theory.htm

Baron, R. (1996). Interpersonal relations in organizations. In K. Murphy (Ed.), *Individual differences* (pp. 334–370). San Francisco, CA: Jossey Bass.

Bierema, L. L. (1999). *The process of the learning organization: Making sense of change*

Bollinger, A. S., & Smith, R. D. (2001). Managing organizational knowledge as a strategic asset. *Journal of Knowledge Management*, *5*(1), 8–18. doi:10.1108/13673270110384365

Bolman, L. G., & Deal, T. E. (2003). *Reframing organizations: Artistry, choice, and leadership* (3rd ed.). San Francisco, CA: Jossey Bass.

Bolman, L. G., & Deal, T. E. (2006). *The wizard and the warrior: Leading with passion and power*. San Francisco, CA: Jossey-Bass.

Bolman, L. G., & Deal, T. E. (2009). Battles and beliefs: Rethinking the roles of today's leaders. *Leadership in Action*, *29*(5), 14–18. doi:10.1002/lia.1306

Burgess, R. L., & Huston, T. L. (2013). *Social exchange in developing relationships*. New York, NY: Academic Press.

Buselli, E. F. (1999). The stress response. *The Journal of Cardiovascular Nursing*, *13*(3), 60–72. doi:10.1097/00005082-199904000-00006 PMID:10098006

Cameron, G. D. (2012). *A cross-sectional study to examine occupational stress between online and on-ground educators* (Doctoral dissertation).

Campbell, M., Baltes, J., Martin, A., & Meddings, K. (2007). *The stress of leadership*. Colorado Springs, CO: Center for Creative Leadership.

Colligan, T. W., & Higgins, E. M. (2005). Workplace stress: Etiology and consequences. *Journal of Workplace Behavioral Health*, *21*(2), 89–97. doi:10.1300/J490v21n02_07

Collins, J., & Porras, J. (1991). Organizational vision and visionary organizations. *California Management Review*, *34*(1), 30–51. doi:10.2307/41166682

Cosma, D., & Gilceava, S. A. (2014). How important is money as an incentive to motivate employees in the higher education sector? *Analele Universitatii Constantin Brancusi din Targu Jiu. Seria Economie*, *2*(2), 116–122.

Covey, S. M. R. (2010). How can workplace learning and performance professionals instill trust in an organization's leaders? *T+D, 64*(10), 10-11.

Cowherd, D. M., & Levine, D. I. (1992). Product quality and pay equity between lower-level employees and top management: An investigation of distributive justice theory. *Administrative Science Quarterly*, *37*(2), 302. doi:10.2307/2393226

Cowley, E., & Smith, S. (2014). Motivation and mission in the public sector: Evidence from the world values survey. *Theory and Decision*, *76*(2), 241–263. doi:10.1007/s11238-013-9371-6

Davenport, N., Schwartz, R. D., & Elliott, G. P. (2005). *Mobbing: Emotional abuse in the American workplace*. Ames, IA: Civil Society.

Deming, W. E. (1986). *Out of the crisis*. Cambridge, MA: Massachusetts Institute of Technology.

Dickerson, S., & Kemeny, M. (2004). Acute stressors and cortisol responses: A theoretical integration and synthesis of laboratory research. *Psychological Bulletin*, *130*(3), 355–391. doi:10.1037/0033-2909.130.3.355 PMID:15122924

Dobbs, J. M. (2014). *The relationship between perceived toxic leadership styles, leader effectiveness, and organizational cynicism* (Doctoral dissertation).

Doty, J., & Fenlason, J. (2013). Narcissism and toxic leaders. *Military Review*, *93*(1), 55–60.

Drucker, P. (1998). *Managing and leadership*. Retrieved from http://web.mit.edu/mbarker/www/ideas/drucker.html

Duffy, M., & Sperry, L. (2014). *Overcoming mobbing: A recovery guide for workplace aggression and bullying*. New York, NY: Oxford University Press.

Educational Testing Service. (2014, October 10). ETS to host experts for innovative assessment of collaboration. Retrieved from https://www.ets.org/newsroom/news_releases/ets_host_experts

Edwards, B. D., Franco-Watkins, A., Cullen, K. L., Howell, J. W., & Acuff, R. E. Jr. (2014). Unifying the challenge-hindrance and sociocognitive models of stress. *International Journal of Stress Management*, *21*(2), 162–185. doi:10.1037/a0034730

Flum, H. (2015). Relationships and career development: An integrative approach. In P. J. Hartung, M. L. Savickas, & W. B. Walsh (Eds.), *APA handbook for career intervention* (pp. 145–158)., doi:10.1037/14438-009

Forman, S. G. (2015). *Leadership for implementation and change. Implementation of mental health programs in schools: A change agent's guide* (pp. 55–69). Washington, DC: American Psychological Association; doi:10.1037/14597-005

Garfield, C. (1992). *Second to none: How our smartest companies put people first*. Homewood, IL: Business One Irwin.

Garvin, D. A., Edmondson, A. C., & Gino, F. (2008). Is yours a learning organization? *Harvard Business Review*, *86*(3), 1–11. Retrieved from http://mfi.caifos.com/wp-content/uploads /2013/03/Is-Yours-a-Learning-Organization.pdf PMID:18411968

Gilbert, J. (2011). The millennials: A new generation of employees, a new set of engagement policies. *Ivey Business Journal*, *75*(5), 26–28.

Gilbert, J. A., Carr-Ruffin, N., Ivancevich, J. M., & Konopaske, R. (2012). Toxic versus cooperative behaviors at work: The role of organizational culture and leadership in creating community-centered organizations. *International Journal of Leadership Studies*, *7*(1), 24–46.

Goffee, R., & Jones, G. (2006). *Why should anyone be led by you? Harvard Business Review*. Boston, MA: Harvard Business School Press.

Goleman, D. (2004). *What makes a leader? Harvard Business Review*. Boston, MA: Harvard Business School Press.

Graham, S., & Weiner, B. (1996). Theories and principles of motivation. In D. C. Berliner & R. C. Calfee (Eds.), *Handbook of educational psychology* (pp. 63–84). New York, NY: Macmillan.

Greenleaf, R. K. (1970). *The servant as leader*. Indianapolis, IN: Greenleaf Center.

Gregory, B., Harris, S., Armenakis, A., & Shook, C. (2009). Organizational culture and effectiveness: A study of values, attitudes, and organizational outcomes. *Journal of Business Research*, *62*(7), 673–679. doi:10.1016/j.jbusres.2008.05.021

Guillén, M., Ferrero, I., & Hoffman, W. M. (2015). The neglected ethical and spiritual motivations in the workplace. *Journal of Business Ethics*, *128*(4), 803–816. doi:10.1007/s10551-013-1985-7

Haas, B. W., Anderson, I. W., & Filkowski, M. M. (2015). Interpersonal reactivity and the attribution of emotional reactions. *Emotion (Washington, D.C.)*, *15*(3), 390–398. doi:10.1037/emo0000053 PMID:25706827

Hall, G. E., & Hord, S. M. (2015). *Implementing change: Patterns, principles, and potholes* (4th ed.). Upper Saddle River, NJ: Prentice-Hall.

Hawthorne Effect. (n.d.). *Harvard Business School Baker Library Collections*. Retrieved from http://www.library.hbs.edu/hc/hawthorne/09.html

Hendrickson, R., Lane, J., Harris, J., & Dorman, R. (2013). *Academic leadership and governance of higher education*. Sterling, VA: Stylus.

Herzberg, F. (2003). One more time: How do you motivate employees? Retrieved from https://hbr.org/2003/01/one-more-time-how-do-you-motivate-employees

Hodgkinson, G. P., Sadler-Smith, E., Burke, L. A., Claxton, G., & Sparrow, P. R. (2009). Intuition in organizations: Implications for strategic management. *Long Range Planning*, *42*(3), 277-297. doi:10.1016/j.lrp.2009.05.003

Howard, D. Z. (2003). *Stress@work: An exploration of the impact of information and communication technology on Canadian workers* [Master's thesis]. Concordia University, Montreal, Quebec, Canada.

Huang, T. Y. (2012). Intuition and emotion: Examining two nonrational approaches in complex decision making (Unpublished doctoral dissertation). London, England: City University; Retrieved from http://openaccess.city.ac.uk/2072/1/Huang,_Tori_Yu-Wen.pdf

Huitt, W. (2007). Maslow's hierarchy of needs, educational psychology interactive. Retrieved from http://www.edpsycinteractive.org/topics/cponation/maslow.html

Human Resources, U. C. S. F. (n.d.). Chapter 14: Team building. Retrieved from http://ucsfhr.ucsf.edu/index.php/pubs/hrguidearticle/chapter-14-team-building/

Jaramillo, F., Locander, W. B., Spector, P. E., & Harris, E. G. (2007). Getting the job done: The moderating role of initiative on the relationship between intrinsic motivation and adaptive selling. *Journal of Personal Selling & Sales Management, 27*, 59-74. doi:10.2753/PSS0885-3134270104

Juli, T. (2011). *Leadership principles for project success*. New York, NY: CRC Press.

Katsapis, C. C. A. (2008). *Incidence and types of occupational role stress among university research administrators* [Doctoral dissertation].

Kim, C. H., & Scullion, H. (2013). The effect of corporate social responsibility on employee motivation: A cross-national study. The Poznan University of Economics Review, 13(2), 5-30.

Krishna, V., & Marquardt, M. J. (2007). *A framework for the development of organizational commitment using action learning.*

Kumpakaite, V. K. (2008). Human resource development in learning organization. *Journal of Business Economics and Management*, *9*(1), 25–31. doi:10.3846/1611-1699.2008.9.25-31

Lazarus, J. (2000). *Stress relief & relaxation techniques*. Los Angeles, CA: Keats.

Lazarus, R. S. (1966). *Psychological stress and the coping process*. New York, NY: McGraw-Hill.

Lee-Chai, A. Y., & Bargh, J. A. (2001). *The use and abuse of power: Multiple perspectives on the causes of corruption*. Philadelphia, PA: Taylor & Francis Group.

Lencioni, P. (2002). *The five dysfunctions of a team: A leadership fable*. San Francisco, CA: Jossey-Bass.

Liao-Troth, M., & Dunn, C. P. (1999). Social constructs and human service: Managerial sensemaking of volunteer motivation. *Voluntas, 10*(4), 345-361. doi:10.1023/A:1021486408619

Lindh, D. (2013). *Workplace stress, Mindfulness Based Stress Reduction (MBSR) and Gas Discharge Visualization (GDV): Innovative practical measurements in Organization Development (OD) and employee wellness* [Doctoral dissertation].

Locke, E. A., & Latham, G. P. (2002). Building a practically useful theory of goal setting and task motivation: A 35-year odyssey. *The American Psychologist*, *57*(9), 705–717. doi:10.1037/0003-066X.57.9.705 PMID:12237980

Magnusson, D. (1996). Interactionism and the person approach in developmental psychology. *European Child & Adolescent Psychiatry*, *5*(S1), 18–22. doi:10.1007/BF00538538 PMID:9010658

Marquardt, M. J. (2011). *Building the learning organization: Achieving strategic advantage through a commitment to learning* (3rd ed.). Boston, MA: Nicholas Brealey.

Maslow, A. H. (1943). A theory of human motivation. *Psychological Review, 50*(4), 370–396. doi:10.1037/h0054346

McClelland, D. C. (1961). *The achieving society*. Princeton, NJ: D Van Nostrand; doi:10.1037/14359-000

McCleskey, J. (2013). The dark side of leadership: Measurement, assessment, and intervention. *Business Renaissance Quarterly, 8*(2), 35–53.

McEwen, B. S. (2005). Stressed or stressed out: What is the difference? *Journal of Psychiatry & Neuroscience, 30*(5), 315–318. PMID:16151535

McVicar, M. (2015). Decisions in crisis - An examination. *Comparative Strategy, 34*(1), 14–43. doi:10.1080/01495933.2015.994403

Mehta, M. (2012). Situational leadership and personal effectiveness: Managers in Indian development organizations. *Foundation for Organizational Research & Education, 30*(1), 23–34.

Merrifield, J. (2012). *Ecologies of learning: How culture and context impact outcomes of workplace literacy and essential skills*. Montreal, QC, Canada: Centre for Literacy of Quebec.

Metcalf, J. A. (2014). *The challenges of replicating human resource (HR) practices in a global environment: A qualitative study of HR leaders in a manufacturing company* (Order No. AAI3602346).

Millan, R. O. (2008). *Examining emotional intelligence differences among nursing students at a college in South Texas* (Doctoral dissertation).

Mink, M. (2012, October 17). Gain the right direction. *Investor's Business Daily.*

Moberg, C. R., & Leasher, M. (2011). Examining the differences in salesperson motivation among different cultures. *American Journal of Business, 26*(2), 145–160. doi:10.1108/19355181111174525

Muo, I. (2013). Motivating and managing knowledge workers: Evidences from diverse industries and cultures. *Journal of Management and Sustainability, 3*(2), 119-131. doi:10.5539/jms.v3n2p119

Muscalu, E., & Muntean, S. (2013). Motivation a stimulating factor for increasing human resource management performance. *Review of International Comparative Management, 14*(2), 303–309.

Namie, G., & Namie, R. (2003). *The bully at work: What you can do to stop the hurt and reclaim your dignity on the job*. Naperville, IL: Sourcebooks.

Němečková, I. (2012). Education as employee motivation and retention factor of the companies operating in the Czech Republic. *Central European Business Review, 1*(1), 33–37. doi:10.18267/j.cebr.6

Northouse, P. G. (2012). *Introduction to leadership: Concepts and practice*. Los Angeles, CA: Sage.

Pink, D. H. (2009). *Drive: The surprising truth about what motivates us*. New York, NY: Riverhead Books.

Raye, J. (2014). Fractal organisation theory. *Organisational Transformation and Social Change, 11*(1), 50–68. doi:10.1179/1477963313Z.00000000025

Riaz, M. N., Riaz, M. A., & Batool, N. (2014). Managerial decision making styles as predictors of personal and organizational outcomes of in-service employees. *Journal of Behavioural Science*, *24*(2), 100–116.

Robbins, S. P., DeCenzo, D. A., & Wolter, R. (2013). *Supervision today?* (7th ed.). Upper Saddle River, NJ: Pearson.

Rosenbach, W. E., Taylor, R. L., & Youndt, M. A. (2012). *Contemporary issues in leadership*. Boulder, CO: Westview Press.

Ross, D. B., Matteson, R., & Exposito, J. A. (2014, December). Servant leadership to toxic leadership: Power of influence over power of control. *Paper presented at the Fifth Annual Virtual Conference on Moral Leadership: Narcissism and Toxic Leadership*, Regent University. Paper retrieved from http://www.regent.edu/acad /global/conferences/virtual/2014/papers/2014_Moral_Leadership_Conference _Ross_Matteson_Exposito.pdf

Ruiz-Mercader, J., Merono-Cerdan, A. L., & Sabater-Sanchez, R. (2006). Informational technology and learning: Their relationship and impact on organizational performance in small businesses. Retrieved from papers.ssrn.com/sol3/papers.cfm?abstract_id=1501588

Russell, L. M. (2014). An empirical investigation of high-risk occupations. *Management Research Review*, *37*(4), 367–384. doi:10.1108/MRR-10-2012-0227

Schmidt, A. A. (2014). *An examination of toxic leadership, job outcomes, and the impact of military deployment.*

Schultz, J. R. (2014). Creating a culture of empowerment fosters the flexibility to change. *Global Business and Organizational Excellence*, *34*(1), 41–50. doi:10.1002/joe.21583

Senge, P. (2006). *The fifth discipline: The art and practice of the learning organization*. New York, NY: Currency Doubleday.

Shambrook, J. (2007). Results from the 2007 research administrator stress perception survey. *Research Management Review*, *15*(2), 12.

Smith, M. K. (2009). Jean Lave, Etienne Wenger and communities of practice: The encyclopedia of informal education. Retrieved from www.infed.org/biblio/communities_of _practice.htm

Southard, S. (1993). *Total quality management (team building and cross training): From business to academe and back again to business.*

Thomas, J. R., & Holley, R. P. (2012). Management versus repetitive tasks-avoiding "working for the weekend". *New Library World, 113*(9), 462-473. doi:10.1108 /03074801211273939

Thompson, H. L. (2007). Catastrophic leadership failure: An overview. Retrieved from https://www.hpsys.com/PDFs/CatastrophicLeadershipFailureOverviewv2_18SEP2007 .pdf

Thompson, H. L. (2010). *The stress effect: Why smart leaders made dumb decisions and what to do about it* (1st ed.). San Francisco, CA: Jossey-Bass.

Verner, J. M., Babar, M. A., Cerpa, N., Hall, T., & Beecham, S. (2014). Factors that motivate software engineering teams: A four country empirical study. *Journal of Systems and Software*, *92*, 115–127. doi:10.1016/j.jss.2014.01.008

Villarreal, J. (2014). Addressing narcissistic leadership through organizational leadership and systematic implementations. *Paper presented at the Fifth Annual Virtual Conference on Moral Leadership: Narcissism and Toxic Leadership*, Regent University. Paper retrieved from http://www.regent.edu/acad/global/conferences/virtual/2014/papers/2014_Moral_Leadership_Conference_Villarreal.pdf

Vranova, S. (2012). Identifying the specifics of motivating different groups of employees. *Journal of Global Science and Technology Forum*, *2*(2), 98–104. doi:10.5176/2010-4804_2.2.188

Wang, Y., Ph, D., Yang, C., Ph, D., Wang, K., & Ph, D. (2012). Comparing public and private employees' job satisfaction and turnover. *Public Personnel Management*, *41*(3), 557–573. doi:10.1177/009102601204100310

Welch, D. M. (2006). *Occupational stress, self-efficacy and symptom relationships among medical-surgical hospital nurses* [Doctoral dissertation].

Weldy, T. G., & Gillis, W. E. (2010). The learning organization: Variations at different organizational levels. *The Learning Organization*, *17*(5), 455-470. doi:http://dx.doi.org.ezproxylocal.library.nova.edu/10.1108/09696471011059831

Wilenius, M. (2014). Leadership in the sixth wave-excursions into the new paradigm of the Kondratieff cycle 2010-2015. *Eur J Futures Res*, *2*(1), 36. doi:10.1007/s40309-014-0036-7

Yadav, S. (2014). The role of emotional intelligence in organization development. *ICFAI Journal of Knowledge Management*, *12*(4), 49.

Zhou, J., & Fischer, K. W. (2013). Culturally appropriate education: Insights from educational neuroscience. *Mind. Brain & Education*, *7*(4), 225–231. doi:10.1111/mbe.12030

KEY TERMS AND DEFINITIONS

Biopsychosocial Model: The biopsychosocial model provides a theoretical framework for understanding how the human body is impacted by biological, psychological, and sociological factors. It provides the foundation for the theory of mind/body interaction and how stress impacts an individual at a physiological and psychological level.

Healthy Leadership: This positive approach of leadership creates an inspirational, healthy, and collaborative workplace culture and promotes the sharing of ideas, embraces diversity and diverse thinking, and spreads spiritual and emotional health among others. Healthy leadership reduces stress and helps people reach their potential to move to the next goal.

Motivation: motivation helps a leader create an environment to inspire action, challenge and stimulate the mind, and promote a person's psychological well-being. People who find work important, interesting, and useful will be motivated to be productive and successful. Intrinsic motivation leads to a reduction in stress.

Stress: Stress involves two factors: (a) the stressful stimulus, and (b) the organism's response to that stimulus. When exposed to a stressful stimulus, whether physical or psychological, a series of neuroendocrine and neuronal responses occur, which lead to a distinctive set of physiological responses.

Toxic Leadership: This type of abusive leadership involves an individual who negatively influences others and exerts his or her power by placing a hardship on the corporate culture. The psychological, physiological, and emotional hardship harms others and adds stress within the organization, diminishes leadership efficacy, decreases organizational morale and productivity, and has a negative financial impact on the organization.

Workplace Culture: The culture within the workplace structure is created by leaders who are concerned with the ethical and moral behaviors and the emotional well-being of the entire staff and leadership teams who share the same mission, vision, expectations, beliefs, and values.

Chapter 11
Framework of Indian Healthcare System and its Challenges:
An Insight

Prashant Mehta
National Law University, India

ABSTRACT

India, one of the oldest civilizations and second most populous country is ethnically, linguistically, geographically, religious, and demographically diverse is poorly ranked due to complex public healthcare system, which suffers from insufficient funding, poor management. Poor health intertwined with poverty, affordability, accessibility, burden of infectious and non-communicable affecting lives of most Indians. Healthcare ecosystems are complex and still evolving, investments in service delivery system, infrastructure, and technology, are still being experimented and explored. India's booming population; increasing purchasing power; rising awareness of personal health and hygiene; and significant growth in infectious, chronic degenerative, and lifestyle diseases are driving the growing market. In this chapter we will explore accessible and affordable healthcare system, state of public healthcare, healthcare reforms, governance (Constitutional Provisions, Law, and Policy framework) in healthcare delivery, and Opportunity offered by market drivers.

INTRODUCTION

India is a highly heterogeneous country in ethnicity, religion, and language. It is also diverse in its demographics, given the presence of an extremely large rural population. The country covers only a little over 2 percent of the earth's land surface, yet its population is approaching 20 percent of the world total. Because of its scale, strengths, and vulnerabilities, the future of India and its ability to safeguard the health and wellbeing of its citizens raises issues of importance to the entire world community. The growing demand for quality healthcare and the absence of matching delivery mechanisms pose a challenge as well as opportunity for healthcare service providers, to design and engineer a sustainable healthcare system with customizable delivery formats to benefit demanding and health conscious Indian population (Sreenu, 2011).

DOI: 10.4018/978-1-5225-0640-9.ch011

The relationship between health and poverty or health and development is complex, multi-faceted and multidirectional. Notwithstanding sixty-eight years of existence as an independent republic, large sections of the Indian population do not as yet have reliable and affordable access to good quality healthcare. This is because of poverty, which in its various dimensions could be a manifestation, as well as a determinant of an individual's health. In its most basic form — as a state of food deprivation and nutritional inadequacy — poverty has a direct bearing on the morbidity and longevity of people.

Defining health has become more complex and diversified than ever before as it does not have much to do with the state of having a disease, or absence of it, but it is to do with a person's integrated ability to perform and function efficiently with a productive value conducive to the well-being of self, his family, and society at large. This notion also correlates with the definition of health given in preamble of constitution of World Health Organization (WHO), which states that "*Health is a state of complete physical, mental, and social well-being and not merely the absence of disease or infirmity*" (WHO, 1948a). Attainments on other dimensions of human development, especially educational and economic wellbeing, reinforce the transition towards better health and longevity.

Further the idea of integrating health to a duo of a disease free state and a sound social, psychological, and spiritual combination was recognized as early as 2000 years ago, when Sushruta who lived between 600 to 1000 BC (a surgeon and teacher of Ayurveda) compiled the medical treatise "Sushruta Samhitain" containing multiple detailed references to diseases and medical procedures in Vedic Sanskrit. He is also considered to be the 'Father of Surgery' who defined health as a physiological balance added with psycho sensual happiness (Shasthri, 2007). Sushruta goes further to state that health is also affected by one's moral, social, and spiritual values. Ayurveda holds that Dharma (spiritual gains), Artha (monetary gains), Kama (sensual gains), and Moksha (liberation), the four primary objectives of human life, are possible only for a healthy human being. This is possible when ideal healthcare system as defined by Ayurveda is one which cures a disease without causing or precipitating other illnesses (Tripathi, 1983). In today's era, healthcare covers not merely medical care but also all aspects -preventive care too. Nor can it be limited to care rendered by or financed out of public expenditure within the government sector alone but must include incentives and disincentives for self-care and care paid for by private citizens to get over ill health.

STRUCTURE AND RESOURCES OF HEALTHCARE SYSTEM

The structure of India's healthcare system is multifaceted, consisting of various types of providers practicing in different systems of medicine and facilities, and within federal structure. There are about 600000 hospital beds in more than 13550 Hospitals; 27400 Dispensaries; 717860 Registered Medical Practitioners; 295000 Nurses; 227000 Auxiliary Nurses; and Midwives. This includes multi-layered rural healthcare system having District hospitals usually with bed strength of over 300 beds located at district headquarters, Sub-district hospitals usually with bed strength of 100-300 located at divisional headquarters in each district, Community Health Centre (3043 in no.) is a 30 bed hospital, acts as a referral unit for four Primary Health Centres (PHCs), and each Primary Health Centre (22842 in no.) is a referral unit for six sub-centres has around 4-6 beds. Sub-centre (137311 in no.) is the most peripheral contact point between the PHC and the community.

The central government policies, though well-intentioned, have mostly failed to deliver intended outcomes, as under the Indian Constitution, health and family welfare has been identified as a State subject. The main responsibility of infrastructure and manpower building rests with the different State Governments. The states spend more than 80 percent of the total expenditure on curative cure. The Central Government spends more than 70 percent of the total expenditure on preventive and promotive health care. These decisions have introduced policies and fiscal incentives that have inadvertently enabled states to prioritize medical services and single-issue programs over broader public health services, and reduced the capacity of the public health workforce to deliver public health services.

Persistent gaps in manpower and infrastructure, with wide inter-State differences, especially at the primary health care level, disproportionately impacts less developed rural areas. This is due to low public spending on health, rural healthcare infrastructure is ailing or severely depleted were nearly three quarters of Indian population resides. The Primary Healthcare Approach was never implemented in its full form as it was considered too idealistic and expensive, and it was replaced with disease focussed selective model. Thus selective vertical programmes were pushed as a substitute for comprehensive health system development as it has not responded adequately to the interrelationship between health and socio-economic development. It only indicates than the approach to development of health sector in the country has not been sufficiently integrated with the overall process of development. What India needs is a healthcare system that can meet the demands of over 1.28 billion people, most of whom are unable to bear the burden of rising healthcare costs. Thus the federal structure has impacted healthcare policy in such a large, diverse, and fragmented country leaving healthcare system in disarray.

According to Mann, et.al., WHO recognizes health as a human right and the common denominators for ensuring social well-being (as cited by Golechha, 2015), however combination of poor social policies, unfair economic planning, and bad political mechanisms over a period had led to inequality, social stratification, socio-economic disparities based on visible circumstances of people's lives -. their access to healthcare and education, their conditions of work and leisure, their homes, communities, towns or cities, and - their chances of leading a flourishing life (WHO, 2008b).Therefore impact of healthcare system on population derives from social determinants like living conditions, nutrition, safe drinking water, sanitation, education, early child development, providing financial security using social security measures etc. Together, the structural determinants and conditions of daily life constitute the social determinants of health. Lack of adequate progress on these underlying social determinants of health has been acknowledged as a glaring failure of the Indian healthcare system.

CURRENT HEALTHCARE SCENARIO

India encapsulates a paradox; its relatively unimpressive performance in healthcare despite high economic growth of 7 percent. India's public health expenditure is currently 1.26 percent of GDP is very lowest among BRICS countries and far less from the WHO recommended level of 5 percent. Continuous budgetary cuts and neo liberal policies meant that private sector spending on health as a percentage of GDP is higher than that of public sector. The Government (Central and State Governments combined) expenditure on health was 1.36 percent of the GDP, as a percentage of total expenditure, the expenditure on health was 4.8 percent, as per social services expenditure, the expenditure on health was 19.2 percent as per budget estimates in 2012-13.

As per the (World Health Statistics 2011), in case of India, the total expenditure on health as percent of GDP was 4.6 percent in 2000 this came down to 4.2 percent in 2008. The government expenditure on health as percentage of total expenditure on health was 27.5 percent in 2000 which rose to 32.4 percent in 2008. The out-of-pocket expenditure as percent of private expenditure on health was 92.2 percent in 2000 which reduced to 74.4 percent in 2008. The draft National Health Policy, 2015 has proposed target of raising public health expenditure to 2.5 percent from the present 1.36 percent of GDP. The consequences of low public spending and poor access to public healthcare facilities, and the burden of high health costs is felt disproportionately by the poorest income class resulting in a huge out-of-pocket (OOP) expenditure, pushing 40 million people below poverty line every year (Ramachandran, 2015). The unequal geographic distribution of doctors and lack of hospitals infrastructure makes it difficult for low-income families to seek treatment and access quality medical facilities, leading to delays and aggravating health problems.

The proposed Universal Health Coverage (UHC) includes provisions for 50 free essential drugs, health coverage for the poor and competitively priced premium health insurance for all. In simplest terms UHC means access to quality, effective and affordable health services for all, without imposing financial burden (O'Connell, Rasanathan & Chopra, 2014). Notwithstanding the goals of UHC in the 12th plan document, the government had reduced its role to merely providing preventive aspects like immunization and practically handing over all clinical part to unorganized private sector which provides 80 percent of healthcare services. Thus the phase of privatization and liberalisation of economy in 1990, has witnessed staggering health inequities, resurgence of communicable diseases and an even more unregulated drug industry with drug prices shooting up, adding up to the current crisis in public health. Along with the retreat from the goal of universal access, special health needs of women, children and other sections of society with special needs have become further sidelined or are inadequately addressed.

Every healthcare system however old or developed has its own advantages and limitations considering the diversified needs of rural, sub-urban, and urban populations. India needs to focus on giving equitable access to all by overcoming inequity based on religion, caste, and gender. There is also questionable efficiency and distrust in much of the public healthcare system, as it is crippled with inadequate funds, poor surveillance of health programs, lack of trained manpower, and other resources. The Ministry of Health and Family Welfare (MoHFW) can play a crucial role in guiding India's public health system by regulating clinical establishments, professional and technical education, food safety, medical technology products, research, clinical trials, implementation of policies and health related laws. Each of these areas needs urgent reforms which will entail moving away from reactive, voluminous, poorly implemented regulatory regimes, cobbled up in an ad-hoc manner to a more effective, rational, transparent and consistent regime (MoHFW, 2014a). Healthcare must be made a core priority for the next decade, to enable transformation of the healthcare system, while promoting pro-health policies in other sectors.

The largest gains in health status will come from preventive measures (Joumard & Kumar., (2015). Integration of traditional practices and home remedies with modern advancements in healthcare technology and associated services will be key differentiator. However we need to protect our highly diversified traditional healthcare systems without devaluing or delineating the essential framework on which it rests. There is every possibility where one system may work better than another under certain conditions which can be further improved by utilization of traditional skills in combination with the innovative technological breakthroughs made by the modern science (Alex, 2005) resulting in development of healthcare system which just ideal.

Determining the right mix of factors like *Availability* (what type of services exists), *Accessibility* (how they can be reached), *Adequacy* (does it meets consumers' requirements), *Affordability* (what is direct and indirect cost), *Acceptability* (does providers explain treatment with empathy) and balancing it will appropriate resource allocation will determine the success or failure of healthcare system in India.

Thus government and the society have to make concerted efforts together for improving the quality of life of people by redefining the health system on three key dimensions of health delivery: *Access, Cost,* and *Quality*.

The rise in the number of vehicles on the road and chaotic behaviour of drivers has resulted into increase in accidents, injuries, and road fatalities which are amongst the highest in the world. A National Crime Records Bureau (NCRB) report revealed that every year, more than 135,000 traffic collision-related deaths occur in India. Road traffic injuries are the sixth leading cause of death in India with a greater share of hospitalization, deaths, disabilities, and socio-economic losses in the young and middle-aged population (MoHFW, 2004b). Road traffic injuries also place a huge burden on the health sector in terms of pre-hospital, acute care, and rehabilitation (Gururaj, 2006). The nonexistence of "911" like system, poor public awareness of the Emergency Medical System (EMS), inadequate availability of right equipment's at emergency and trauma centres has placed big burdens on a healthcare delivery system in India. In most cases people help themselves during times of emergency as the current emergency response system is not appropriate. It has been observed that people call up emergency number, normally police helpline 100, only to get diverted to other departments, which delays response time. The Ministry of Home Affairs has also been pushing for a single emergency helpline number (police, fire, medical and other kind of emergencies services) in India in its bid to prepare effective and timely response in event of emergency.

As India seeks to become a global power, there is perhaps nothing more important than the health and well-being of its citizens. This is ensured in part through an effective, comprehensive healthcare system which needs to be strengthened further. The National Rural Health Mission (NRHM) and Rashtriya Swasthya Bima Yojana (RSBY) launched by the Government of India is a forward step in establishing effective integration and convergence of health services, reducing the out of pocket spending on tertiary healthcare, and affecting architectural correction in the healthcare delivery system in India. Health profiles published by the government should be used to help communities prioritize their health problems and to inform local decision making. Primary healthcare should be prioritized, since it is the greatest need of the vast majority and, if effectively delivered, will substantially reduce the demand for secondary and tertiary care. At the same time the government should come up with policy for improving the health status of the urban poor by adopting effective, efficient and sustainable strategic intervention approaches.

With severe shortage of qualified human resources for healthcare delivery, the public health facilities continue to face staff shortage as over 85 percent specialist doctors, 75 percent doctors, 80 percent laboratory technicians, 53 percent nursing and 52 percent ANM (auxiliary nurse midwife) posts are vacant across States (Nandan & Agrawal, 2012). Further health research activities do not match with public health priorities, which is necessary for better health outcomes. Government should make research initiatives more interactive with policies and implementation of health programmes for making health research more relevant to health system and policy. Also there is a need for strengthening research infrastructure and capacity building in the departments of community medicine in various institutes and to foster their partnerships with state health services for effective health outcomes.

Health Transitions

Rapid economic growth, coupled with rapid growth of middle class, is directly responsible for increased 'healthcare innovation', 'healthcare promotion' 'healthcare consumption' and 'health transition'. Healthcare innovation can be defined as "the introduction of a new concept, idea, service, process, or product aimed at improving treatment, diagnosis, education, outreach, prevention, and research with the long term goals of improving quality, safety, outcomes, efficiency, and costs" (Omachonu & Einspruch, 2010). Healthcare industry is experiencing a steady and stable transformation the world over, majorly with Information Technology (IT) playing a primary role in every aspect of healthcare value chain ensuring faster adaptability of advanced technologies, reduction of service costs and provision of quality healthcare at affordable prices. IT is increasingly penetrating the healthcare service delivery in India as well, driven by the need to reduce costs, efficiency imperatives, interoperability of existing fragmented hospital systems and increased health awareness among citizens. The technology shift has cast itself over the field of healthcare, bringing with it a digital transformation in the way doctors and patients interact. However adoption of same has been restricted due to factors like affordability, knowledge about its clinical utility, distribution, service, funding etc.

Within the context of health promotion, health has been considered less as an abstract state and more as a means to an end which can be expressed in functional terms as a resource which permits people to lead an individually, socially, and economically productive life. Health promotion is defined as "a process for initiating, managing, and implementing change, a process of personal, organizational, and policy development" (Kickbusch, 1994). It can be achieved by actionable strategies like building healthy public policy, creating supportive environments, strengthening community action, developing personal skills, and re-orientation of health services. Revival of public health regulation by the government is possible through updating and implementation of public health laws, in consultation stakeholders and increasing public awareness of existing laws and their enforcement procedures must be implemented universally across the country. India needs to reshape the paradigm of care by creating a culture of health and wellness. The National Accreditation Board for Hospitals & Healthcare Providers (NABH) defines wellness as "a state of a healthy balance of the mind and body that results in overall well-being". As per a recent study by the Stanford Research Institute International, Indian wellness industry valued at USD 9.8 billion is less than 2 percent of the global wellness industry valued at USD 2 trillion.

The new agenda for Public Health in India includes the epidemiological transition, demographical transition, environmental changes and social determinants of health. Yet the slowness of India's demographic and epidemiological adaptation means that at the beginning of the 21st century the nation's population is still challenged by a high prevalence of infectious disease, alongside an already large and growing non-communicable illness burden. The complex range of factors that interact to determine the nature and course of this epidemic needs to be understood in order to adopt preventive strategies to help developing societies like India deal with these burgeoning problem Non Communicable diseases (NCDs) (Shetty, 2000). Major healthcare transitions are described below.

Shifting Demographics

India continues to be in the middle of its demographic transition. It justifiably claims to be the first country to adopt an official policy to slow population growth, beginning with the country's first Five Year Plan in 1952 (Jain, 1998). The first National Population Policy (NPP) proposed in 1976, contained a comprehensive socio-demographic program covering 14 topics such as reducing infant and maternal mortality, banning child marriage, universal immunization of children, and preventing the spread of HIV. The National Population Policy, 2000 affirms the commitment of government towards voluntary and informed choice and consent of citizens while availing of reproductive health care services, and continuation of the target free approach in administering family planning services. It is based upon the need to simultaneously address issues of child survival, maternal health, and contraception, while increasing outreach and coverage of a comprehensive package of reproductive and child health services by government, industry and the voluntary non-government sector, working in partnership (National Population Policy, 2000).

With population of nearly 1.28 billion, India represents almost 17.31 percent of the world's population, which means one out of six people on this planet live in India (India's Population, 2015). Three factors, namely, a large segment of the population in the reproductive age group; high fertility due to considerable unmet need for contraception; and high desired level of fertility due to prevailing high IMRs have been found to influence the population momentum and, hence, its current growth rate. India is predicted to have more than 1.53 billion people by end of 2030. India's demographic transition is also visible through population pyramids which provide data on a nation's age structure (Trovato, 2009). More than 50 percent of India's current population (Census India, 2011) is below the age of 25 and over 65 percent below the age of 35 offering a demographic '*window of opportunity*' where the growth in the working-age population is greater than the growth in the total population in 2015. This increase in the share of the working-age population in total population is referred to as the '*demographic dividend*' (Bloom, Canning, & Sevilla 2002). If working-age people can be productively employed, India's economic growth stands to accelerate.

As per Registrar General, government of India figures (as cited by Haub, & Sharma, 2006), about 72.2 percent of the population lives in some 638,000 villages and the rest 27.8 percent lives in about 5,480 towns and urban agglomerations. With almost 55 percent population moving to cities by 2050, India is experiencing largest rural-urban migration of the century. Health is instrument of social and economic development. It has resulted in significant improvements of health indicators showing that India is well positioned in its demographic transition.

Statistics released by the MoHFW shows that life expectancy has increased at an average pace of 4.5 years per decade since 1950, pegged at 67.3 years (males) and 69.6 years (females) in 2011-2015. The fertility rate has declined sharply from approximately 6 children per woman in the 1950s to 2.7 children per woman today. Infant mortality rate has experienced a 70 percent decline from over 165 deaths per thousand live births in the 1950s to around 50 today. Maternal mortality ratio has declined from 301 per 100,000 live births in 2001-03 to 212 in 2007-09. With the population growth rate at 1.58 percent (birth rate is 20 births per 1,000 people per year and death rate are 8 deaths per 1,000 people per year between 2010-2014) (World Bank, 2015).

An important concern in the present stage of India's demographic transition relates to persisting adverse sex ratio, defined as number of females to thousand males (approx. ratio is 933/1000 live births). There is a significant variation in sex ratio across states. The sex ratio also varied between the rural and urban areas, as well as among different sections of the society. This points to the possibility of widespread prevalence of pre-natal sex determination and sex selection practices. The government has redoubled efforts to enforce the ban in recent years in the face of growing alarm at the frequency of female feticide (Gender tests, 2006; Neelam, 2006). The National Family Health Surveys (NFHS), a part of the global Demographic and Health Survey (DHS) program, have provided a wealth of information on a wide variety of socio-demographic topics. The NFHS produce measures of fertility, contraceptive use, childbearing desires, the status of women, infant mortality, immunization coverage, use of iodized salt, reproductive health, knowledge of HIV and AIDS, housing, and other valuable data.

Socio-Economic Transitions

India's society is deeply rooted in religion, language, tradition, and caste system. Demand for qualitative healthcare services will be fuelled by the growing literacy and affluence of the Indian middle-class. Following economic liberalization, India's GDP growth averaged 6.6 percent between 1990 and 2010. As a result, the incidence of poverty was nearly halved from 51.3 percent in late 1970s to 28.6 percent in late 1990s. India has the largest illiterate population in the world and the literacy rate of India as per 2011 population census is 74.04 percent, with male literacy rate at 82.14 percent and female at 65.46 percent (Lawton, 2014a). Notwithstanding the diversity of this experience of change, one can also say rather confidently that there would be hardly any pocket of India today that has been left untouched by the process of development and democratization.

However, despite the economic growth, resultant increase in personal incomes, and collected tax revenues, India is the only country which has seen a fall in public spending on healthcare form 4.6 percent in 2000 to 4.2 percent in 2008 as percentage of GDP (World Health Statistics, 2011). To manage budget deficit, central government reduced spending on healthcare failed to benefit the disabled, drug addicts, street children, child labourers, and the poor without extended family. Private sector mostly catered to needs of urban rich and middle class. The Central and State governments combined expenditure on health was 1.26 percent of the GDP as a percentage of total expenditure, 4.8 percent as per social services expenditure, 19.2 percent as per budget estimates in 2012-13, and out-of-pocket expenditure as percent of private expenditure on health was 92.2 percent in 2000 which reduced to 74.4 percent in 2008 (SAARC Development Goals, 2013). The draft National Health Policy (NHP), 2015 has proposed target of raising public health expenditure form current 1.36 to 3 percent of GDP, however it is yet to be realized.

Epidemiologic Transitions

Credits given to the success stories post-independence are far and few. For a country of size and population of India, the emerging infections remain a real and present danger. A meaningful response must approach the problem at the systems level. A comprehensive national strategy on infectious diseases cutting across all relevant sectors with emphasis on strengthened surveillance, rapid response, partnership building and research to guide public policy is needed.

With rapidly changing disease profile (infectious and chronic degenerative diseases) has resulted into an epidemiological transition across its diverse and young population, which is reflected as growing burden of Non Communicable Diseases NCDs like cardiovascular diseases (like heart attacks and stroke), cancers, chronic respiratory diseases (such as chronic obstructed pulmonary disease and asthma) and diabetes especially in rural India (Joshi, Cardona, & Iyengar, 2006). Diseases that have declined in many developing countries continue to be common here. India accounts for 21 percent of the world's global burden of disease (WHO, 2013c). The increasing problem of emerging and re-emerging communicable diseases (drug-resistant TB, malaria, dengue, viral hepatitis, SARS, avian flu, H1N1, Kalaazar, and Japanese Encephalitis) exerts immense pressure on the already overstretched health systems. Many research studies have shown India stands to lose nearly six percent of its GDP annually due to premature deaths and preventable illnesses (World Bank Report, 2010) and nearly USD 6.2 trillion by 2030 due to NCDs.

NCD's are rapidly increasing in many developing countries, largely due to demographics and lifestyle changes (Lopez, Mathers, Ezzatti, Jamison, & Murray, 2006). With increase in the number of elderly, there will be higher incidence and prevalence of NCDs like Hypertension, Cardiovascular diseases,

Obesity, Stroke, Diabetes, Cancers, and the whole range of geriatrics problems. Health service users are facing increasing challenges associated with the prevention and treatment of such chronic diseases (Patel, et. al., 2011). The estimated number of cancer cases in India is two million, seven lakh new cases are detected, and three lakh die due to cancer every year. Various studies put the prevalence of diabetes from 0.95 percent to 3.8 percent in urban areas and 0.6 to 1.93 percent in rural areas of the country. About 40 million are estimated to suffer from coronary vascular diseases, 5.1 million suffer from HIV/AIDS, 14 million suffer tuberculosis, 12.5 million blind (80 percent of this blindness is due to cataract), nearly 60 million suffer from endemic goiter, and an estimated 8.8 million have mental or psychomotor handicap due to iodine deficiency (Kapilasrami, 2000). Significant contribution to these epidemics also resulted from environmental degradation, excessive food adulterations, and toxic contaminants leading to increase incidence of allergic, respiratory, neoplastic, and latrogenic diseases.

In 2004, chronic diseases accounted for an estimated over 50 percent of the 10 million deaths, compared to 37 percent of deaths due to communicable diseases and other disorders. Disparities in treatment for chronic disease are enormous between urban-rural and rich-poor population. Episodes of hospital care for chronic disease are twice those for infectious disease and expenditures on chronic diseases accounted for 45 and 70 percent of average monthly income for the highest and lowest income group respectively. The relative frequency of treatment for lifestyle and chronic illness conditions varies between inpatient and outpatient settings. It is hard to tackle diseases as healthcare is more biased towards curative care, with a significant drop-off in number of patients along the treatment cycle, due to under-diagnosis and inappropriate care.

The rise in NCDs in urban areas will spur an increase in inpatient hospital admissions and related costs. It is projected to account productivity loss of USD 236 billion by 2015. Compounding effect of both trends is longer life expectancy and the growth of the elderly population (Lawton, 2014b). India also has very low coverage to key health interventions like oral rehydration therapy, antibiotic treatment for childhood pneumonia, and immunization. As many as a third or more of the country's children still do not receive the full set of immunizations which is one of the most cost-effective health interventions. Several infectious and vaccine-preventable childhood diseases still contribute 30 percent of the disease burden in India (John, Dandona, Sharma, & Kakkar, 2011). The direct interaction of these two transitions namely urbanization and chronic illness will have enormous effects on India in future.

ANALYZING HEALTHCARE SYSTEM

The healthcare system and its specific institutional architecture are the results of policy decisions and policy devices like financing, payment, organizational, regulatory, and behavioural initiatives are conditioned by the country's economic, social, and cultural context. Though government has attempted to define standards for healthcare facilities through legislation such as the Clinical Establishment Act, 2010, National Accreditation Board for Hospitals and Healthcare Providers (NABH), 2006, and Indian Public Health Standards (IPHS), 2007 (revised 2012), the rapid growth of healthcare is supported by few entry barriers, poorly enforced regulations and lack of single authority to ensure that people have access to appropriate and cost-effective care. The Central government addresses issues related to health policies, regulatory matters, and disease control measures whereas State governments deals with healthcare delivery, financing, and training of personnel. As health is a State responsibility, these issues are left for them to manage. Given the weak starting position and complex realities of healthcare in India, researchers at the World Bank and the WHO have developed a 'Control Knobs' framework that analyses the policy devices like how healthcare is financed, provided, regulated, and what are the outcomes of different government plans which directly impact the transitional outcomes of cost, access, and quality of healthcare.

The *National Rural Health Mission* (NRHM), 2005 was accelerative step towards integration and convergence of health services, besides affecting architectural correction in the healthcare delivery system in rural India. Its vision envisaged provision of effective healthcare to rural population throughout the country, to begin with special focus on 18 states in 2005, which had weak public health indicators and weak infrastructure. The mission seeks to provide accessible, affordable, and quality healthcare to vulnerable and underserved rural populations across the country by adopting synergistic approach by relating health to determinants of good health viz. nutrition, sanitation, hygiene, and safe drinking water. This will have cascading effect on ultimate outcomes like improved health status, protection from the financial risks of illness, and consumer satisfaction (Hsiao, 2003).

Devising such a framework of policy levers of the health system, there are structural parameters that directly or indirectly affect health and healthcare (as shown in Figure 1) and it is also supportive in our understanding of the broader societal and regulatory constraints within which our healthcare system operates. The much anticipated increase in fund allocation for making healthcare reform a national priority has taken a backseat in budget 2015. The massive mismatch between the declared objective of

Figure 1. Policy levers, intermediate outcomes, and ultimate ends of health system

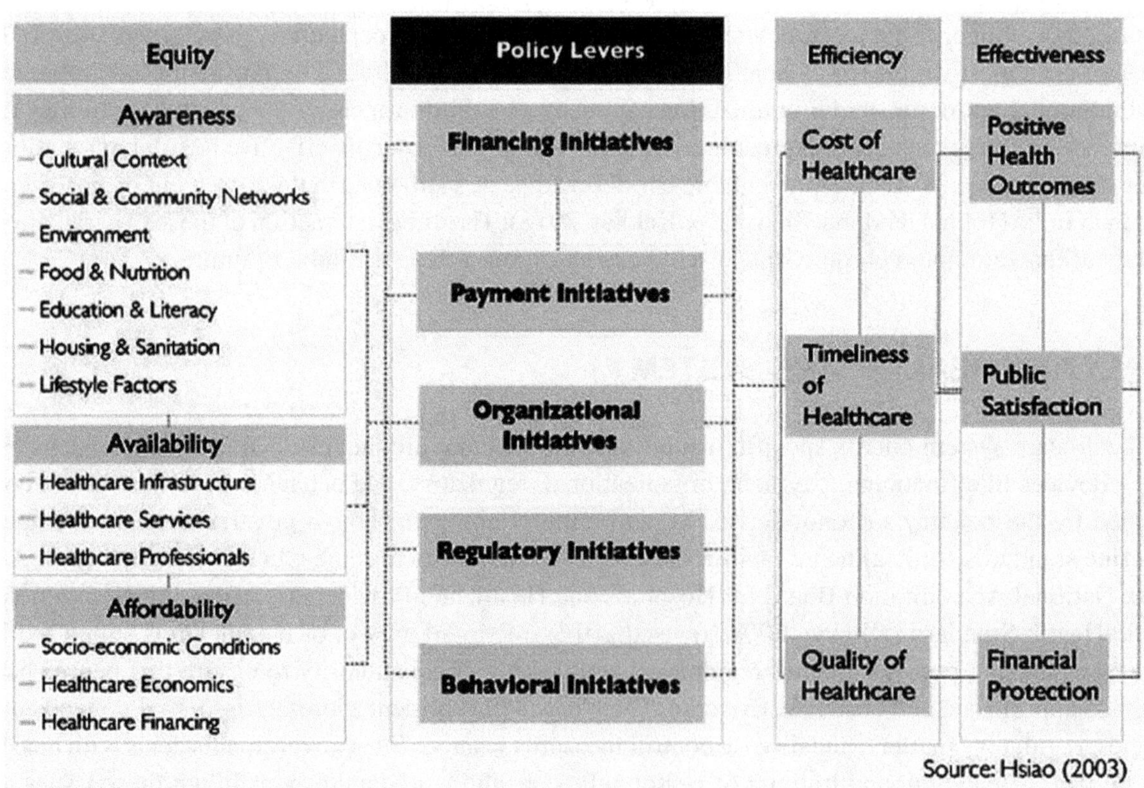

UHC through the public health system and the actual level of expenditure thus remains a serious concern (Kacchap, 2015). According to Harvard scholars (Pritchett & Natarajan, 2015), "The unfortunate fiscal fact is that India may not be able to have anything like UHC where all people can have all medically effective treatments for all diseases".

HEALTHCARE CHALLENGES

Today public health is enabling a paradigm shift to healthy living, with emphasis on disease prevention. Bain analysis defined India's healthcare aspirations as "A healthy India, where citizens are health aware and engaged, and have equitable access to affordable health coverage with a focus on prevention, early diagnosis, and assured minimum quality of care, offered by a vibrant and sustainable ecosystem of public and private players" (as cited by Singh & Ghosh, 2015). A High-Level Expert Group constituted by Planning Commission of India in 2011, defined UHC for purpose of report as

Ensuring equitable access for all citizens, resident in any part of the country, regardless of income level, social status, gender, caste or religion, to affordable, accountable, appropriate health services of assured quality (promotive, preventive, curative and rehabilitative) as well as public health services addressing the wider determinants of health delivered to individuals and populations, with the government being the guarantor and enabler, although not necessarily the only provider, of health and related services.

State should not only provide health and related services, but should also address the wider determinants of health to effectively guarantee health security. It must make clear choices regarding the role of government for addressing these challenges, achieving health equity, including how the government will prioritize and fund Universal Healthcare by 2022. The focus of innovations will shift from the product arena to healthcare delivery and a demand will surge in an environment that favors delivering care using the power of information technology. A good system of regulation is fundamental to successful public health outcomes with constant focus on development of healthcare infrastructure and facilities. However, dis-aggregated data reveals that health status, distribution of healthcare resources, and health outcomes differs significantly across different states as well as urban-rural settings due to population pressure, faulty health policy, inequity, and too many governments run national health programs.

When it comes to healthcare, there are two Indias: The situation in urban India is close to developed country averages where private hospitals provide high-quality medical care to rich and middle class (access to healthcare services at a rate that is double of the rural poor and 50 percent more than national average), urban poor and rural population has access to public health system having inadequate hospital beds, lack of diagnostic equipment's, doctors, paramedics etc. Heterogeneity in the form of culture diversity, education, income, language, religion, social status, system of castes and tribes, high incidence of gender disparity, quacks and faith healers, alternative remedies among others also limit the access of rural population to urban private healthcare services for advanced treatments. Social and economic inequality is detrimental to the health of any society, especially when the society is diverse, multicultural, overpopulated, and undergoing rapid but unequal economic growth (Deogaonkar, 2004).

Access Difficulty

There are three main access difficulties described in the following.

Geographic Distance

It becomes critical with poor rural infrastructure, limited means of transport, people's access, and equipping supplies at remote healthcare facilities. Direct effect of distance on a given population from primary healthcare center on the childhood mortality is well documented in India (Bimal, 1991), Effects of difficult access to health centers are more pronounced for mothers with less education (Caldwell, 1979) and the distance from private hospitals does not affect the health parameters but the distance from public health center does. Difficulties in accessing healthcare facilities is an important factor, along with gender discrimination, as it contributes to higher maternal mortality in women who live in remote areas especially the tribal women in India (Basu & Jindal, 1990). Maternal mortality is clearly much higher in rural areas (United Nations, 2001) due to shortage of trained medical or paramedical staff who can handle complicated cases, as incentives to move to rural locations are generally insufficient and ineffective.

Socio-Economic Distance

Even though majority of healthcare facilities are overwhelmingly concentrated in urban areas, the '*socio-economic distances*' prevent access to economically weak urban poor living in slums and exposed to infectious diseases like HIV/AIDS, tuberculosis, hepatitis, dengue fever, pneumonia, cholera, malaria that easily spread in highly concentrated populations where water and sanitation services are almost non-existent (WHO,1996d). National Urban Health Mission (NUHM), 2005 with allocation of USD 3.78 billion was set up to address the healthcare needs of 46 million slum dwellers spread across 640 towns whereas NRHM, has also sanctioned more than USD 10 billion for capacity enhancement and upgradation of healthcare facilities. Socio-economic barriers also include cost of healthcare, lack of culturally appropriate services, language, ethnic barriers, and prejudices on the part of service providers. All these factors lead to an inability to identify symptoms and seek appropriate care on the part of the poor (WHO, 2001e).

Gender Distance

It is said that the health of society is reflected by health of its female population which is completely disregarded in India. Women in India are socially, culturally, and economically dependent on men (Narayan, Patel, Schafft, Rademacher, & Koch-Schulte, 2000). Whatever the socio-economic status of the family might be, woman in India is less likely to seek appropriate and early care for disease. It's hard to miss the fact that poor women are disproportionately affected by India's public health crisis. Gender discrimination in healthcare access becomes more obvious when women are illiterate, unemployed, widowed or dependent on others (Prakash, 1997). Poor women eat less; have weaker phenotype; they marry young; they give birth quickly, and often find it harder to access medical care making them more vulnerable to various diseases, associated morbidity, and mortality. Statistics shows that one in three Indian women did not receive an antenatal check-up during their pregnancy, 45 percent delivered their babies without the support of trained personnel, 58 percent of children did not complete their immunization schedule, 14.4 percent did not receive a single vaccine, and only one in two women seeks treatment for illness. Thus combination of perceived ill health and lack of support mechanisms (access difficulty and affordability) contributes to a poor quality of life for woman in India.

Infrastructure Shortcomings

India faces severe shortfall of both hard infrastructure and skilled talent both at rural and urban areas. Despite the existence of primary, secondary, tertiary health centers, and public hospitals, the healthcare system is seriously broken due to poor quality of facilities, lack of an organized delivery system, inadequate supplies, ineffective managerial skills, poor planning, monitoring, and evaluation of services. Although rural India accounts for about 70 percent of the population, it has less than one third of the nation's hospitals, doctors, and beds, resulting in huge disparities in health outcomes across states. According to report published by IPHS, 2014, there is short fall of Sub-center's (SCs), Primary health center's (PHCs), Community health center's (CHCs) by 20, 23, and 32 percent respectively in India. It needs to add 1.7 million beds, double its medical manpower and increase its paramedical manpower three-fold to match WHO standards. With such gap, it becomes imperative to create an environment conducive to facilitate infrastructure creation and increase investments across the healthcare ecosystem (Bali, 2015). The foremost priority is to rebuild the public healthcare system using alternative financing and appropriate taxation, as it is single-handedly responsible for basic minimum care, national health programs etc.

Out of Pocket Financing

Health financing is one of the building blocks of health systems and proper allocation of funds is crucial for strong infrastructure and delivery systems. However lack of risk pooling and insurance could be argued as the main reasons for health-related impoverishment in developing nations (WHO, 2000f). National health accounts cell study in 2009 (as cited by Bhojani, et.al., 2012) said that 71.1 percent of healthcare is financed through out-of-pocket (OOP) payments by households in India and such payments act as the primary barrier to access healthcare services in India. (Berman, Ahuja & Bhandari, 2010) reported that approximately 6.2 percent of Indians fell below the poverty line due to OOP payments for healthcare; a greater proportion of them for outpatient care (4.9 percent) than for inpatient care (1.3 percent), and expenditure for medications constituted the greatest share (71.2 percent). High OOP payment for chronic conditions, even for outpatient care, accentuates socioeconomic inequalities. Healthcare costs worsen poverty, pushing an additional average of 39 million people into poverty every year (Balarajan, Selvaraj, & Subramanian, 2011). Strong public healthcare system would be crucial for the establishment of UHC and control OOP spending.

Fragmented Healthcare Industry

A vibrant and dynamic healthcare sector is imperative for the new human resource intensive world and quality healthcare is vital for the growth of any nation. India has largest private healthcare delivery systems in the world which nearly accounts for more than 80 percent of total healthcare spending of USD 38 billion in 2012. Such preponderance of the unorganized private sector in healthcare is not because of a preferred choice, but more because of functional imperatives like absence of affordable, convenient, and quality public healthcare delivery systems. Thus private sectors success is attributed less to its own efficiency and more to government's failure (Chirmulay, & Gupte, 1997). Although there is a big divide between the demand and supply of healthcare services across rural and urban India, off late the overall healthcare infrastructure in India is fast improving with initiatives like Public Private Partnership (PPP) and funding from international donor agencies. Healthcare system is broadly classified by using three dimensions which creates a complex plurality making development of an organized system difficult. These dimensions are:

1. Ownership styles:
    a. Public sector includes government-run hospitals, dispensaries, clinics, PHCs, SCs etc.
    b. Non Profit Sector includes voluntary health programs, charitable institutions, trusts, and missionaries.
    c. Organized private sector (for profit) includes qualified registered general practitioners, private hospitals, nursing homes, and dispensaries.
    d. Private informal sector includes practitioners not having any formal qualifications (e.g., faith healers, herbalists, priests, tantriks, hakims, and vaidyas).
2. Types of delivery structures (hospitals, dispensaries, and clinics).
3. Systems of medicine (Allopathic, Ayurveda, Homeopathic, Unani, and Siddha):
    a. **Allopathy:** The system of medical practice which treats disease by the use of remedies which produce effects different from those produced by the disease under treatment.
    b. **Ayurveda:** It aims to keep structural and functional entities in a functional state of equilibrium, which signifies good health. Any imbalance due to internal and external factor causes disease and restoring equilibrium through various techniques, procedures, regimes, diet and medicine constitute treatment.
    c. **Homeopathy:** It believes in a specialized method of treatment of curing diseases by administration of potency drugs, which have been experimentally proved to possess the power of producing similar artificial systems on human beings.
    d. **Siddha:** It emphasize that medical treatment is oriented not merely to disease, but also has to take into account the patient, environment, age, habits, physical condition.
    e. **Unani:** It is based on established knowledge and practices relating to promotion of positive health and prevention of diseases. It emphasise the use of naturally occurring, most herbal medicines, though it uses ingredients of animal and marine origin.

Bio-Medical Waste

Hospitals are complex institutions normally inhabited with patients, staff, and frequented by people without any distinction between age, sex, race, and religion. The main drivers of growth in the healthcare sector are India's growing economy; booming population; increasing literacy; awareness of personal health; increasing purchasing power; low treatment cost; technology adaption; and government supportive programs (social and food security), expansion of healthcare infrastructure, high patient turnout, growing burden of diseases and re-emerging infections due to infectious, chronic degenerative, and lifestyle diseases; have resulted in excessive use of medicines and disposables leading to unprecedented growth of bio-medical and hospital waste. According to Ministry of Environment and Forests (MoEF) gross generation of bio-medical wastes in India is 4,05,702 kg/day of which only 2,91983 kg/day is disposed, which means that almost 28 percent of the bio-medical and hospital waste is left untreated. Ostensibly, such infectious and often toxic waste, is littered around hospitals and it end up in our drainage system, which in turn has the potential to become ideal breeding grounds for vectors and spread infection.Improper acts of waste disposal pose a huge risk to the healthcare personnel who handle these wastes at the point of generation, health of the public, patients, professionals, and to persons involved in segregation, storage, transport, treatment, and disposal of such wastes (Joseph & Krishnan, 2004).

MAJOR HEALTH POLICY INITIATIVES

India's political leadership had made substantial contributions for advancing good health for people through National Health Policy (NHP) that covers pertinent dimensions of healthcare financing, healthcare delivery system, roles of public and private sectors, equity and affordability across rich and poor, phenomenon of convergence, divergence, and two-way causation between human development and income and the impact of increased longevity on social security. In India until 1982-1983 there was no formal health policy statement. The policy was part and parcel of the planning process and various committees appointed from time to time, which provided most of the inputs for the formulation of health programme designs. It was not until 1983 that India adopted a formal or official NHP with the goal of achieving "Health for All" by 2000 through stressing the creation of a strong primary health infrastructure, increasing the involvement of volunteer organizations and NGOs, and providing quality health-related serviceswhich are relevant to the actual needs and priorities of the community at a cost which people can afford (MoHFW, 1983c). Reappraisal and reformulation of the NHP in 2002 became necessary with changing context of healthcare, since it's over stated goals 'Universal, Comprehensive, PHCs'was not achieved.

Policy revision ensured that a reliable and relevant policy framework was available not only for improving healthcare but also measuring and monitoring the healthcare delivery systems and health status of the population in the next two decades. The main objective of NHP 2002 is to achieve an acceptable standard of good health amongst the general population of the country. It also needs to be praised for its concern for regulating the private health sector through statutory licensing and monitoring of minimum standards by creating a regulatory mechanism. Subsequently the primary aim of the NHP, 2015, is to "inform, clarify, strengthen, and prioritize the role of the government in shaping health systems in all its dimensions, investment in health, organization and financing of healthcare services, prevention of diseases, promotion of good health through cross sectorial action, access to technologies, developing human resources, encouraging medical pluralism, building the knowledge base required for better health, financial protection strategies, and regulation and legislation for health" (MoHFW, 2014d).

However new policy lacks vision to address issues of the larger majority and succumbs to pressure that push forward the pre-existing policies of dependence on markets, big business, and the corporate sector. In addition to above mentioned NHP, numerous policies having health related component were framed as prescriptions for achieving stated health outcomes through National Health Mission and to improve the health of India's population. These policies are: National AIDS Prevention & Control Policy, 1992, National Nutrition Policy, 1993, National Policy on Older Persons, 1999, National Population Policy, 2000, National Policy for Empowerment of Women, 2001, National Blood Policy, 2002, National Health Policy, 2002, National Policy on Indian System of Medicine & Homeopathy, 2002, National Environment Policy, 2006, National Pharmaceutical Policy, 2012, National Water Policy, 2012, National Policy for Children 2013, National Youth Policy, 2014.

India has built up a vast health infrastructure and initiated several NHP (aimed at increasing the standard of health of the people and decreasing the incidence of disease and death due to illness) over last five decades in government, voluntary, and private sectors under the guidance and direction of various committees (Bhore (1946), Mudaliar (1962), Kartar Singh (1973), Srivastava (1975), the Constitution, the Planning Commission, the Central Council of Health and Family Welfare, and Consultative Committees attached to the MoHFW. However most NHP functioned almost independently of each other and allocations for disease control programs was driven more by donor organizations will than by the country's epidemiological realities. The government has increased the plan allocation for public health spending to USD 5.96 billion in 2011–12 from USD 4.97 billion in 2010–2011. Extra funding of USD 293.35 million is allocated to develop institutions like AIIMS. However, neglect of the public health sector is an issue larger than government policy formulation and with 20 percent cut in healthcare budget 2014-15 is putting at risk key disease control initiatives in a country whose public spending on health is already among the lowest in the world.

Government have prioritized healthcare sector in the 12th plan from 2012-17 and has initiated several steps like reduction in import duties, higher depreciation on life-saving medical equipment, tax exemption of 5 years on hospitals located in Tier II, Tier III cities, and rural areas, and 100 percent Foreign Direct Investment (FDI) under automatic route for healthcare services. Adoption of Public Private Partnership (PPP) model has resulted in growth of private healthcare facilities and private sector has emerged as a new avenue of reforms. There is a growing realisation that, given their respective strengths and weaknesses, neither the public sector nor the private sector alone can operate in the best interest of the healthcare system, rather public and private healthcare sectors can potentially gain from one another (ADBI, 2000; Bloom, Craig, & Mitchell, 2000; Agha, Karim, Balal, & Sossler, 2003).

Tier-II and tier-III cities are seeing more growth as more villagers around tier-II cities are expected to visit these healthcare centres for access to quality health service. Through partnerships, government has created a state-funded healthcare insurance program to provide basic healthcare services to poor. National Sample Survey Organization (NSSO, 42 round 1986-1987 & 52 round 1995-1996) puts the number of people who could not seek medical care because of lack of money increased significantly between 1986 and 1995. About 3.5% of the population fall the below the poverty line and 5% households suffer catastrophic health expenditure due to unaffordable health cost (Sahrawat, & Rao, 2011). It is the people belonging to the lower income classes or poor who suffer the most. This re-emphasizes the role socio-economic inequality in healthcare delivery. Involvement of the private sector is, in part, linked to the wider belief that public sector bureaucracies are inefficient and unresponsive, and the market mechanisms will promote efficiency, ensure cost effective, and good quality services (WHO, 2001g).

This unregulated growth of private healthcare sector also adds to an ever increasing social dichotomy. The dominance of the private sector not only denies access to poorer sections of society, but also skews the balance towards urban-biased, tertiary level health services, with profitability overriding equality, and rationality of care often taking a back seat. In the absence of an effective regulatory authority over the private healthcare sector the quality of medical care is constantly deteriorating (Mudur, 2004). Powerful medical lobbies prevent government from formulating effective legislation or enforcing the existing ones. A recent World Bank report acknowledges the facts that, doctors over prescribe drugs, recommend unnecessary investigations, promote longer treatments, deliver poor quality of services that are overpriced. Commissions for recommending investigation, gifts and other expenses provide to doctors from pharmaceutical companies to prescribe expensive medicines makes a hole in the system which is difficult to fill. Thus, the solution for satisfying the health needs of the people, we need structural changes in the political economy that can facilitate implementation of progressive health policies and plans.

KEY RECOMMENDATIONS

Mentioned below are critical steps that can help bring a successful transformation of India's ailing health system.

1. **Inclusive Growth:** It is now on the political and economic agenda of most nations around the world. Public policy and public sector forms only one part of the equation to achieving inclusive growth, the other part of the equation is private sector component having inclusive business models, is considered to have stronger and more sustainable potential to achieve inclusive growth. For India to improve the quality and affordability of healthcare services in both the public and private sectors, the country will need to intervene in each sector appropriately by developing inter-sectorial linkages, especially in promotive and preventive services which can immensely benefit from accessibility, equity, and efficient allocation of healthcare resources.
2. **Compliance:** A healthcare establishment needs to comply with numerous laws and the current regulatory mechanism is extremely weak due to fragmented structure. For example, The Quality Council of India (NAHB) comes under Ministry of Commerce and Industry, IPHS and Clinical Establishment Act comes under MoHFW, Medical Insurance (IRDA) comes under Ministry of Finance, Bureau of Indian Standards (BIS) and Consumer Protection Act comes under Ministry of Consumer Affairs, Food, and Public Distribution besides governing bodies like Medical Council of India and Dental Council of India. It is time that central government develops a framework for an India-centric healthcare system and assigns *National Priority Status* to the healthcare sector.
3. **Healthcare Financing**: Given the huge skew in health expenditure in the country with private sector contributing 80 percent of the total expenditure, government should introduce a host of financing mechanisms to improve our health infrastructure and realise its economic aspirations. The 12th plan has envisaged 150 percent increase in spending (2.5-4 percent) of GDP by 2025 from present 1.26 percent and restore balance in the long run as we know that public healthcare facilities which are burdened beyond capacity, under-equipped, underfunded, and understaffed.
4. **Bridging the Gap:** With huge differences in health outcomes across states, government should drive policy consensus and bring in uniformity in health regulations among the central and various state governments. It needs to create enabling regulations to foster private enterprise in healthcare in delivery infrastructure, medical education, R&D and domestic manufacturing and encourage development of healthcare infrastructure into underserved areas; optimize existing infrastructure by restoring non-functional capacity; and relax norms for expansion within existing facilities with enhanced Central government support.
5. **Universal Healthcare Coverage:** The government should institutionalize UHC as a way to remove barriers to good health and expand access to quality, affordable care. In the UHC model, all citizens should be entitled to a comprehensive package of healthcare services, and have access to public

health and accredited private facilities for attaining services such as diagnostics, medicine, vaccines or surgeries as an entitlement, without having to pay at the point of use (Planning Commission of India, 2011). Anticipated demand growth following implementation of UHC will require substantial measures to enhance supply-side infrastructure particularly in rural areas.

6. **Disease Transition**: Current healthcare programs focus disproportionately on specialist care rather than primary care, which is arguably more important in meeting the treatable everyday needs of the poor, as country is saddled with a high burden of preventable illnesses. According to the NCD country profiles of 2014 released by WHO, diseases like cancer, chronic respiratory problems and cardiovascular diseases are the biggest global killers accounting for 38 million deaths every year with a whopping 28 million in low and middle income countries, including India. As per WHO estimates, NCDs account for almost 60 percent of the total mortality reported annually in India. Enabling a paradigm shift to healthy living, by developing a vision and roadmap for NCDs, India should roll out high-impact public-health interventions by ensuring multi-stakeholder engagement and apportion of greater share of public spending on prevention of such diseases.
7. **Research Initiative**: Government should focus on research capacity building and institutional strengthening by making research initiatives more interactive with policies and making health research more relevant to Indian health system. Stakeholders can also encourage innovation in care models, shifting from hospital-centred delivery and procedure-centred, to fee-for-service models to low-cost delivery and so on.
8. **Control Out of Pocket Expenditure**: According to MoHFW, each year nearly 63 million people face poverty due to "catastrophic" healthcare expenditure, which neutralizes any gains made due to rising income. Various government schemes aimed at reducing poverty as the cost of seeking treatment even at public hospitals had increased five-fold (simultaneously, the cost of treatment in private hospitals increased nearly seven-fold), though the purchasing power of the poorer classes had not changed in any substantial way. Government should establish systems to rationally determine the pricing of publicly funded health products and services.
9. **National Medical Device Authority (NMDA):** Although India has a growing domestic medical device manufacturing sector the country still imports more than half of its high technology healthcare equipment. The draft policy issued by the central Department of Pharmaceuticals proposes an autonomous NMDA tasked with promoting the local industry and ensuring adherence to safety standards designed for the country's USD 4 billion medical device industries. It is assumed that efficient regulatory system will not only help benefit healthcare sector but it will support the development of India's domestic industry through 'Make in India' program and transforming India into an export hub for medical products and equipment.
10. **Controlling Private Sector**: The predominance of the private sector in healthcare in India is largely a consequence of the Indian government's failure to keep pace with the growing healthcare needs of its population. Although the growth of private-sector healthcare has generally increased access to healthcare services, there are concerns about cost of treatment which is way too expensive. Urgent steps need to be taken to enact legislation and institutionalize minimum standards, standard management protocols, patient's rights, ceiling on fees, and licensing based on need of the private sector. Further there is an urgent need to eliminate widespread irrational medical practices including unnecessary medications and procedures both in public and private sector organizations.

11. **Quality of Personnel:** Investments in training and educating a skilled workforce by encouraging the adoption of minimum standards, enhancing the skills and capabilities of doctors, nurses, paramedics, and allied personnel through training, career progression, and continuing medical education (CME) for professionals. Expanding the supply of healthcare talent in critical roles, increasing post graduate medical seats, bringing them at par with undergraduate levels, and encouraging public and private investment for establishing more medical colleges and training institutes will go a long way in providing healthcare services to all. Besides this competitive pay, and attractive living conditions (especially in rural India) will ensure that public health facilities are staffed by qualified people.
12. **Rejuvenating Traditional System:** The important resource of traditional and alternative healing systems needs to be encouraged, reasonable regulations and standards need to be introduced, and it should be integrated with the modern medical system based on reasonable standards. This would entail rejuvenating and enhanced public system support to AYUSH (Ayurveda, Yoga and Naturopathy, Unani, Siddha, and Homeopathy).

CONCLUSION

Since independence, India has undergone a slow but sustained demographic, social, economic, agricultural, nutrition, and health transition, its massive public healthcare service does not provide enough incentives for improvement in efficiency and quality services. The existing health system in India is fraught with many inequities (between states, urban-rural areas, and rich-poor) segments of the population, attempted efforts towards building a provider and patient-friendly public healthcare system is lost under the burden of weak regulations. It is no secret that many government programmes suffer from lack of focussed outcomes, implementation failures, and quality deficiencies due to low public spending. However, this would require large scale changes in the way that healthcare in the country is organised. Keeping the interests of the general public paramount, powerful vested interests would have to be curbed, regulated and made accountable health system having efficient disease surveillance mechanism, focus on primary, preventive, and affordable programs in conjunction with improved access to the entire spectrum of health determinants (food, water, sanitation, education, housing, environmental, and working conditions). There has to be a mix of public and private initiatives in healthcare in secondary and tertiary segments of healthcare leading to a system where everyone enjoys their 'Right to Health'.

As discussed India does not have a strong health infrastructure and has several weaknesses in its health system. Delivering affordable healthcare to billion-plus presents enormous challenges and opportunities for the medical community, insurers, and other service providers. Healthcare gap can be overcome by creating incentives for local companies, roping in support from global players having enormous potential in terms of their technological prowess, improvise overall process efficiency, work to build infrastructure to reach underserved rural areas, create innovative financing mechanism to deliver healthcare to the underprivileged, putting in place effective public-private partnerships program. Developing people-based initiatives like community health worker programs using resources from the public health system, appropriate use of traditional healing systems, and low-cost models of healthcare delivery will reshape healthcare outcomes. India needs to embark on the path of urgent reforms for strengthening health systems and provide UHC in accordance with the WHO framework, which includes the following six discrete "building blocks": (i) service delivery; (ii) health workforce; (iii) information; (iv) medical products and technologies; (v) financing; and (vi) leadership and governance (WHO, 2007h).

With regards to quality, there is little regulation of providers, treatments, and medical products, considerable variation in the training and education of providers, little or poor enforcement of laws, and separate regulations at central and state level. All this translates into poor health outcomes among the larger section of Indian population. Ensuring accountability of service providers through medico-legal instruments, that are agreed upon and implemented along with standardized protocols, as well as continuously enhancing consumer awareness at all levels about their rights to quality healthcare, may improve the current status of healthcare system in India. It was a glorious past, but the future of a healthy India lies in mainstreaming the public health agenda in the framework of sustainable development (Lakshminarayanan, 2011). The costs are huge, but there are enormous payoffs in long-term investment in healthcare. Such investments can not only raise quality of life for all citizens but also make the healthcare industry in India a great force for economic growth.

To achieve the required spectrum of changes of course demands a much wider social process. A powerful people's movement on health issues is needed, to enable people to more actively claim their health rights and to push for changes in the health sector. The ultimate goal of great nation would be one where the rural and urban divide has reduced to a thin line, with adequate access to clean energy and safe water, where the best of healthcare is available to all citizens, where the governance is responsive, transparent, and corruption free, where poverty and illiteracy have been eradicated and crimes against women and children are removed and so on. A reorganised, strengthened and accountable healthcare system in conjunction with improved access to the entire spectrum of health determinants - food, water, sanitation, education, housing, environmental and working conditions – could lead to an India where everyone enjoys their Right to Health, and we are able to achieve the dream of Health For All.

REFERENCES

Agha, S., Karim, A. M., Balal, A., & Sossler, S. (2003). A Quasi Experimental Study to Assess the Performance of a Reproductive Health Franchise in Nepal. Commercial Market Strategies (CMS) Country Research Series Paper No. 14, Washington DC

Alex, H. (2005). The scientific value of Ayurveda. *Journal of Alternative and Complementary Medicine (New York, N.Y.)*, *11*(2), 221–225. doi:10.1089/acm.2005.11.221 PMID:15865485

Asian Development Bank Institute (ADBI). (2000). *Public Private Partnerships in Health, Executive Summary Series No. S34/01, Executive Summary of Proceedings (30 October to 3 November)*. Thailand: Ayutthaya.

Balarajan, Y., Selvaraj, S., & Subramanian, S. V. (2011). India: Towards Universal Health Coverage for Healthcare and Equity in India. *Lancet*, *377*, 505–515. doi:10.1016/S0140-6736(10)61894-6 PMID:21227492

Bali, V. (2015). Union Budget 2015 fails to deliver on healthcare. *Business Today*. Retrieved from http://www.businesstoday.in/union-budget-2015-16/india-inc-on-budget/union-budget-2015-fails-to-deliver-on-healthcare-vishal-bali/story/216411.html

Basu, S. K. & Jindal, A., (1990). Genetic and socio-cultural determinants of tribal health: A primitive kuttiya kondhs tribal group of Phulbani district. ICMR Final Report, NIHFW, Orissa.

Berman, P., Ahuja, R., & Bhandari, L. (2010). The impoverishing effect of healthcare payments in India: New methodology and findings. *Economic and Political Weekly*, *xlv*(16), 65–71.

Bhojani, U., Thriveni, B. S., Devadasan, R., Munegowda, C. M., Devadasan, N., Kolsteren, P., & Criel, B. (2012). Out-of-pocket healthcare payments on chronic conditions impoverish urban poor in Bangalore, India. *BMC Public Health*, *12*(1), 990. doi:10.1186/1471-2458-12-990 PMID:23158475

Bimal, K. P. (1991). Health Service Resource as a Determinant of Infant Death in Rural Bangladesh: An Empirical Review. *Social Science & Medicine*, *32*(1), 43–49. doi:10.1016/0277-9536(91)90125-V PMID:2008620

Bloom, D. E., Canning, D., & Sevilla, J. (2002). *The Demographic Dividend: A New Perspective on the Economic Consequences of Population Change. MR-1274*. Santa Monica, CA: Rand.

Bloom, D. E., Craig, P., & Mitchell, M. (2000). Public and Private Roles in Providing and Financing Social Services: Health and Education.

Caldwell, J. (1979). Education as a factor in Mortality Decline: An Examination of Nigerian Data. *Population Studies*, *33*(3), 396–413. doi:10.2307/2173888

Census India. (2011) Office of the Registrar General and Census Commissioner, India. Retrieved from http://www.censusindia.gov.in/2011census

Chirmulay, D., & Gupte, A. (1997). Factors Affecting Health Seeking and Utilization of Curative Healthcare, Pune: Bharatiya Agro Industries Foundation (BAIF) Development and Research Foundation.

Cyber Laws in India and Technology Laws and Regulations in India. (2014). Retrieved from http://perry4law.org/cyberlawsinindia

Deogaonkar, M. (2004). Socio-economic inequality and its effect on healthcare delivery in India: Inequality and healthcare. *Electronic Journal of Sociology*, 8(1). Retrieved from http://www.sociology.org/content/vol8.1/deogaonkar.html

Gender Tests. (2006), Actions Sought Against 35 Doctors, The Hindu (Delhi), May 14, 2006.

Golechha, M. (2015). Health agenda for Indian government. *The Indian Journal of Medical Research*, *141*(2), 151–153. doi:10.4103/0971-5916.155541 PMID:25900948

Gururaj, G. (2006). Road traffic injury prevention in India. National Institute of Mental Health and Neuro Sciences, Bangalore, Publication No. 56.

Haub, C., & Sharma, O. P. (2006). India's Population Reality: Reconciling Change and Tradition. *Population Bulletin*, 61(3), 8. Retrieved from http://www.prb.org/pdf06/61.3indiaspopulationreality_eng.pdf

Hsiao, W. (2003). *What Is A Health System? Why Should We Care?* Cambridge, MA: Harvard School of Public Health.

India's Population. (2015). Retrieved from http://www.indiaonlinepages.com/population/india-current-population.html

Jain, A. (Ed.), (1998). Do Population Policies Matter? Fertility and Policies in Egypt, India, Kenya, and Mexico. New York: Population Council.

John, T. J., Dandona, L., Sharma, V. P., & Kakkar, M. (2011). Continuing challenge of infectious diseases in India. *Lancet*, *377*(9761), 252–269. doi:10.1016/S0140-6736(10)61265-2 PMID:21227500

Joseph, J., & Krishnan, A. (2004), Hospital Waste Management in the Union Territory of Pondicherry: An exploration. Retrieved from www.pon.nic.in/citizen/science/ppcc-new/joe.pdf

Joshi, R., Cardona, M., Iyengar, S., Sukumar, A., Raju, C. R., Raju, K. R., & Neal, B. et al. (2006). Chronic diseases now a leading cause of death in rural India: Mortality data from the Andhra Pradesh Rural Health Initiative. *International Journal of Epidemiology*, *35*(6), 1522–1529. doi:10.1093/ije/dyl168 PMID:16997852

Joumard, I., & Kumar, A. (2015). *"Improving health outcomes and health care in India", OECD economics department working papers, No. 1184*. OECD Publishing. Doi:10.1787/5js7t9ptcr26-en

Kacchap, N. M. (2015). Budget 2015: In search of an effective healthcare system. Retrieved from http://www.financialexpress.com/article/healthcare/cover-story-healthcare/budget-2015-in-search-of-an-effective-healthcare-system/62145/

Kapilashrami, M. C. (2000). Review of the present health status of India, emerging, health problems and their Solutions. *Health and Population; Perspectives and Issues*, *23*(1), 1–10.

Kickbusch, I. (1994). Tell me a story. In A. Pedersen et al (Eds.), Introduction to Health Promotion in Canada (pp. 8-17). Provincial, National and International Perspectives Canada, WB Saunders.

Lakshminarayanan, S. (2011). Role of government in public health: Current scenario in India and future scope. *J. Family Community Med.*, *18*(1), 26–30. doi:10.4103/1319-1683.78635 PMID:21694957

Lawton, R. B. (2014a). A System Perspective on India's Healthcare Industry, Global economy, Healthcare Reform, India, World Development. *The World Financial Review*. Retrieved from http://www.worldfinancialreview.com/?p=2604

Lawton, R. B. (2014b). A system perspective on India's healthcare delivery, Industry, Global economy, Healthcare Reform, India, World Development. *The World Financial Review*. Retrieved from http://www.worldfinancialreview.com/?p=2604

Lopez, A. D., Mathers, C. D., Ezzatti, M., Jamison, D. T., & Murray, C. J. L. (2006). Global and regional burden of disease and risk factors, 2001: Systematic analysis of population health data. *Lancet*, *367*(9524), 1747–1757. doi:10.1016/S0140-6736(06)68770-9 PMID:16731270

Ministry of Health & Family Welfare (MoHFW). (2014a). Draft National Health Policy, 2015, Government of India, New Delhi.

Ministry of Health & Family Welfare (MoHFW). (2004b). *Integrated Disease Surveillance Project: Project Implementation Plan 2004–09*. New Delhi: Government of India.

Ministry of Health & Family Welfare (MoHFW). (1983c). *National Health Policy*. New Delhi: Government of India.

Ministry of Health & Family Welfare (MoHFW). (2014d). *Draft National Health Policy, 2015*. New Delhi: Government of India.

Mudur, G. (2004). Inadequate Regulations Undermine India's Healthcare. British Medical Journal (BMJ), 2004, 124, 328.

Nandan, D., & Agarwal, D. (2012). Human resources for health in India: Urgent need for reforms. *Indian Journal of Community Medicine*, *37*(4), 205–206. doi:10.4103/0970-0218.103464 PMID:23293430

Narayan, D., Patel, R., Schafft, K., Rademacher, A., & Koch-Schulte, S. (2000). Changing gender relations in the household. In *Voices of the Poor: Can Anyone Hear Us?* New York, NY: Oxford University Press. doi:10.1596/0-1952-1601-6

National Population Policy. (2000). National Health Portal, Government of India, New Delhi. Retrieved from http://www.nhp.gov.in/national-population-policy-2000_pg

National Sample Survey Organization (NSSO), Department of Statistics: Government of India, 42nd round (1986-87).

National Sample Survey Organization (NSSO), Department of Statistics: Government of India, 52nd round (1995-96).

Neelam, R. (2006, March 29). Sex Selection is High-Volume, Low-Risk Biz. *The Times of India* (New Delhi).

O'Connell, T., Rasanathan, K., & Chopra, M. (2014). What does universal health coverage mean? *Lancet*, *383*(9913), 277–279. doi:10.1016/S0140-6736(13)60955-1 PMID:23953765

Omachonu, V.K. & Einspruch, N.G., (2010), Innovation in Healthcare Delivery Systems: A Conceptual Framework. The Innovation Journal: The Public Sector Innovation Journal, Volume 15(1), Article 2

Patel, V., Chatterji, S., Chisholm, D., Shah, E., Gopalakrishna, G., Mathers, C., & Reddy, K. S. et al. (2011). Chronic diseases and injuries in India. *Lancet*, *377*, 413–428. doi:10.1016/S0140-6736(10)61188-9 PMID:21227486

Planning Commission of India. (2011). High level expert group report on universal health coverage for India. Retrieved from http://planningcommission.nic.in/reports/genrep/rep_uhc0812.pdf

Prakash, I. J. (1997). Women and Ageing. *The Indian Journal of Medical Research*, *106*, 396–408. PMID:9361474

Pritchett, L., & Natrajan, G. (2015), Putting the 'Universal in Healthcare' Retrieved from http://indianexpress.com/article/opinion/columns/putting-the-universal-in-healthcare/

Ramachandran, R. (2015, October 16). For private plunder. Frontline, 16-20.

Developmental Goals, S. A. A. R. C. India Country Report (2013), Central Statistics Office Ministry of Statistics and Programme Implementation. Government of India.

Shashtri, A. D. (Ed.), (2007). *Sushruta Samhita*. Varanasi: Chaukambha Sanskrit Sansthan.

Shetty, P. S. (2000). Diet and life-style and chronic non-communicable diseases: what determines the epidemic in developing societies? In K. Krishnaswami (Ed.), *Nutrition Research: Current Scenario and Future Trends. New Delhi* (pp. 153–167). Oxford: IBH Publishing Co.

Sahrawat, R., & Rao, D. K. (2011). Insured yet vulnerable: Out-of pocket payments and India's poor. *Health Policy and Planning*, 2011, 1–9.

Singh, K., & Ghosh, P. (2015). *Aarogya Bharat India Healthcare Roadmap for 2025*. New Delhi: Bain and Company.

Sreenu, N. (2011). A study of healthcare infrastructure financing and economic growth in India. In A. S. Lather & D. Gakhar (Eds.), *Contemporary issues in corporate finance* (p. 164). New Delhi: Excel Books.

The World Bank working for world free of poverty, (2015). Retrieved from http://data.worldbank.org/indicator

Tripathi, B. N. (Ed.). (1983). *Charaka Samhita*. Varanasi: Nidana Sthana, Chaukhambha Surbharti Prakashana.

Trovato, F. (2009). *Canada's Population in a Global Context: An Introduction to Social Demography*. Oxford University Press Canada.

United Nations. (2001). World Population Monitoring, Population, Environment, and Development (ESA/P/WP.164). Population Division, Department of Economic and Social Affairs, New York, United Nations.

World Health Organization (WHO). (1948a), Preamble to the Constitution of the World Health Organization as adopted by the International Health Conference, New York, 19-22 June, 1946; signed on 22 July 1946 by the representatives of 61 States (Official Records of the World Health Organization, no. 2, p. 100) and entered into force on 7 April 1948.

World Health Organization (WHO). (2008b). Closing the gap in a generation. Health equity through action on the social determinants of health. Geneva. Retrieved from http://apps.who.int/iris/bitstream/10665/43943/1/9789241563703_eng.pdf

World Health Organization (WHO). (2013c). Country cooperation strategy at a glance. Retrieved from http://www.who.int/countryfocus/cooperation_strategy/ccsbrief_ind_en.pdf

World Health Organization (WHO). (1996d). Creating Healthy Cities in the 21st Century Background Paper, *UN Conference on Human Settlements: Habitat II*, Istanbul

World Health Organization (WHO). (2001e). Private Sector Involvement in City Health Systems proceedings of a WHO conference meeting, Dunedin, New Zealand.

World Health Organization (WHO). (2000f). *Who Pays for the Health System? The World Health Report*. Geneva: WHO.

World Health Organization (WHO). (2001g). Making a Public-Private Partnership Work: An Insider's View. *Bulletin of the World Health Organization*, *79*(8), 795–796.

World Health Organization (WHO). (2007h). Everybody's business: strengthening health systems to improve health outcomes: WHO's framework for action. Geneva.

KEY TERMS AND DEFINITIONS

Communicable/Infectious/Contagious Diseases: It spread from one person to another or from an animal to a person via airborne viruses or bacteria, through blood or other bodily fluids.

Demographic Dividend: A country with both increasing numbers of young people and declining fertility has the potential to reap a 'demographic dividend'. It boosts economic productivity, when there are growing numbers of working people relative to the number of dependents.

Epidemiological Transition: It characterized by a shift in patterns of disease and mortality from primarily infectious diseases to chronic diseases (NCDs).

Health: It is "a state of complete physical, mental, and social well-being and not merely the absence of disease or infirmity."

Health Promotion: "A process for initiating, managing, and implementing change, a process of personal, organizational, and policy development."

Non Communicable Diseases (NCDs): Non-infectious, non-transmissible (chronic diseases) which last for long periods of time and progress slowly like cancer, diabetes, cardiovascular diseases, chronic respiratory diseases etc.

Universal Health Coverage (UHC): "Ensuring equitable access for all citizens, resident in any part of the country, regardless of income level, social status, gender, caste or religion, to affordable, accountable, appropriate health services of assured quality (promotive, preventive, curative and rehabilitative) as well as public health services addressing the wider determinants of health delivered to individuals and populations, with the government being the guarantor and enabler, although not necessarily the only provider, of health and related services."

Wellness: "A state of a healthy balance of the mind and body that results in overall well-being."

Chapter 12
Incognito:
The Neuroscience of Grief and Grieving

Linda Ellington
Southern New Hampshire University, USA

Valerie Bryan
Florida Atlantic University, USA

ABSTRACT

In this chapter, we explore the neuroscience of grief and grieving. Even though the cognitive portion of the initiation into loss implores us to see a correlation between what is expected of us and the concept of reality as we move toward the outcome, the brain is meaning-driven, attempting to match new information with prior understanding. And as neural connections continue to develop and change throughout grief and grieving the "emotional monster" may not be capable of being quieted through support, whether professional or personal. The resistance from a cognitive approach is taken over by our effort to tame that "emotional monster" and images and feelings that are unique to the loss process stunt the capability of the brain to provide rational thinking. We end by picturing how our relentless search began, as we are in awe of what we intuitively know to be true, and that we are not fixed in toxicity, but can change the most challenging neurological situation. Our search was to understand the process of cognition as we move through grief and grieving. We wrote this chapter hoping it would shed a well-lit conversation on the most difficult time we will experience in our lives, the initiation into loss. The light shines on the neuroscience of this journey – as it would not honor 'self' if we did not look at 'self 'in a wholesome way. We frame this chapter through four focus lenses: self and self-discovery focus; emotion focus; social context and role identity focus; and cognitive focus.

INTRODUCTION

Grief and grieving come in many forms. Not just through the death of family and friends, but also in the feelings of loss that come with the inevitable life changes we all endure (Kubler-Ross & Kessler, 2005, p. xi). For example, loss of employment and its accompanying status (such as, loss of finances or social circle due to change or loss of the employment with its accompanying loss of home and memo-

DOI: 10.4018/978-1-5225-0640-9.ch012

ries associated with the home); change in marital status with loss of partner's social circle; lessened ability to function (whether due to being disabled later in life, suffering memory-impaired aged, being severely handicapped with a disease such as cancer or Lupus, or loss of a body part due to accident or injury); loss of way (e.g., transitions from high school to college, college to life, and so forth); and loss of financial status due to retirement, theft, death of a spouse, or catastrophic situation, etc. During loss, our world may take on a slowness or a surrealness that propels us to see ourselves as an observer rather than a participant. It seems strange to each of us that the clocks in the world continue when our inner clock does not (Kubler-Ross & Kessler, 2005, p. 29). To understand the grief and grieving process this chapter is written to hopefully shed a well-lit conversation of neuroscience when we are initiated into loss.

The chapter will address common manifestations of grief and how it may affect us physically, mentally, and emotionally, and how each of these may not be the same in two individuals or even occur in the same stage from person to person. The perspective used is as individual as is the person and may cause the differences in manifestations of the grief and grieving. Yet, knowing what is feasible in terms of possible occurrences may help us to allow the person either the support or comfort that he or she needs or the time and space he or she needs, to heal and move on individually. Grief alone has the power to heal (Kubler-Ross & Kessler, 2005, p. 227). Grief is a normal process and each person has their own way to grieve. Each person also has a different timetable to allow grief to help them find a new sense of self.

Like everything physiological, our brains have limitations. Mayer & Moreno (2003) point out limitations are based on cognitive overload (as cited in Bruning, Schraw & Norby, 2011, p. 29). Going through the loss progression requires substantial cognitive processing using all sensory channels available. However, the brain has limited processing capacity available at any moment, thus it may become overloaded and miss part of the grief and grieving leading to incomplete or incorrect thinking, and thus not being able to tame the "emotional monster". Regardless of whether the loss is an actual loss or a symbolic loss of the events related to the loss, grief can affect your sense of self. Grief is actually there to help us to heal and regrow our sense of self (Patricelli & Dombeck, 2015). The grief generally ends when the person has healed and regrown their sense of self.

How do we apply neuroscience research and derived principles to grief and grieving? Possibly by maximizing cognition and reducing emotional overload: (1) find personal space, (2) allow all senses to be applied, (3) tell supportive people that they need to allow your individualized path, (4) create an environment for the monster emotion to take over once in a while; (5) engage in self-discovery; and, (6) allow for self-determination (Eagleman, 2011).

The cognitive abilities have a presence unlike any other during this time of loss, but the presence may be undermined by emotions. We are fragile human beings during the progression through loss and we must have a realization that we will not come out unscathed; it may be an incomplete story for years in the future, and 'self' as we once knew it may no longer exist; our world of self has changed.

SELF AND SELF-DISCOVERY FOCUS

Extended consciousness inevitably leads to the phenomenon of the self. Taken from Dai and Sternberg (2004) we paraphrase Gazzaniga (2000), we are constantly running an autobiographic narrative and this is not trivial as researchers suggest the self is not only of extended consciousness but also by emotional feeling, a position reminiscent of James (1997) who described the phenomenal self as a person's emotional center. James (1997) commented "All we know is that there are dead feelings, dead ideas, and cold beliefs, and there are hot and live ones; and when they grow hot and alive within us, everything has to re-crystallize about it" (as cited in Dai & Sternberg, 2004, p. 14). This re-crystallization has a direct bearing on a wide range of intellectual activities in our concept of change (Dai & Sternberg, 2004, p. 15).

Focusing on the process of 'self' it may fit into the Kubler-Ross change curve, thus expanding knowledge on the curve characteristics. Are we witnessing a new respect for a rather classical form of change as we progress through the grief and grieving functioning as seen through physiological self, psychological self and spiritual self? Are the various models intentional in their experiences of self through this loss process or should we be asking--can anyone produce real conscious experiences who has not walked in the shoes of a person in peril due to loss? The limitation may be in the inability to include sincere support that is characterized as helping, but may be an omission of legitimate experience. Thus, the importance of integrating the perspective of self.

From physiological self not only, do we feel and know in the present tense, but can we anticipate further physical functioning in future tense while immersed in the grief and grieving process? The focus on our physiological self is not a selfish act, but one that could be devastating if not spotlighted upon by the individual going through the loss as this is a crucial piece of experience that motivates adaptive adjustment to the loss. Dai and Sternberg (2004) pointed out that almost all human activity, including thinking of self, serves not one but a multiplicity of motives at the same time (p.5). Thus, knowing this then grief and grieving should not be discounted going through loss being focused on oneself.

From a psychological self, there is an intimate association with emotion and feelings which are never entirely lost. There must be awareness that 'self' is not free of emotion and that during the grieving process, even though there may appear to be mechanical and rational movement, we must not negate reality knowing that this is a reduction in psychological functioning. There needs to be a conscious effort to let the grieving tenet cover all spectrums of human emotions that contribute to the richness and complexity of working through the loss process (Dai & Sternberg, 2004).

The emergence of spiritual self can appear very early in the process or may need time and space to allow it to be internalized as a relational construct to the loss. This particular self can be directly boosted by the immediate initiation into the loss, or present itself as it affects the physiological and psychological functions in an unpredicted time table. The awareness of spiritual self may activate two schemes, each separately in order to reach the objective to heal.

First scheme is that of motivating oneself for independence, showing strength, and not weakness in the time of loss. The second scheme is that of involving coordination of the "quasi-needs"; spirituality just in time. If we take a view of 40K feet above, we can visualize that deep, intellectual, disciplined thinking with attention regulation, thinking, body awareness, emotion regulation, and a sense of self changes our brain positively (Leaf, 2013, p. 172). What are the intersection in this change curve as it relates to neuroscience in grief and grieving (Figure 1)?

There is a radically different story about our existence than had previously been experienced when confronted with loss (Eagleman, 2011). For many the fall from our familiar will cause profound unease and the challenge for us is to challenge our thinking and emotions so we come out on the other side intact, but a different self. We are moving between accessible and inaccessible parts of our being and perhaps many of us move deeper into those caverns inside ourselves. Against this cave backdrop, the rigor of the support may overwhelm our senses, or could provide us with an accurate representation of the outside world. During this time, we are not aware of the outside world, but instead only of the signals in our nervous system (Eagleman, 2011) which tell us that something is out there, but it may be real or not.

Figure 1. Kubler-Ross change curve

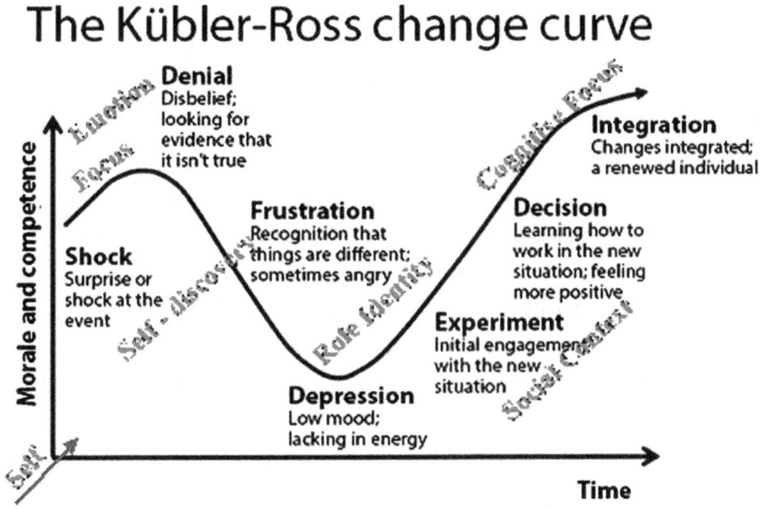

Against this backdrop, a German physician named Ernst Heinrich Weber (1795-1878) grew interested in bringing the rigor of physics to the study of the mind. His new field of "psychophysics" (Eagleman, 2011, p. 14) aimed to quantify what people can detect, how fast they can react, and what they perceive and yet, 200+ years later, it is obvious that our senses give us a perception of the outside world and we consider the physical brain a relationship with perception (Eagleman, 2011). So again, if our perception is to be incognito, (e.g., disguised) how well do we handle the continued movement through loss? We are not at the center of ourselves but out on a distant edge, hearing little of what is transpiring (Eagleman, 2011). Is being in disguise deconstructing the experience for us and thus engendering a 'new' self? (Eagleman, 2011, p. 19-20)

In self-discovery we want to open our eyes and voila the world is beautiful with reds and golds, but yet what we see are lightning storms as we do not know what is coming next or making decisions about what to do now; our brain is going through a great deal of trouble to disambiguate the information hitting us all at once (Eagleman, 2011, p. 23). We tell 'self' that we are seeing through a frosted shower door and what we are experiencing is just an illusion (Eagleman, 2011, p. 23). This limited cone of reality becomes wider and clearer as the progression moves forward and our perception of self begins to construct a world for us that represents our different self. We can begin to see small changes in our lives and no guarantee but the discovery should allow the brain processes to show the bigger picture and how our new self fits into the larger landscape of our life. Not only is the perception of our 'new' world a construction that does not accurately represent the outside of what is occurring around us, but we additionally have a false impression of a picture when in fact we see only what we need to know and see, and no more (Eagleman, 2011, p. 28). What is important at this point in time, is to explore the loss in a slow, gradual exploration which could engender the brain to move deeper and uncover another layer of tenacity which we may not have known is available to us (Eagleman, 2011, p. 100).

EMOTION FOCUS

If our brain is the mission control center that drives the whole operation" then how do, we chug through the emotional darkness"? (Leaf, 2011, p. 1). In grief we often have a deep well of different emotions occurring at the same time, which is what makes grief confusing (Kubler-Ross & Kessler, 2005, p. 33). We are not accustomed to the emotional upheaval that accompanies a loss. People experience a wide array of emotions after a loss. We can go from feeling okay to feeling devastated in a minute without warning. We can have mood swings that are hard for anyone around us to comprehend, because even we do not understand them. That is how grief works (Kubler-Ross & Kessler, 2005, p. 34).

We cannot tuck messy emotions into neat packages (Kubler-Ross & Kessler, 2005, p. xiv). There is not a typical response to loss as there is no typical loss. Our grief and grieving is as individual as our lives. We often times move through the experiences of loss, trying to make sense of the losses, without any guidance or framework for how to understand them (Kubler-Ross & Kessler, 2005, p. xi). We have a sense that we are the only ones that have gone through the experience and that no one can understand what we are actually experiencing in part because it is unique to us, but also because we are not in control of the experience ourselves. The psychological effects of having consciousness and self-awareness of feelings and emotions are obvious, but often get neglected (Dai & Sternberg, 2004, p. 12). Thoughts are driven by the power of feelings which are the designers of the landscape of our brains (Leaf, 2013, p. 104). Eagleman identifies the pretending as he states, "There is someone in my head, but it is not me" (2011, p. 1)

The manner in which our brain interrogates the world during loss is to gather details and then the "unexpected visitor" comes in – that being the "emotional monster" (Eagleman, 2011, p. 28). During this time of loss, our life seems to be a series of snapshots rather than a movie. Our picture is 'painted on' our views of the 'new' world, and yet we must consider we do not need to explicitly represent the new until the point that introspection has more time for meaningful insight into what is happening. A misstep or a hiccup is magnified through our emotional lens. When we think, we also feel. This is because thoughts have an emotional component in addition to the information, or what the actual memory is about. That means that when we bring a thought into consciousness, we also bring up the attached emotion. When the thought along with its emotions bubble up into the conscious mind, we feel the emotions (Leaf, 2013, p. 161).

Attitude is a state of mind – a thought plus its attached emotions – and it influences what we say and do. If the attitude that is activated is negative (toxic), then the emotional response will naturally be negative or stressful feeling. If the attitude is positive, the feeling will be peaceful. The truth is that our attitude will be revealed no matter how much we try to hide it (Leaf, 2013, p. 161). Question for us then is, can we determine the attitude of the thoughts that move through our conscious mind during grief and grieving? Our attitudes – positive or toxic – not only cannot be hidden from others, but they have a profound impact on our own brain and body (Leaf, 2013, p. 161). And yes, although we may not be able to control our environment during this time of loss, we can try to control how it affects our mission control center – our brain.

Steeped in grief is an incredibly lonely experience. Our world, as we knew it, stops, while everything around us continued on around us. Feeling grief can make us feel like we are crazy because our heart is shattered into a thousand tiny pieces. But everyone wants us to say we are "okay", so we do. We live in a culture that does not know how to grieve, we do not know how to experience pain, or how to understand its process. We live in a society that wants us to get back to normal as soon as possible. We are expected to go back to work immediately, keep moving, to "get on with our lives". But it does not work that way. We need time to move through the pain of loss. We need to step into it, get to know it, in order to learn how to live with it. That is what grief is. It is the opening up to the exquisite pain of absence. It is the moment when we stop trying to change how much it hurts. Grief is the intense emotional response to the pain of a loss. It is the reflection of a connection that has been broken and most importantly, grief is an emotional and psychological journey to healing (Kubler-Ross & Kessler, 2005, p. 227).

THE CONTRIBUTION OF THE HEART

When talking about thinking and understanding we need to also consider the contribution the heart makes to thinking and decision making (Brackett, Lopes, Ivcevic, Mayer & Salovey, as cited in Dai & Sternberg, 2004, p. 175). Our heart is not just a pump, it helps with decision making and choices, acting like a checking station for all the emotions generated by the flow of chemical from thoughts. In fact, every single cell is connected to our heart and, because our heart responds to and is controlled by our brain, every single cell in our body is affected by our thoughts in some way regardless of whether those thoughts are conscious or unconscious (Leaf, 2013, p. 177).

Our heart is in constant communication with our brain and the rest of our body, checking the accuracy of our thought life. As we are about to make a decision, our heart pops in a quiet word of advice. And because of the deep hurt we experience during loss, it is well worth listening to our heart's advice, because when we listen to our heart, is secretes a hormone that is produced by the heart that regulates blood pressure, thus in turn a feeling of some peace (Leaf, 2013). Doctors, nursing, therapists, and clerical personnel often give the sage advice that "time will heal", but the reality is that all of them need to be advising us to listen to our heart and allow it be calm us and to lessen our pain threshold.

We have the opportunity to rethink and reevaluate what our reaction to the information of loss should be and to evaluate how toxic the thought is and then re-transcribing it to be a healthy and strong part of our memory library (Leaf, 2013, p. 189). How do we do this? By consciously becoming aware of our "thought life" we are re-transcribing and changing our underlying neuronal networks. We need to uncover the negative thoughts that create such powerful internal conflicts in our mind and that are capable of causing electrochemical imbalances that, when taken to the extreme, cause parts of ourselves to be cut off from the rest of us. It is not unheard of for people to have a stroke or a heart attack when faced with a great loss. If these individuals carried with them the tools to reevaluate our "thought life" we may be able to avoid these extremes.

But we certainly do not have to solve everything on day one – and in fact that would not be wise, and yet during a death or an extreme loss that is exactly what the outside world expects of us as humans, particularly in the American culture (Leaf, 2013, p. 190). Dai and Sternberg pursue an integrative approach which views motivation, emotion, and cognition as inextricably related, for good or ill (2004, p. xi). In this type of emphasis, it puts perception and cognition back in the context of human adaptive efforts to effect changes in their environments, as well as in themselves, and related emotional reactions and affective experiences (2004, p. xi).

As Neisser (1963) pointed out a long time ago:

1. Human thinking begins in an intimate association with emotion and feelings which is never entirely lost;
2. Almost all human actions, including thinking, serve not one but a multiplicity of motives at the same time (as cited in Dai and Sternberg, 2004, p. 5).

Efforts for integrating motivation, emotion and cognition have been made by those pioneers of cognitive psychology (Bruner, 1986; Norman, 1980; Simon, 1967, 1979, 1994, as cited in Dai and Sternberg, 2004) and yet it is "an all too narrow focus on cognition if we place restrictions on cognitive science (2004, p. 8). The notion that basic mental processes, such as attention, perception, and cognition never occur as neutral events containing raw data of whatever we are registering in our thought minds, is not new (Bartlett, 1932, as cited in Dai & Sternberg, 2004, p. 8-9). In the early years of the cognitive revolution, Abelson (1963) challenged cognitive simulation researchers to simulate cognition with an affect or attitude (Dai & Sternberg, 2004, p. 9).

EMOTION AND COGNITION INTEGRATION

Emotional intelligence is crucial. It is one of the primary forms of information that human beings process. That does not mean that everybody has to process it well. But it does mean that it is circulating around us, and thus we need this component to help us through our emotionally demanding times in our lives (Mayer, 2005, as cited in Snyder & Lopez, 2007, p. 159).

The Stoic philosophers of ancient Greece argued that emotions were unreliable and idiosyncratic sources of information (Lloyd, 1978, as cited in Dai and Sternberg, year). They emphasized the superiority of reason, cognition and intelligence (Kerferd, 1978, as cited in Dai & Sternberg, 2004). The presence of an emotional component, or emotional intelligence, would likely have seemed inconceivable to them – an oxymoron. Two millennial later psychologists and philosophers still debate whether emotions are disorganized interruptions or whether they contribute to logical thought (Dai & Sternberg, 2004, p. 175). For example, Woodworth (1940) viewed emotions as disorganizing interruptions of thought, whereas Leeper (1948) suggested that emotions contribute to logical thought. Whether during the Ancient Greece time or today, for those who are experiencing grief and grieving, emotions indeed interact with thought. The cognitive loop connects emotions to judgement (Dai & Sternberg, 2004, p. 175). The research shows that thought processes are affected by emotions (e.g., Forgas & Moylan, 1987; Mayer & Breer, 1985; Salovey & Birnbaum, 1989; Singer & Solovy, 1988 as cited in Dai and Sternberg, 2004, p. 176). During stressful times of loss, the emotional components include recognition, understanding and importantly the management of one's own and others' emotional states to solve emotion-laden problems (Dai & Sternberg, 2004, p. 176).

In 1960, Mowrer addressed the prevailing thoughts about emotions undermining intelligence by suggesting that emotion was, in fact, "high order of intelligence" (Snyder & Lopez, 2007, p. 154). Peter Salovey of Yale University and John Mayer of the University of New Hampshire shred Mowrer's sentiment and theorized that adapting to life circumstances required cognitive abilities and emotional skills that guide behavior (Mayer, DiPaolo, & Salovey, 1990; Salovey & Mayer, 1990, as cited in Snyder & Lopez, 2007, p. 154). Even though the term, emotional intelligence (EI) was introduced in the 1990s, it was mostly unknown to lay people until Goleman (1995) popularized the term in his book, *Emotional Intelligence* (Dai & Sternberg, 2004, p. 176). From thence, researchers have now claimed that EI is as powerful and at times more powerful than IQ (Dai & Sternberg, 2004, p. 176). Today however, the field of emotional intelligence is filled with both empirical articles and popular books on the topic and therefore, making it difficult to decipher what EI actually is, and how it plays into the environment of loss (Dai & Sternberg, 2004, p. 177).

Sternberg (1999) states that "practical emotional intelligence" helps one to implement solutions effectively, drawing on previous experience and tacit knowledge. His view of practice EI encompasses social and emotional skills, and emphasizes the notion of common sense (Dai & Sternberg, 2004, p. 183). The authors of this chapter respectfully disagree with his view, because of the personal experience of grief and grieving, there is no drawing on previous familiarity if one has never experienced a death of a loved one or loss of a lifestyle or even a loss of a limb or ability to function as a whole human being.

There is no common sense that comes to the front of the mind – and should not be expected. The conflict enters at this point, as the external world expects emotional and practical abilities to reflect attunement to social norms and expectations; however, those who are experiencing the loss, there is a minimal, at most a modest, correlation between the understanding and managing of emotions (Dai & Sternberg, 2004, p. 183). The ability to manage emotions and their expressions is vital for coping with loss challenges, and EI theory posits that a person's ability to accurately perceive, use, understand and regulate emotions may help to prevent involvement in potentially harmful behaviors, such support through alcohol or medication or even excess physical exercise (Dai & Sternberg, 2004, p. 187). Dweck, Mangels & Good (as cited in Dai & Sternberg, 2004) find in their research that motivation affects attentional processes, cognitive strategies, and cognitive performance in the face of challenge and setbacks. Their research speaks to the ways in which motivation, emotions and neuroscience work together and to the idea that cognition in isolation cannot yield a full or valid picture of the workings of the mind (p.53).

SOCIAL CONTEXT AND ROLE IDENTITY FOCUS

The social support structure by contrast may be damaging to our capacity to understand, because often they "steal our tongue" as we are unsure of how to maneuver through the complexity of our brain as it too is telling us what to do, how to act, make decisions, and get back into living (Eagleman, 2011). At particular stressful times, the griever may find others "talking" for them and yet, not saying what the griever is feeling at that time. At times during the 20th century, psychology research and practice sullied the reputation of emotions (Snyder & Lopez, 2007, p. 149). At worst, helping professionals characterized emotions as detrimental to rational decision-making. At best, emotions had been portrayed as signals of specific daily actions that needed to be taken are of (Snyder & Lopez, 2007, p. 149). Research popularized in the 21st century demonstrates that both positive and negative emotions may determine how adaptive we are in grief and grieving (2007, p. 149).

The power of emotions traditionally is described in such negative terms as "the beast within" (Averill, 1990 as cited in Snyder & Lopez, 2007, p. 150). Intense emotions were seen as dysfunctional and opposed to rationality. But when Annette Stanton, a positive psychologist at the University of California at Los Angeles, considered the adaptive potential of emotion-focused coping (e.g., regulating the emotions surrounding a stressful encounter) her research found that there was a problem in how emotions were defined. Wide disparity was apparent in the emotion-focused coping phenomenon and this led to unclear associations between what was referred to as "emotion-focused coping" and "cognitive adjustment" (Snyder & Lopez, 2007, p. 150). Stanton and her colleagues have spent the last decade researching the idea that "emotional-focused coping" may depend on the situational context, the interpersonal milieu, and attributes of the individual (p.150). They identify emotional approaches which involve active movement toward, rather than away from a stressful encounter, such as loss.

Identity plays a critical role in the way we address environmental pressures and expectations of change. During grief and grieving we are compelled to simultaneously abide by different "rules of the game", each prescribing a different, and at times contradictory, set of normative guidelines (Kraatz & Block, 2008, p. 243; Reay & Hinings, 2009, as cited in Kodeih and Greenwood, 2014). There is potentially an importance in the role of identity in the process of loss. This 'new' identity may affect how we respond and interpret not only internal signals, but external as well. Our understanding of an unexpected emerging new identity may cause conflict in navigating and assimilating in a logical world; one that does not exist for those experiencing grief and grieving. An integral part of who we are, that it emanates from our sense of self and thus self-determination may be in conflict with the new role as the participant in loss. The integration of an identification with other aspects of oneself, that is with other identifications such as new the role of a widow or of the amputee or the person with cancer; may demonstrate itself in non-traditional social behaviors (Gagne and Deci, 2005). Others may try to console us in the only way they know. But our loss stands alone in its meaning to us, in its painful uniqueness (Kubler-Ross & Kessler, 2005, p. 29).

As difficult as this may be, what matters is not how an external force sees us but how we see ourselves in our 'new' role. Do we simply unpack our old self or do we find opportunities to see how the role of our identity has changed because of the loss? Can the scale of those changes help us as we transition through the loss process? Despite this shift in attention in our identity, there is a need to actually cope with the present and the demands of the new reality. There is an incomplete feeling of how we cope with the complexity posed by the loss that embodies our new identity. From this newness of a new role in self there may be an emerging appreciation, of the importance of identity because it "functions as a filter for interpreting and responding to changes occurring around us" (Glynn, 2008; Kraatz & Block, 2008; Yu, 2013, as cited in Kodeih & Greenwood, 2014, p. 10). Although, there is a re-framing of the new role, there may be an opportunity for reconfiguration that offers a slightly nuanced picture of identity. Because our preprogramming is deeply involved in social exchange the way humans interact with each other, the picture of our identity may be expanding rather than shrinking. Social interaction has been critical to our species for millions of years, and as a result the social aspect has worked its way deep down into the neural brain circuitry (Eagleman, 2011, p. 84).

We do not enter loss with a blank slate brain, but a system that may be unable to quickly learn the new complex rules in our 'new' world and without social interaction, we may fail. "We know this from the long history of failure of artificial neural networks that start off knowledge free and attempt to learn the rules of the world" (Eagleman, 2011, p. 84). The vast networks of neurons underpinning the social interactions are so well turned that we fail to be aware of their normal interaction, until we are initiated into grieving and grief. This explosion of awareness is now no longer effortless and the hidden network of neurons is disguised as not reality, but a momentary force that will change if only we can imagine the end game, which may be obvious to everyone but us, who enter the loss involuntarily. Additionally, during this time, we cannot always elicit a straight answer from the unconscious brain, and therefore how can we access its knowledge? Sometimes the important part is to assess our "gut" feelings and then rely on those feelings to help in making the right choice instead of relying on the social networking to choose options.

Human beings can be engaged or alienated, largely as a function of progressing through the grief and grieving process. Research guided by self-determination theory has focused on the social contextual conditions that facilitate versus forestall the natural processes of self-motivation (Ryan & Deci, 2000). Broadly defined, self-determination or motivation, is indicated by the intensity, direction and persistence of the action. In other words, motivation does not just kick start a mental act, with the rest of the action carried out by cognitive processes. The attentional focus on the self or on the task frames the mindset and can significantly influence the allocation of attentional resources and emotional reactions to difficulties in the face of loss (Dai & Sternberg, 2004, p. 11). Healing from grief is often an overwhelming and lonely experience (Kubler-Ross & Kessler, 2005, p. 204). We do not have any real framework to help us and because we live in a grief-dismissing world now, our work society allows three to four days of grieving, very few will tell us, "Take as much time as you need . . . ." (Kubler-Ross & Kessler, 2005, p. 206). This type of societal attitude expects everyone to grieve the same way and in the same time (Kubler-Ross & Kessler, 2005, p. 206). It is as ridiculous as expecting every child to learn how to walk at the exact same chronological age.

In today's culture there are so few models of grief. It is invisible to the untrained eye (Kubler-Ross & Kessler, 2005, p. 228). While some mourners have access to grieving counselors and other health care professionals, most people today feel very alone in their grief. They long for a pathway through their pain and isolation (Kubler-Ross & Kessler, 2005, p. 228). We unconsciously seek models, which are few and far between. Because we may not know how to handle the pain of grief, we avoid it. Yet by avoiding grief, we turn our backs to the help that grief occurs, thus prolonging the pain (p.229). Research has supported that sudden unexpected losses are generally harder to navigate than expected losses. With anticipated losses, people generally have time to prepare, both by feeling grief before the fact of the loss and also by planning ways to minimize the negative impact of the loss when it does occur. But even this may be offset if the loss is for an immediate family member (spouse, child, parent, best friend).

COGNITIVE FOCUS

The term thinking has its roots in philosophy. However, the general notion that good thinking involves detecting and acting on occasions is found in many accounts of complex cognitive activity (Dai & Sternberg, 2004, p. 354). Thinking is a powerful force, both a blessing and a curse, and should not be taken lightly (Leaf, 2013, p. 124). Achieving positive thinking and health is not accomplished by putting on a brave face, nor are they attained by adopting an ostrich mentality and pretending that the loss does not exist (Leaf, 2013, p. 139). We must wire in a positive thought networks that can fill us with the power to get us on track (Leaf, 2013, p. 140). As difficult as this sounds as we journey through loss. We do control our brain; our brain does not control us (Leaf, 2013, p. 140).

How do we turn the chore of cognitive translation into seeing reality – this data comes in from the brain, as it works its way up the sensory hierarchy and makes sense to us (Eagleman, 2011, p. 44). A surprising aspect of this translation is that the internal data is not generated by external sensory but merely modified by it. LeDoux (1996) reveals that a particular brain structure, the amygdala, plays a significant role in processing matters of emotional significance. Specifically, LeDoux suggest that, under stress-free circumstances, our thinking is governed by the hippocampus, but during stressful times such as during grief and grieving, our thought processes – hence aspects of our emotional coping are ruled by the amygdala (Snyder & Lopez, 2007, p. 152). To date, numerous amalgamations of psychological constructs have been conceptualized as reflective of emotional intelligence (Bar-On, 1997; Schutte, 1998, as cited in Snyder and Lopez, 2007, p. 153). For example, Bar-On (1997, 2000) defines emotional intelligence as an array of non-cognitive capabilities, competencies and skills that help us deal with the demands of emotional experiences, such as loss (Snyder & Lopez, 2007, p. 154).

The perception of time is a construction of the brain and our perception of the world lags behind the real world. And so it is with our conscious life, it collects a lot of information before it airs it live (Eagleman, 2011, p. 51). Thus, the space between our thinking and action during loss needs to be understood that it is our brain catching up to itself, even though we may appear 'brain dead'. There is a looming chasm between what your brain knows and what your mind is capable of accessing (Eagleman, 2011, p. 55). When we are forced to access it consciously, we are flummoxed (Eagleman, 2011, p. 55). To the context that consciousness is useful, it is useful in small quantities and for very particular kinds of tasks. Thus, the feeling of putting one foot in front of the other is a simple task as we travel the lonely path of loss. For those who wish to help, be aware that your support efforts only lower the timing of seeing reality – it does not remove it.

We often do not know whether to turn inward or away from what our brain is telling us because there are several little sets of hands on the steering wheel of our behavior (Eagleman, 2011, p. 108). If we begin to withdraw we may not find the courage to begin again. We are conflicted at this point and find ourselves stuck at the point where the 'pull' matches the 'push' and in reality we get nowhere (Eagleman, 2011, p. 108). What is important at this point in time, is to explore the loss in a slow, gradual exploration which could engender the brain to move deeper and uncover another layer of courage which we may not have known is available to us (Eagleman, 2011, p. 100).

According to Leaf, "Neuroscientific research is confirming daily what we instinctively knew all along: What we are thinking becomes a physical reality in the brain and body, which does affect our optimal mental and physical health" (2013, pp.13-14). So how does this influence our state of mind during times of loss? Leaf tells us that the influence is not our DNA, but rather the electromagnetic, quantum and chemical flow in the brain that switches groups of genes on or off in a positive or negative direction based on our choices and subsequent reactions (Leaf, 2013, p. 14).

Does our social support network know this? Before they give us their 'best' advice, maybe they should gain the knowledge that the brain, all our brains, respond to our minds by sending these neurological signals throughout the body, which means that thoughts and emotions are transformed into physiological and spiritual effects, and then physiological experiences transform into mental and emotional states (Leaf, 2013, p. 14). Eric Kandel, a Nobel Prize winning neuropsychiatrist, showed how thoughts, even our imaginations, get 'under the skin' of our DNA and can turn certain genes on and certain genes off, changing the structure of the neurons in the brain (Leaf, 2013, p. 32). So, as we think and imagine, we change the structure and function of our brains. This tells us that while we can imagine moving through the loss and into our new reality, we have the power to redesign the landscape of our brain. Even Freud speculated back in the 1800s that thought leads to changes in the brain (Leaf, 2013, p. 32).

During grief and grieving, we need to understand our brain is being rewired for a moment in time, and that with love and patience, we can get back control of our thoughts and renew the direction we are heading in. Based on Leaf's research on the brain and her clinical experiences we can once again learn how thoughts impact our spirit, soul and body, and to learn how to detox our fear-driven thoughts and thus strive to choose our mind to make changes and decisions to create a quality and positive 'new' world we have been forced into (Leaf, 2013, p. 15). This may then be the path toward a mindful determination to pull ourselves up, renew the mind, and move beyond what we thought we were not capable of during the initiation into loss.

As we move through grieving we react to the events and circumstances, which does have an enormous impact on our mental and physical health. But, as we continue to think we change the physical nature of our brain. If we are able to direct our thinking during this time, we can wire out toxic patterns of thinking and begin to replace them with healthier thoughts, and new thought networks then grow. This transition brings a healing to our brains, minds, and physical bodies (Leaf, 2013, p. 20). Our mind and body's response to toxic thinking is normal stress gone wrong. Even a little bit of these negative levels of stress from a little bit of toxic thinking has far reaching consequences for mental and physical health (Leaf, 2013, p. 36).

As we react to circumstances during the grief and grieving process, our brains become shaped by the process in either a positive or negative direction. So, it is the 'quality' of our thinking and decisions during this difficult time and our reactions that determine our "brain architecture" the shape or design of the elastic brain and resultant quality of the health of our minds and bodies during this time of stress (Leaf, 2013, p. 34).

When we feel shut down by our introduction to the "emotional monster", our body feels this too, which in turn reduces the quality of our expressions which are often mistaken for less than capable of making decisions, so the support team feels they must make the decisions. This type of interaction with the support puts the brain into protection mode and stress then manifests itself into our bodies. But the good news is, that scientists basically have proven we can rewire and renew our minds (Leaf, 2013, p. 36). Knowing this, our 'reset button' can demonstrate hope through our positive language and healthy decisions. According to Luthans and Avolio (2003), "The force multiplier throughout history has often been attributed to an ability to generate hope" (p. 42). The thinking component of hope exerts a strong influence on flexibility possibly accommodating new routes of thinking during the grief and grieving process.

In our determination to know how our thoughts influence our movement through loss, we understand through neuroscience research that the frontal lobes are how we enable ourselves in a sense to stand outside ourselves and observe our own thinking. If we have the ability to do this, we may be able to bring all thoughts into captivity and feel less anxious when we realize we have the equipment and knowledge to do so (Leaf, 2013, p. 45). Does this then allow us to see things from many different angles – like different perspectives? Our perception of the environment, plus how we manage our environment, controls our bodies and lives. So, according to Leaf, if you change your perception, you change your biology (2013, p. 66). During this period of loss, our perception is in conflict with itself, and there is a disconnect between what is real and what we feel deep down, that may not seem real to us. This is called *cognitive dissonance* and we need to focus our attention on real choices, not what we wish would be true. This then affects how the chemicals and wiring of our brain changes and functions.

Scientists are proving that the relationship between you and how you understand and perceive inner thought has a significant impact on how your brain works (Leaf, 2013, p. 66). Paying attention to our thoughts and purposefully focusing our mind leads to transformation, in time (Leaf, 2013, p. 67). What influences our perception is whatever we immerse ourselves in, our beliefs and the beliefs of those around us. How we interact with those people, our inner faith, our ability to control our bodies (through exercise or reflective techniques) and what we expose ourselves to, all leads to differences in the way we focus our attention, which has a direct effect on how our neurochemicals work together (Leaf, 2013, p. 67).

What does this mean? It helps explain that with the elimination of toxic thinking we can renew our mind over time, and often intervention changes the brain physically, chemically, structurally, and functionally. If we agree with that premise, then we need to pay attention and understand how neuroplasticity works for and against us as we move forward to rewire healthy new circuits in our brain (Leaf, 2013, p. 71).

How do we quiet our mind, focus our attention on the present issue, and dismiss the distractions that are in front of us during grief and grieving? One could answer this, as Leaf did, that research dating back to the 1970s shows that capturing our thoughts in a disciplined way rather than letting them chaotically run rampant can bring about notable changes in how we feel and think. The change is evidenced in cognitive, emotional functioning, as well as at the neural level. Her research shows that controlled focused thinking leads to improvement in cognitive functioning and emotional balance (Leaf, 2013, p. 72). So, getting our thoughts disciplined and under control is one of the first steps in freeing ourselves of the burden of loss, and we can begin to diminish the negative impact of toxic thinking and thus begin rewiring healthy new circuits into our brain (Leaf, 2013, p. 72.). Purposefully catching our thoughts can control the brain's sensory processing, the brain's rewiring, the neurotransmitters, the genetic expression, and cellular activity in a positive direction. A simple way to do this is to say, "I can do this" – "I will come through my grief" – "I know there will be sunshine again" – and so forth. Self-affirmations are strong guideposts for healing.

We are thinking beings, and as we think, we are making a way to a decision of some kind, and during times of stress, that thinking process becomes more complex and we may choose several different courses of action we face, and the fear is then living with those actions. The fear can paralyze our thinking which then creates the cycle of toxicity which generates a powerful signal that may change the landscape of our brain, and out of the fear and toxicity we become wrapped in a cocoon that 'protects' us.

Somehow in this maze of thinking and feeling, we must initiate signals that get the ball rolling again that will signal for the healthy thoughts to outmaneuver the negative and ill-will thinking. Leaf identities this as the switch gene called the 'creb gene' which we can switch on with our thoughts (2013). The significance of the creb gene is that it can activate the making of proteins, thus we grow protein branches that allow thoughts, healthy thoughts, to permeate our brain, protein synthesis happens and a new branch grows, thus making a healthy connection at a synapse to other branches (Leaf, 2013, p. 50). So what does this mean to us who are mired in the grieving process? Scientists have discovered that we have a profound healing and regenerative impact on our bodies and minds by affecting our genetic expression (creb gene) that can help escort us through the precise pathways by which we voyage through the grief process (Leaf, 2013, p. 50).

This all sounds like a vicious cycle, doesn't it? Not catching and stopping toxic and fearful thoughts leads to those thoughts being wired into the brain; which can lead to depressive thoughts, which can then cause the body to go into stages of high level stress (Leaf, 2013, p. 74). All of this is from not catching the negative and fear driven thoughts. How do we fix this? Recent research has shown that teaching strategies to handle and control stress, the body's reaction to toxic thinking, could help individuals who have involuntarily been initiated into grief and grieving (Leaf, 2013, p. 75). This teaching strategy could be part of the Hospice experience, or even the earlier medical experience before the final step into Hospice. And yet, why not use these strategies to teach how to look at job loss, or divorce, or for that matter, all types of loss? Where are the psychologist, medical personnel, career trainers, or adult educators in providing these strategies?

Just possibly this may be where conflict with our support members occurs because if we switch into a mode of a deeply thinking state, which is focused more on introspective and tunes out the outside world, this may cause a cessation from an active external component; thus, our brain functioning is seen as shuffling, limited conscious, and cognitive weakness. The support network wants us to deal with reality as it currently presents itself to us, and yet we who are internalizing the loss, cannot expectedly change our brain quickly into a positive way when internally is where our attention is focused. And the shuffling, limited conscious and cognitive weakness may be exactly what is occurring, and therefore we are plagued with 'hurry sickness' and being bombarded with stimulation. We may need to ask for 'space in time' in order to be able to capture and control our thoughts that would then improve our brain function as well as mind, body and spiritual health (Leaf, 2013, p. 91).

Balance is an oxymoron during loss, there is no balance, nor should there be an expectation of such. We are skimming the surfaces of multiple pieces of information, which of course could have a detrimental effect on our well-being as we haphazardly dash back and forth between tasks. The 'space in time' approach will not only increase our understanding of our new reality, but will provide us with more deeply intellectual thinking patterns which once we get on a healthier thinking path, it will continue upward in a cascading fashion to our physical and emotional health, as well as cognitive effectiveness (Leaf, 2013, pp.97-98).

We cannot control the events and circumstances of life, but we can control our reactions to those events and circumstances; however, controlling our reactions requires flexibility in our thinking (Leaf, 2013, p. 82). Bernardes and Hanna (2009) defined flexibility as the "inherent property in our thinking which allows us to change within pre-established parameters" (p. 30). This then may lead to positive thinking as stated by Youssef & Luthans (2007), "What is good about life is as genuine as what is bad and what is bad, therefore deserves equal attention in our thinking" (p. 774). The concept of flexibility may be that we switch off from the outside world and move into a state of focused mindfulness (Leaf, 2013, p. 83). When we focus inward, we appear to slow down, but actually, our mental resources speed up and our thinking moves onto a higher level. When we think this way, we will emerge far ahead of where we would have been if we just operated within the realms of a shifting, shuffling, limited conscious, cognitive mind (Leaf, 2013, p. 83). In fact, research shows that if we do not engage in this 'slow down' we may get stuck, unable to cope, and have a tendency to focus on the problem and not the solution (Leaf, 2013, p. 85).

In their research study by Pascual-Leone & Johnson (Dai & Sternberg, 2004, p. 197) they state there are dynamic interactions between emotive processes and modes of cognitive processing possibly related to constraints already built into the brain's processes (Beck, 1996; Damasio, 1994, 201; Greenberg, 2002; Kuhl, 2000, as cited in and Sternberg, 2004, p. 224)? So, should we ask, "What is good thinking"? To ask this is to pose one of the most venerable questions. Aristotle's (350 BCE analysis of syllogisms, Bacon's (1620/1878) account of scientific inquiry, Kant's (1785/1994) categorical imperative, Von Neumann and Morgentern's (1944) exposition of game theory, Inhelder and Piaget's (1958) notion of formal operational thinking, Wertheimer's (1945) formulation of productive thinking (p.351). Contemporary work expands, ramifies, and refines the analysis into many particular kinds of thinking (e.g., Baron, 1985; Basseches, 1984; Case, 1992; Elgin, 1996; Langer, 1989; Paul, 1990; Toulmin, 1958, as cited in Dai and Sternberg, 2004, p. 351).

But why ask that question during the grief and grieving journey? How can this even be measured, as psychologists typically try to look for consistent levels of performance, and yet we, the authors of this chapter, would posit that there is no practical gauge in the domain of loss. The tasks asked of those experiencing loss are unfamiliar and varied, which may show in time a general capacity for handling, complex challenges, but to correlate this to what is good thinking, is a jump into a field of study that links levels of, or patterns of, cognitive thinking to grief and grieving.

Perkins and Ritchhart (Dai & Sternberg, 2004, p. 352) posit that it is assumed people usually think about as well as they can whenever they need to. When they do not, it is mostly because they cannot. To compare with rowing across a rushing river, it is not that people miss the boat or decline to take it. It is that they simply cannot row well enough. Suppose just the opposite: It is not that people cannot row well enough, but that they often miss the boat or decline to take it. Occasions that call for thinking pass them by and they choose not to engage those occasions. This would yield a very different account of how thinking works and what it is to be a good thinker (Dai & Sternberg, 2004, p. 352). If one has never been initiated into loss, the good thinking may be a choice, whether subconscious or conscious, to be oblivious to the sensitive drama occurring around them, or displaying an aversion to the complexities and ambiguities of thinking that, "may make my heart and heart hurt." Our judgement at this time may not serve us well because our experiences do not reflect a rich base of relevant experience, and thus shortfalls into our thinking.

Dewey (1922) emphasized the importance of good habits of mind, which can carry people past moments of distraction and reluctance. He asserted that the word habits having their roots in knowledge, motivation and attitudes, indicates their complex nature and situatedness (Dai & Sternberg, 2004, p. 355). This is why Scheffler (1991) accentuates the role of cognitive emotions in guiding thought (Dai & Sternberg, 2004, p. 353). In linking thought, choice, and science, quantum theory is a concept that is important to understand from a cognitive aspect of grief and grieving. So what does that have to do with grief and grieving?

Quantum theory converts science's conception of humans from being mere cogs in a gigantic, mechanical machine to being free thinking agents whose conscious choices affect their physical world (Leaf, 2013, p. 105). For example, our first initiation into loss, we are faced with a multitude of possibilities to choose and there is an endless array of these choices we think we need to make at any one moment in time, but during loss we collapse all the possibilities into one choice, "I cannot do this today" and so we choose collapse (Leaf, 2013, p. 106). Quantum physics enters into this collapse by its basic ingredients free will, directed attention as a result of the choices, and the effects and consequences of those choices (Leaf, 2013, p. 106). Let's take a simple example as we apply the basic ingredients of quantum physics: paying attention, thinking and choosing, and consequences.

1. **Information:** We are initiated into the loss.
2. **Thoughts:** Multiple thoughts are now swirling around in our head. Option one is fear. Option two is denial. Option three is unimaginable murmurs.

3. **Choice:** We choose an option. For instance, if we choose fear, our brain responds by wiring in the thought, "Because of the loss, I cannot make it through this day."
4. **Consequence:** We suddenly see life through a smoky fog.

So our brain becomes what we focused on (body carries out the will of the spirit and soul), and what our brain has become produces what we say and do, and how we feel physically and mentally (Leaf, 2013, pp106-107). Quantum physics has multiple definitions, but basically it is, "The way we experience our feelings, the way we interface with our thoughts, and the kind of attention we give them will change how our brain functions (Leaf, 2013, p. 107). Quantum physics, and neuroscience for that matter, do not provide ultimate answers; they are simply stepping stones in the development of our understanding (Leaf, 2013, p. 118). A question we may want to ponder for ourselves is: once we are aware that thoughts are unstable and changeable when they are in our conscious mind, can we focus on one in particular and change it? (Leaf, 2013, p. 174). Leaf answers this by saying, "A constant change means that the deeper we think, the more change we can make. This change is real and happens via electromagnetic and quantum forces, as well as neurotransmitters activating protein synthesis" ((Leaf, 2013, p. 175). And, she reminds us that proteins are made and used to grow new branches to hold our thoughts. In other words, if we do not get rid of the thought, such as a negative thought, we reinforce it (Leaf, 2013, p. 175). If you say, "I can't" we are bringing that into captivity which then remodels our mind (Leaf, 2013, p. 175). In simplistic words, what is bad about life is as genuine as what is good and therefore deserves equal attention (Peterson, 2006 as cited in Youssef & Luthans, 2007).

PLASTIC PARADOX

If, after wiring out a toxic thought, you have stopped using the healthy new thought and revert back to the toxic thought, you reverse the process you went through in the first place, breaking down the healthy thought and rebuilding the toxic thought, which Leaf defines as a plastic paradox (2013, p. 153). This is why we need to make a choice to be alert to creating the ability of renewing the mind (Leaf, 2013, p. 153). So how do we relate this to our grief and grieving? Just possibly, if we know it takes 21 days, then just possibly our support should know the time frame, and not pressure us to make quick decisions or expectations that are not going to be met, thus our 'putting on the brave face" (Leaf, 2013, p. 155). In America particularly, the griever may be expected to "take a few days or even a week", but 21 days are not likely.

We have to develop disciplined thought lives and part of that is increasing our awareness of what we are allowing into our minds by becoming aware of the signals that are coming in our mind from the external environment and understanding the internal environment of our mind (Leaf, 2013, p. 157). The process of being aware prior to a loss means we begin the process of bringing rogue thoughts into captivity (Leaf, 2013, p. 157). Leaf tells us that, "a simple awareness can be developed to the point where we learn not to let any thought go through our mind unchecked (p.158). However, this simple step is an intricately development process, before initiation into grief and grieving. An example of our brain as we engage in the 'simple' step is described by Leaf as 'breeze through the trees" (Leaf, 2013, p. 160). According to her research and clinical experiences, our thoughts in our brain look like trees in a forest.

And as the signals sweep through those these trees like a wind, research shows they will activate around four to seven thought trees (memories) that will then move into the conscious and we will become aware of them (Figure 2) (Leaf, 2013, p. 160).

Through modifying our practices of thought toward a more disciplined, focused and reflective thought life, before we are initiated into loss, we can build up 'healthy neural real estate' that is better able to bring our thoughts into captivity and deal with the demands of grief and grieving in a more positive way (Leaf, 2013, p. 90).

In our brain, building a foundation is called having 'integrity', which means we are using words and actions to line up the thought. We can be presented with all the reason, logic, scientific evidence, and just plain common sense in the world, but we will not believe something is true unless our brain's limbic system – the central location of our emotions – allows us to feel that it is true (Leaf, 2013, p. 196). So if we are on a collision course with the "emotional monster", and we are acting one way and speaking something different, there will be a lack of integrity operating in our brain, which will leave an overwhelming feeling of 'being out of control'. An example is if we are working on a toxic thought of saying, out loud or in our mind – could have, should have, if only statements, then we are telling ourselves that the issue will disappear in a puff of smoke, Thus, our speaking is in conflict with what we need to do, our way of acting, in the process of loss.

Real world cognitive functioning operates in concert with motivation and emotional processes, sometimes harmoniously and sometimes discordantly (Dai & Sternberg, 2004, p. 143). Traditionally, intellectual functioning is seen as a high-level cognitive processes; however, during loss we do not have the conventional ability to think pragmatically at making decisions or solving problems, thus stress is experienced which then causes disturbances in cognition (e.g., worry) and we enter the transient state (Dai & Sternberg, 2004, p. 144-145). This state construct is best known from studies of affect, that is,

Figure 2. Google pics

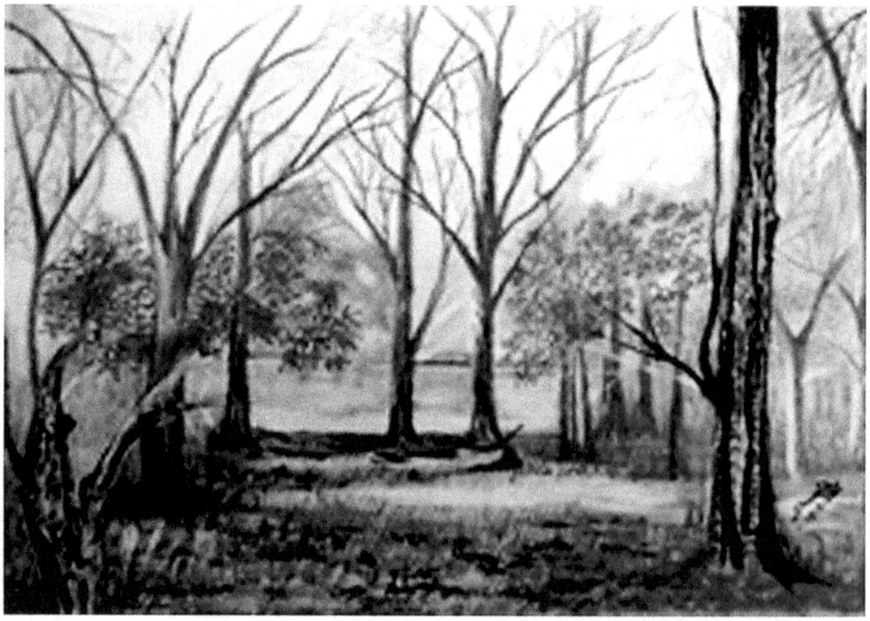

differentiated emotions (p.144). Anticipation heightens the senses and unfortunately can also magnify the possibility or reality of a loss (Kubler-Ross & Kessler, 2005, p. 1). A deep 'anticipatory grief' occurs when someone we love has a terminal illness, and 'anticipatory grief' is the "beginning of the end" in our minds (Kubler-Ross & Kessler, 2005, p. 1). We now operate in two worlds, the safe world that we are used to and the unsafe world of loss. Anticipation may help us brace ourselves for what is to come, but we should be aware that the anticipation of an event may be just as powerful as the event itself (Kubler-Ross & Kessler, 2005, p. 4).

Forewarned is not always forearmed. Experiencing anticipatory grief may or may not make the grieving process easier or shorten it. It may bring only feelings of guilt that we were grieving before the loss actually occurred (Kubler-Ross & Kessler, 2005, p. 4). Not everyone experiences 'anticipatory grief', and if they do, certainly not in the same way (2005, p. 4). What is important for us to know is that anticipatory grief stands alone from the grief we feel after the loss. For many, anticipatory grief is just a prelude to the painful process we face; however, a double grief that will ultimately bring healing (2005, p. 5).

Recognizing our new reality is the permanent reality. We may never like this reality or make it okay, but eventually we accept it. We learn to live with it. It is the new norm with which we must learn to live. This is where our healing and adjustment takes a firm hold, despite the fact that healing often looks and feels like an unattainable state (Kubler-Ross & Kessler, 2005, p. 25). Our past has been forever changed and we must readjust. We must learn to reorganize roles, and we start the process of reintegration, trying to put back the pieces that have been ripped away (Kubler-Ross & Kessler, 2005, p. 25). Little by little we withdraw our energy from the loss and begin to invest it in life. Instead of denying our emotions, we listen to our needs; we move, we change, we grow, we evolve. We begin to live again, but we cannot do so until we have given grief its time (Kubler-Ross & Kessler, 2005, p. 28).

CONCLUSION

Grief is one of life's passages we all experience. It is one of life's equalizers. But though it is not a similar experience for every person, most of us go through it as little islands of pain (Kubler-Ross & Kessler, 2005, p. 229). And, yet the sadness, anger, and emotional pain sit on our doorstep with a deeper range than we have ever felt. This intensity is beyond our normal range of human emotions. Our defenses are no match for the power of the loss. We often stand alone with no precedent or emotional repertoire for the loss (Kubler-Ross & Kessler, 2005, p. 230). We probably do not know that these foreign, unwelcome, intense emotions are part of the healing process. How can anything that feels so bad ever help to heal us? (Kubler-Ross & Kessler, 2005, p. 231). So why grieve? For two reasons. First, those who grieve well, live well. Second, grief is the healing process of the heart, soul, and mind; it is the path that returns us to wholeness (p.229). It should not be a matter of if you will grieve; the question is when will you grieve. And until we do, we suffer from the effects of that unfinished business (p.229).

We all grieve differently and are comforted differently. We look for reassurance when our world of logic can offer us none. While we try to comprehend and make sense of something incomprehensible and our heart feels the pain of loss, our mind lags behind, trying to integrate something new into our thinking. At this moment though, heart and mind are joined in one state, pain remembering pain (Kubler-Ross & Kessler, 2005, p. 63).

You have entered an abnormal, lonely, and unwelcoming new world where you are nothing but an island of sadness. And so far, there is no way out, no matter what anybody else wants for you (Kubler-Ross & Kessler, 2005, p. 82). Isolation feels like being in a room with no doors or windows – a place with no way out. Healing can get further and further away the longer you stay isolated. Isolation too much and for too long can result in your world becoming tighter and closer, until you can literally become emotionally paralyzed (Kubler-Ross & Kessler, 2005, p. 83). However, isolation is a very important stop on the path of grief, but usually, it should only be a step along the way; we should not stay too long in the walled garden. A lack of an expressive outlet is one of the toughest parts of isolation. Grieving groups may allow you to maintain a sense of privacy and aloneness while at the same time, they offer the opportunity for connection in a safe and controlled way. In time, you will find a bridge back to the outside world (Kubler-Ross & Kessler, 2005, p. 83).

Why do people tell us to be strong? Putting on a brave face does not mean being unfeeling (p.101). In our society it has become confused with keeping a 'stiff upper lip'. At what cost do we then camouflage our grief? When we shelve our pain, it does not go away. Rather, it festers in a myriad of ways (Kubler-Ross & Kessler, 2005, p. 102).

Mourning is the external part of loss. It is the actions we take, the rituals and the customs. Grief is the internal art of loss, how we feel. The internal work of grief is a process, a journey. It does not end on a certain day or date. It is as individual as each of us. Life and grief are made up of good days and bad days (Kubler-Ross & Kessler, 2005, p. 115). How long does it take to journey through Ross change curve, as it relates to loss? You might be asked, "Isn't it time to move on and get over your loss?" Grief is not just a series of events, stages, or timelines. Our society however, places enormous pressure on us to get over loss, to get through the grief (Kubler-Ross & Kessler, 2005, p. 203). Each grief has its own imprint.

In his 1991 book, *Head First: The Biology of hope and the healing power of the human spirit*, Cousins wrote the following description of the brain and thinking:

Brain researchers believe that what happens in the body can affect the brain, and what happens in the brain can affect the body. Emotions, such as hope, have electrochemical connections that play a large part in the workings of the total human organism. (Synder & Lopez, 2007, p. 192)

REFERENCES

Bernardes, E. S., & Hanna, M. D. (2009). A theoretical review of flexibility, agility and responsiveness in the operations management literature: Toward a conceptual definition of customer responsiveness. *International Journal of Operations & Production Management*, *29*(1), 30–53. doi:10.1108/01443570910925352

Bruning, R. H., Schraw, G. J., & Norby, M. M. (2001). *Cognitive psychology and instruction*. Boston, Mass: Pearson.

Dai, D. Y., & Sternberg, R. J. (2004). *Motivation, Emotion, and Cognition*. Mahwah, New York: Lawrence Erlbaum Associates.

Eagleman, D. (2011). *Incognito: The Secret lives of the brain*. New York, NY: Pantheon Books.

Gagne, J., & Deci, E. L. (2005). Self-determination theory and work motivation. *Journal of Organizational Behavior*, *26*(4), 331–362. doi:10.1002/job.322

Kodeih, F., & Greenwood, R. (2014). Complexity: The Role of identity. *Organization Studies*, *35*(1), 7–39. doi:10.1177/0170840613495333

Kubler –Ross. E. & Kessler, D. (2015). On Grief & Grieving: Finding the meaning of grief through the five stages of loss. New York, NY: Simon and Schuster.

Leaf, C. (2013). *Switch on your brain*. Grand Rapids, Michigan: Baker Books.

Luthans, F., & Avolio, B. J. (2003). Authentic leadership: A positive developmental approach. In K. S. Cameron, J. E. Dutton, & R. E. Quinn (Eds.), *Positive organizational scholarship* (pp. 241–261). San Francisco: Barrett-Koehler.

Patricelli, K., & Dombeck, M. (Eds.). (2015). Introduction to grief and bereavement issues. *Making a difference in your community every day*. Aroostook, ME: Aroostook Mental Health Center (AMHC). Retrieved from http://www.amhc.org/58-grief-bereavement-issues/article/8441-introduction-to-grief-and-bereavement-issues

Patricelli, K., & Dombeck, M. (Eds.). (2015). Grief is a normal and natural process. *Making a difference in your community every day*. Aroostook, ME: Aroostook Mental Health Center (AMHC). Retrieved from http://www.amhc.org/58-grief-bereavement-issues/article/8442-grief-is-a-normal-and-natural-process

Ryan, R. M., & Deci, E. L. (2000). Self-determination theory and the facilitation of intrinsic motivation, social development, and well-being. *The American Psychologist*, *55*(1), 68–68. doi:10.1037/0003-066X.55.1.68 PMID:11392867

Snyder, C. R., & Lopez, S. J. (2007). *Positive Psychology*. Thousand Oaks, CA: Sage Publications.

Youssef, C. M., & Luthans, F. (2007). Positive organizational behavior in the workplace: The Impact of hope, optimism, and resilience. *Journal of Management*, *33*(5), 774–800. doi:10.1177/0149206307305562

Compilation of References

Aarabi, M. S., Subramaniam, I. D., & Akeel, A. B. (2013). Relationship between motivational factors and job performances of employees in Malaysian service industry. *Asian Social Science*, *9*(9), 301–310. doi:10.5539/ass.v9n9p301

Adams, C. (2013, February27). Character education seen as student-achievement tool. *Education Week*, 2013, 7.

Adams, K. (1990). *Journal to the Self.* New York, NY: Warner Books.

Adler, R., Rosenfeld, L., & Proctor, I. I. R. (2015). *Interplay*. New York, NY: Oxford University Press.

Agarwal, M., Dalal, A., Agarwal, D., & Agarwal, R. (1995). Positive life orientation and recovery from myocardial infarction. *Social Science & Medicine*, *40*(1), 125–130. doi:10.1016/0277-9536(94)E0058-Z PMID:7899916

Agency for Healthcare Research and Quality. (2007). *Health literacy measurement tools (revised).* Retrieved from http://www.ahrq.gov/professionals/quality-patient-safety/quality-resources/tools/literacy/index.html

Agency for Healthcare Research and Quality. (2016). *TeamSTEPPS® strategies and tools to enhance performance and patient safety.* Retrieved from http://www.ahrq.gov/professionals/education/curriculum-tools/teamstepps/index.html

Agency for Healthcare Research Quality. (2016). *Team STEPPS 2.0.* Retrieved from http://www.ahrq.gov/professionals/education/curriculum-tools/teamstepps/instructor/index.html

Agha, S., Karim, A. M., Balal, A., & Sossler, S. (2003). A Quasi Experimental Study to Assess the Performance of a Reproductive Health Franchise in Nepal. Commercial Market Strategies (CMS) Country Research Series Paper No. 14, Washington DC

Albert, A., & Anderson, M. (1997). Dogs, cats, and morale maintenance: Some preliminary data. *Anthrozoos*, *10*(2/3), 121–124. doi:10.2752/089279397787001193

Alcoholics Anonymous. (2001). Alcoholics Anonymous (4th ed.). New York, AA. World Services.

Alexander, E. (2012). *Proof of Heaven.* New York, NY: Simon and Schuster.

Alexander, E. (2014). *The map of Heaven.* New York, NY: Simon and Schuster.

Alex, H. (2005). The scientific value of Ayurveda. *Journal of Alternative and Complementary Medicine (New York, N.Y.)*, *11*(2), 221–225. doi:10.1089/acm.2005.11.221 PMID:15865485

Allen, K. M., Blascovich, J., & Mendes, W. B. (2002). Cardiovascular reactivity and the presence of pets, friends, and spouses: The truth about cats and dogs. *Psychosomatic Medicine*, *64*(5), 727–739. doi:10.1097/01.psy.0000024236.11538.41 PMID:12271103

Allen, K. M., Blascovich, J., Tomaka, J., & Kelsey, R. M. (1991). Presence of human friends and pet dogs as moderators of autonomic responses to stress in women. *Journal of Personality and Social Psychology*, *61*(81), 582–589. doi:10.1037/0022-3514.61.4.582 PMID:1960650

Allen, K., Golden, L. H., Izzo, J. L. Jr, Ching, M. I., Forrest, A., Niles, C. R., & Barlow, J. C. et al. (2001). Normalization of hypertensive responses during ambulatory surgical stress by perioperative music. *Psychosomatic Medicine*, *63*(3), 487–492. doi:10.1097/00006842-200105000-00019 PMID:11382277

Allison, K. (2012). Experiences and perceptions as expressed by adolescent females at a residential treatment center (RTC) [Unpublished Doctoral Dissertation]. Florida Atlantic University, Boca Raton, FL, USA.

American Academy of Physician Assistants. (2006). *Q&A about physician assistants: The most commonly asked questions about PAs*. Retrieved from http://www.gidoctor.net/client_files/file/Physician-Assistants.pdf

American Association of Colleges of Nursing. (2016). *Home page*. Retrieved from http://www.aacn.nche.edu/

American Association of Colleges of Osteopathic Medicine. (2016). *Home page*. Retrieved from https://www.aacom.org/

American Association of Colleges of Pharmacy. (2016). *Home page*. Retrieved from http://www.aacp.org/Pages/Default.aspx

American Dental Education Association. (2016). *Home page*. Retrieved from http://www.adea.org/

American Diabetes Association. (2015). Making healthy food choices. Retrieved from: http://www.diabetes.org/food-and-fitness/food/what-can-i-eat/making-healthy-food-choices/?loc=ff-slabnav

American Heart Association. (2015). Prevention and treatment of high blood pressure. Retrieved from: www.heart.org/HEARTORG/Conditions/HighBloodPressure/PreventionTreatmentofHighBloodPressure

American humane operational guide. (2010). Retrieved from http://www.americanhumane.org/assets/pdfs/animals/operational-guides/op-guide-humaneed.pdf

American Music Therapy Association (AMTA). (2015). About Music Therapy & AMTA. Silver Spring, MD: AMTA. Retrieved from http://www.musictherapy.org/about/musictherapy/

American Pharmacists Association. (2014). *Pharmacists' patient care processes*. Retrieved from http://www.pharmacist.com/sites/default/files/files/PatientCareProcess.pdf

American Recovery and Reinvestment Act (ARRA) of 2009, Pub. L. No. 111-5, 123 Stat. 115, 516 (2009).

American Society of Health-System Pharmacists, & the American Pharmacists Association. (n.d.). *ASHP-APhA medication management in care transitions best practices*. Retrieved from http://media.pharmacist.com/practice/ASHP_APhA_MedicationManagementinCareTransitionsBestPracticesReport2_2013.pdf

American Society of Health-System Pharmacists. (2010). *2015 ASHP health-system pharmacy initiative*. Retrieved from http://www.ashp.org/doclibrary/policy/2015/2015goals.aspx

American Society of Health-System Pharmacists. (2016). *Transitions of care resource center*. Retrieved from http://www.ashp.org/menu/PracticePolicy/ResourceCenters/Transitions-of-Care

Americans with Disabilities Act (ADA). (1990). Washington, D.C.: U.S. Department of Justice.

Anderson, G. (2005). *U.S. still spends more on health care than any other country* [Press release]. Retrieved from http://www.jhsph.edu/news/news-releases/2005/anderson-health-spending.html

Anderson, C. M., & MacCurdy, M. M. (2000). Introduction. In C. M. Anderson & M. M. MacCurdy (Eds.), *Writing and healing* (pp. 1–22). Urbana, IL: National Council of Teachers of English.

Andrykowski, M. A., & Brady, M. J. (1994). Health locus of control and psychological distress in cancer patients: Interactive effects of context. *Journal of Behavioral Medicine*, *17*(5), 439–458. doi:10.1007/BF01857919 PMID:7877155

Ángeles Ruiz, M.; Sanjuan, P.; Pérez-García, A.M.; Rueda, B.& (2011). Relations between life satisfaction, adjustment to illness, and emotional distress in a sample of men with ischemic cardiopathy. *Spanish Journal of Psychology*, 14(1), 356.

Anh, S., Basu, R., Smith, M. L., Jiang, L., Lorig, K., Whitelaw, N., & Ory, M. G. (2013). The impact of chronic disease self-management programs: Healthcare savings through a community-based intervention. *BMC Public Health*, *13*(1), 1141. doi:10.1186/1471-2458-13-1141 PMID:24314032

Anthony, S. D., Johnson, M. W., & Sinfield, J. V. (2008). Building an engine that produces a steady stream of innovative growth businesses is difficult, but companies that are able to do it differentiate themselves from competitors. Retrieved from sloanreview.mit.edu/article/institutionalizing-innovation

Appel, L.J., Moore, T.J., Obarzanek, E., Vollmer, W.M., Svetkey, L.P., Sacks, F.M., Bray, G.A., Vogt, T.M., Cutler, J.A., & Windhauser, M.M., Lin-P-H, & Karanja, N. (1997). A clinical trial of the effects of dietary patterns on blood pressure. *N ENlg. Journal of Medicine*, *336*, 1117–1124.

Arambašic, L., Keresteš, G., Kuterovac-Jagodíc, G., & Vizek-Vidovic, V. (2000). The role of pet ownership as a possible buffer variable in traumatic experiences. *Studia Psychologica*, *42*(1-2), 135–146.

Armstrong, E. G., Mackey, M., & Spear, S. J. (2004). Medical education as a process management problem. *Academic Medicine*, *79*(8), 721–728. doi:10.1097/00001888-200408000-00002 PMID:15277126

Arterburn, S. (2011). *Healing is a choice*. Nashville, TN: Thomas Nelson.

Ascione, F. R. (2015). 21st Century animal resource and educational services. Retrieved fromhttp://21stcenturycares.org/research.htm

Asian Development Bank Institute (ADBI). (2000). *Public Private Partnerships in Health, Executive Summary Series No. S34/01, Executive Summary of Proceedings (30 October to 3 November)*. Thailand: Ayutthaya.

Association of American Medical Colleges. (2004). *Educating doctors to provide high-quality medical care: A vision for medical education in the United States*. Washington, DC: Author.

Association of American Medical Colleges. (2016). *Home page*. Retrieved from https://www.aamc.org/

Association of Faculties of Medicine of Canada. (n. d.). *The future of medical education in Canada (FMEC): A collective vision for MD education*. Retrieved from https://www.afmc.ca/medical-education/future-medical-education-canada-fmec

Association of Professional Humane Educators. (2011, Summer). Is humane education an endangered species? *The Latham Letter*, *32*(3), 6–9.

Association of Schools of Public Health. (2016). *Home page*. Retrieved from http://www.aspph.org/

Austen, J. (2005). *Pride and prejudice*. New York, NY: Penguin. (Original work published 1813). doi:10.5117/9781904633013

Avoid Readmission through Collaboration. (2013a). How ARC measures improvement. Retrieved from http://www.avoidreadmissions.com/arc-action-network.html

Avoid Readmission through Collaboration. (2013b). *Initiatives.* Retrieved from http://www.avoidreadmissions.com/improving-transitions-of-care/initiatives.html

Aworemi, J. R. (2011). An empirical study of the motivational factors of employees in Nigeria. *International Journal of Economics and Finance, 3*(5), 227-233. doi:10.5539 /ijef.v3n5p227

Baker, M. W. (2013). *A multiple case study of the dark side of leadership: An exploration of executives who led their companies to disastrous results versus exemplary CEOs who did not* (Order No. 3570902).

Baker, B. D. (2014). *America's most financially disadvantaged school districts and how they got that way: How state and local governance causes school funding disparities.* Washington, DC: Center for American Progress.

Balaban, R. B., Weissman, J. S., Samuel, P. A., & Woolhandler, S. (2008). Redefining and redesigning hospital discharge to enhance patient care: A randomized controlled study. *Journal of General Internal Medicine, 23*(8), 1228–1233. doi:10.1007/s11606-008-0618-9 PMID:18452048

Balarajan, Y., Selvaraj, S., & Subramanian, S. V. (2011). India: Towards Universal Health Coverage for Healthcare and Equity in India. *Lancet, 377*, 505–515. doi:10.1016/S0140-6736(10)61894-6 PMID:21227492

Bali, V. (2015). Union Budget 2015 fails to deliver on healthcare. *Business Today.* Retrieved from http://www.businesstoday.in/union-budget-2015-16/india-inc-on-budget/union-budget-2015-fails-to-deliver-on-healthcare-vishal-bali/story/216411.html

Bandura, A. (1973). *Aggression: A social learning analysis.* Englewood Cliffs, NJ: Prentice Hall.

Bandura, A. (1977). Self-efficacy: Toward a unifying theory of behavioral change. *Psychological Review, 84*(2), 191–215. doi:10.1037/0033-295X.84.2.191 PMID:847061

Bandura, A. (1982). Self-efficacy mechanism in human agency. *The American Psychologist, 37*(2), 122–147. doi:10.1037/0003-066X.37.2.122

Bandura, A. (1989). Human agency in social cognitive theory. *The American Psychologist, 44*(9), 1175–1184. doi:10.1037/0003-066X.44.9.1175 PMID:2782727

Bandura, A. (1990). Perceived self-efficacy in the exercise of control over AIDS infection. *Evaluation and Program Planning, 13*(1), 9–17. doi:10.1016/0149-7189(90)90004-G

Bandura, A. (1991). Social cognitive theory of self-regulation. *Organizational Behavior and Human Decision Processes, 50*(2), 248–287. doi:10.1016/0749-5978(91)90022-L

Bao, T. (2014). Integrative oncology: 65+ workshop. Treating symptoms & improving well- being. Memorial Sloan Kettering Cancer Center. Retrieved from: https://www.mskcc.org/cancer-care/treatments/symptom-management/integrative- medicine.

Barasch, M. I. (1994). The amazing power of visualization. *Natural Health, 24*(4), 64.

Barbuto, J., & Wheeler, D. (2007, October). Becoming a servant leader: Do you have what it takes? *NetGuide.* Retrieved from http://www.ianrpubs.unl.edu /epublic/live/g1481/build/g1481.pdf

Barnet, T. (2015). Motivation and motivation theory. Retrieved from http://www.referenceforbusiness.com/management/Mar-No/Motivation-and-Motivation-Theory.htm

Barnett, H. (2001). The Chinatown cornfields: Including environmental benefits in environmental justice struggles. *Critical Planning, 8*, 50–60.

Baron, R. (1996). Interpersonal relations in organizations. In K. Murphy (Ed.), *Individual differences* (pp. 334–370). San Francisco, CA: Jossey Bass.

Barr, V. J., Robinson, S., Marin-Link, B., Underhill, A. D., Ravensdale, D., & Salivares, S. (2003). The expanded chronic care model: An integration of concepts and strategies from population health promotion and the chronic care model. *Hospital Quarterly*, *7*(1), 77. PMID:14674182

Bartholomew, K. (1990). Avoidance of intimacy: An attachment perspective. *Journal of Social and Personal Relationships*, *7*(2), 147–178. doi:10.1177/0265407590072001

Bartholomew, K., & Horowitz, L. (1991). Attachment styles among young adults: A test of a four category model. *Journal of Personality and Social Psychology*, *61*(2), 226–244. doi:10.1037/0022-3514.61.2.226 PMID:1920064

Bartlett, J. (1919). Bartleby Quotations. Retrieved from http://www.bartleby.com/100/707.html

Basu, S. K. & Jindal, A., (1990). Genetic and socio-cultural determinants of tribal health: A primitive kuttiya kondhs tribal group of Phulbani district. ICMR Final Report, NIHFW, Orissa.

Baty, K. (2003). *A girl's gotta do what a girl's gotta do*. New York, NY: Rodale.

Beck, M. (2010, December 21). Beside Freud's couch, a chow named Jofi. The Wall Street Journal. Retrieved from http://online.wsj.com/articles/SB10001424052748703886904576031630124087362

Beck, A., & Katcher, A. H. (1996). *Between pets and people*. West Lafayette, IN: Purdue University Press.

Beck, M. (2001). *Finding your own North Star*. New York, NY: Three Rivers Press.

Beck, M. (2008). *Steering by starlight*. New York, NY: Rodale.

Beck, M. (2012). *Finding your way in a wild new world*. New York, NY: Free Press.

Bedell, W., & Kaszkin-Bettag, M. (2010). Coherence and health care cost-RCA actuarial study: A cost effectiveness cohort study. *The Journal of Alternative Therapies*, *16*(4), 26–31. PMID:20653293

Bedimo-Rung, A. L., Mowen, A. J., & Cohen, D. A. (2005). The significance of parks to physical activity and public health: A conceptual model. *American Journal of Preventive Medicine*, *28*(2), 159–168. doi:10.1016/j.amepre.2004.10.024 PMID:15694524

Bennett, G. G., McNeill, L. H., Wolin, K. Y., Duncan, D. T., Puleo, E., & Emmons, K. M. (2007). Safe to walk? Neighborhood safety and physical activity among public housing residents. *PLoS Medicine*, *4*(10), 1599–1607. doi:10.1371/journal.pmed.0040306 PMID:17958465

Benson, H., & Klipper, M. (1975/2001). *The relaxation response*. New York: HarperCollins.

Benson, H., & Proctor, W. (2010). *Relaxation revolution: Enhancing your personal health through the science and genetics of mind body healing*. New York: Scribner.

Benson, H., Rosner, B. A., Marzetta, B. R., & Klemchuk, H. M. (1974). Decreased blood pressure in pharmacologically treated hypertensive patients who regularly elicited the relaxation response. *Lancet*, *303*(7852), 289–291. doi:10.1016/S0140-6736(74)92596-3 PMID:4130474

Berman, P., Ahuja, R., & Bhandari, L. (2010). The impoverishing effect of healthcare payments in India: New methodology and findings. *Economic and Political Weekly*, *xlv*(16), 65–71.

Bernardes, E. S., & Hanna, M. D. (2009). A theoretical review of flexibility, agility and responsiveness in the operations management literature: Toward a conceptual definition of customer responsiveness. *International Journal of Operations & Production Management*, *29*(1), 30–53. doi:10.1108/01443570910925352

Betensky, M. G. (1995). What do you see? Phenomenology of therapeutic art expression. London: Jessica Kingsley Publishers. Retrieved from http://search.proquest.com/docview/618763898?accountid=4840

Betensky, M. G. (1999). Phenomenological art therapy. In J. A. Rubin (Ed.), *Approaches to art therapy* (2nd ed.). Philadelphia: Brunner-Routledge.

Bhojani, U., Thriveni, B. S., Devadasan, R., Munegowda, C. M., Devadasan, N., Kolsteren, P., & Criel, B. (2012). Out-of-pocket healthcare payments on chronic conditions impoverish urban poor in Bangalore, India. *BMC Public Health*, *12*(1), 990. doi:10.1186/1471-2458-12-990 PMID:23158475

Bierema, L. L. (1999). *The process of the learning organization: Making sense of change*

Bilger, B. (2003). the last meow. Conde Nast Publications, Inc.

Billett, S. (2001). *Learning in the workplace: Strategies for effective practice*. Crows Nest, NSW, Australia: Allen & Unwin.

Bimal, K. P. (1991). Health Service Resource as a Determinant of Infant Death in Rural Bangladesh: An Empirical Review. *Social Science & Medicine*, *32*(1), 43–49. doi:10.1016/0277-9536(91)90125-V PMID:2008620

Bird, J. L. (Ed.). (2015). *Innovative collaborative practice and reflection in patient education*. Hershey, PA: Information Science Reference. doi:10.4018/978-1-4666-7524-7

Bird, J. L., Wanner, E. T., Urenda, R., & Perry, R. (2015). Multigenre medicine. In J. L. Bird (Ed.), *Innovative collaborative practice and reflection in patient education* (pp. 1–19). Hershey, PA: Information Science Reference.

Birmingham Museum of Art. (2014). *Accessibility*. Retrieved from http://www.artsbma.org/access/

Bloom, D. E., Craig, P., & Mitchell, M. (2000). Public and Private Roles in Providing and Financing Social Services: Health and Education.

Bloom, D. E., Canning, D., & Sevilla, J. (2002). *The Demographic Dividend: A New Perspective on the Economic Consequences of Population Change. MR-1274*. Santa Monica, CA: Rand.

Blumenthal, J. A., Babyak, M. A., Hinderliter, A., Watkins, L. L., Craighead, L., Lin, P.-H., & Sherwood, A. et al. (2010). Effects of the DASH diet alone and in combination with exercise and weight loss on blood pressure and cardiovascular biomarkers in men and women with high blood pressure: The ENCORE study. *Archives of Internal Medicine*, *170*(2), 126–135. doi:10.1001/archinternmed.2009.470 PMID:20101007

Bollinger, A. S., & Smith, R. D. (2001). Managing organizational knowledge as a strategic asset. *Journal of Knowledge Management*, *5*(1), 8–18. doi:10.1108/13673270110384365

Bolman, L. G., & Deal, T. E. (2003). *Reframing organizations: Artistry, choice, and leadership* (3rd ed.). San Francisco, CA: Jossey Bass.

Bolman, L. G., & Deal, T. E. (2006). *The wizard and the warrior: Leading with passion and power*. San Francisco, CA: Jossey-Bass.

Bolman, L. G., & Deal, T. E. (2009). Battles and beliefs: Rethinking the roles of today's leaders. *Leadership in Action*, *29*(5), 14–18. doi:10.1002/lia.1306

Bongo therapy. (2011). *Einstein: The Magazine for Alumni and Friends of Albert Einstein College of Medicine*. Summer/fall, 9. Retrieved from https://www.einstein.yu.edu/docs/publications/einstein-magazine/einstein-magazine-summer-fall-2011.pdf

Borgatti, S. P. (2005). *The state of organizational social network research today* [Working paper]. Boston, MA: Department of Organization Studies, Boston College.

Boynton-Jarrett, R., Fargnoli, J., Suglia, S. F., Zuckerman, B., & Wright, R. J. (2010). Association between maternal intimate partner violence and incident obesity in preschool-aged children: Results from the fragile families and child well-being study. *Archives of Pediatrics & Adolescent Medicine*, *164*(6), 540–546. doi:10.1001/archpediatrics.2010.94 PMID:20530304

Boys & Girls Club of America. (2010). *Who we are*. Retrieved from http://www.bgca.org/whoweare/

Bradley, R. T., Galvin, P., Atkinson, M., & Tomasino, D. (2012). Efficacy of an emotional self-regulation program for promoting development in preschool children. *Global Advances in Health and Medicine*, *1*(1), 36–50. doi:10.7453/gahmj.2012.1.1.010 PMID:24278801

Bradshaw, J. (2011). *Dog sense*. New York, New York: Basic Books.

Brandt, B. F. (2015). Interprofessional education and collaborative practice: Welcome to the 'new' forty-year old field. *The Advisor*. Retrieved from https://nexusipe-resource-exchange.s3.amazonaws.com/IPECP%20-%20Welcome%20to%20the%20New%2040-Year-Old%20Field%20-%20Brandt;%20The%20Advisor.pdf

Brazelton, B. (2004). *Altered Books Workshop*. New York, NY: F+ W Media, Inc.

Brennan, K. A., Clark, C. L., & Shaver, P. R. (1998). Self report measure of adult attachment. In J. A. Simpson & W. S. Rhodes (Eds.), *Attachment theory and close relationships* (pp. 46–76). New York, NY: Guilford Press.

Brian, J. W., Chetty, V. K., Anthony, D., Greenwald, J. L., Sanchez, G. M., Johnson, A. E., & Culpepper, L. et al. (2009). A reengineered hospital discharge program to decrease rehospitalization. *Annals of Internal Medicine*, *150*(3), 178–187. doi:10.7326/0003-4819-150-3-200902030-00007 PMID:19189907

Brown, S. (2015). Healing through Self-discovery and Artistic Design Journals. In J.L. Bird (Ed.), Innovative collaborative practice and reflection in patient education (pp. 103-119). Hershey, PA, USA: IGI Global.

Brown, B. (2010). *The gifts of imperfection*. Center City, MN: Hazelden.

Brown, B. (2012). *Daring greatly*. New York, NY: Gotham Books.

Brown, B. (2015). *Rising strong*. New York, NY: Spiegel & Grau.

Brown, K. W., & Ryan, R. M. (2003). The benefits of being present: Mindfulness and its role in psychological well-being. *Journal of Personality and Social Psychology*, *84*(4), 822–848. doi:10.1037/0022-3514.84.4.822 PMID:12703651

Brown, S. (2013). *Teaching art integration in the schools*. Mason, Ohio: Cengage Learning.

Brown, S. G., & Rhodes, R. E. (2006). Relationships among dog ownership and leisure-time walking in western Canadian adults. *American Journal of Preventive Medicine*, *30*(2), 131–136. doi:10.1016/j.amepre.2005.10.007 PMID:16459211

Brownson, R. C., Chang, J. C., Davis, J. R., & Smith, C. A. (1991). Physical activity on the job and cancer in Missouri. *American Journal of Public Health*, *81*(5), 639–642. doi:10.2105/AJPH.81.5.639 PMID:2014869

Bruer, J. (1993). *Schools for thought: A science of learning in the classroom*. Cambridge, MA: MIT Press.

Bruning, R. H., Schraw, G. J., & Norby, M. M. (2001). *Cognitive psychology and instruction.* Boston, Mass: Pearson.

Bryant, B. K., & Donnellan, M. B. (2007). The relation between socio-economic status concerns and angry peer conflict resolution is moderated by pet provisions of support. *Anthrozoos*, *20*(3), 213–223. doi:10.2752/089279307X224764

Buffart, L. M., van Uffelen, J. G., Riphagen, B. J., & Brown, W. J. (2012). Physical and psychosocial benefits of yoga in cancer patients and survivors, a systematic review and meta-analysis of randomized controlled trials. *BMC Cancer*, *12*(1), 559. doi:10.1186/1471-2407-12-559 PMID:23181734

Burdette, H. L., Wadden, T. A., & Whitaker, R. C. (2006). Neighborhood safety, collective efficacy, and obesity in women with young children. *Obesity (Silver Spring, Md.)*, *14*(3), 518–525. doi:10.1038/oby.2006.67 PMID:16648624

Burgess, R. L., & Huston, T. L. (2013). *Social exchange in developing relationships.* New York, NY: Academic Press.

Buring, S. M., Bhushan, A., Broeseker, A., Conway, S., Duncan-Hewitt, W., Hansen, L., & Westberg, S. (2009). Interprofessional education: Definitions, student competencies, and guidelines for implementation. *American Journal of Pharmaceutical Education*, *73*(4), 59. http://www.ncbi.nlm.nih.gov/pmc/articles/PMC2720355/ doi:10.5688/aj730459 PMID:19657492

Burleson, B. R., & Goldsmith, D. J. (1998). Handbook of Communication and Emotion: Research, Theory, Applications, and Contexts.

Buselli, E. F. (1999). The stress response. *The Journal of Cardiovascular Nursing*, *13*(3), 60–72. doi:10.1097/00005082-199904000-00006 PMID:10098006

Byrne, J., Wolch, J., & Zhang, J. (2009). Planning for environmental justice in an urban national park. *Journal of Environmental Planning and Management*, *52*(3), 365–392. doi:10.1080/09640560802703256

Cabana, M. D., & Jee, S. H. (2004). Does continuity of care improve patient outcomes? *The Journal of Family Practice*, *53*(12), 974–980. Retrieved from http://www.jfponline.com/ PMID:15581440

Caldwell, K., Gray, J., & Wolever, R.Q. (2013). The process of patient empowerment in integrative health coaching: how does it happen? *Global advances in health and medicine, 2*(3), 48-57.

Caldwell, L., & Smith, E. (2007). Leisure as a context for youth development and delinquency prevention. In *Pathways and Crime Prevention* (pp. 271-296).

Caldwell, J. (1979). Education as a factor in Mortality Decline: An Examination of Nigerian Data. *Population Studies*, *33*(3), 396–413. doi:10.2307/2173888

Calenda, E. (2006). Massage therapy for cancer pain. *Current Pain and Headache Reports*, *10*(4), 270–274. doi:10.1007/s11916-006-0031-1 PMID:16834941

Calvert, S. B., Kramer, J. M., Anstrom, K. J., Kaltenbach, L. A., Stafford, J. A., & Allen, N. M. (2012). Patient-focused intervention to improve long-term adherence to evidence-based medications. *American Heart Journal*, *163*(4), 657–665. doi:10.1016/j.ahj.2012.01.019 PMID:22520532

Camacho, T. C., Roberts, R. E., Lazarus, N. B., Kaplan, G. A., & Cohen, R. D. (1991). Physical activity and depression: Evidence from the Alameda County Study. *American Journal of Epidemiology*, *134*, 220–231. PMID:1862805

Cameron, G. D. (2012). *A cross-sectional study to examine occupational stress between online and on-ground educators* (Doctoral dissertation).

Cameron, J. (1998). *The right to write*. New York: Tarcher/Putnam.

Cameron, J. (2002). *The artist's way* (2nd ed.). New York, NY: Tarcher/Putnam.

Camic, P. M. (1999). Expanding treatment possibilities for chronic pain through the expressive arts. In C. A. Malchiodi (Ed.), *Medical art therapy with adults* (pp. 43–61). London: Jessica Kingsley.

Camic, P. M., Tischler, V., & Pearman, C. H. (2013). Viewing and making art together: A multi-session art-gallery-based intervention for people with dementia and their carers. *Aging & Mental Health*, *18*(2), 161–168. doi:10.1080/13607863.2013.818101 PMID:23869748

Campbell, M., Baltes, J., Martin, A., & Meddings, K. (2007). *The stress of leadership*. Colorado Springs, CO: Center for Creative Leadership.

Camp, M. M. (2001). The use of service dogs as an adaptive strategy: A qualitative study. *The American Journal of Occupational Therapy*, *55*(5), 509–517. doi:10.5014/ajot.55.5.509 PMID:14601810

Canadian Federation of Humane Societies (CFHS) Ear cropping and tail docking. Retrieved from http://cfhs.ca/athome/ear_cropping_and_tail_docking Regarding Canadian Animal Law, see http://cfhs.ca/features/a_disappointing_day_for_animals_in_canada/

Canadian Interprofessional Health Collaborative. (2016). *CIHC overview*. Retrieved from http://www.cihc.ca/about/overview

Canfield, J. (1999). *Chicken soup for the pet lover's soul: Stories about pets as teachers, healers, heroes and friends.* Deerfield Beach, FL: Health Communications.

Carney, C. P., & Jones, L. E. (2006). Medical comorbidity in women and men with bipolar disorders: A population-based controlled study. *Psychosomatic Medicine*, *68*(5), 684–691. doi:10.1097/01.psy.0000237316.09601.88 PMID:17012521

Carney, C. P., Jones, L. E., & Woolson, R. F. (2006). Medical comorbidity in women and men with schizophrenia: A population-based controlled study. *Journal of General Internal Medicine*, *21*(11), 1133–1137. doi:10.1111/j.1525-1497.2006.00563.x PMID:17026726

Carter, C. (2015). *The sweet spot*. New York, NY: Ballantine.

Carver, C., Pozo, C., Harris, S., Noriega, V., Scheier, M., Robinson, D., & Clark, K. et al. (1993). How coping mediates the effect of optimism on distress: A study of women with early stage breast cancer. *Journal of Personality and Social Psychology*, *65*(2), 375–390. doi:10.1037/0022-3514.65.2.375 PMID:8366426

Casale, P. (2015). Presuppositions in linguistics and NLP. Retrieved from http://www.nlp-secrets.com/nlp-presuppositions.php

Caspari, E. (2003). Animal life in nature, myth and dreams. Wilmette, EL: Chiron.

Cassileth, B. R. (2011). Green Tea (Camellia sinensis). *Oncology (Williston Park)*, *14*, 1432–1433. PMID:22329195

Cassileth, B. R., & Vickers, A. J. (2004). Massage therapy for symptom control: Outcome study at a major cancer center. *Journal of Pain and Symptom Management*, *28*(3), 244–249.

Cecil, J., McHale, C., Hart, J., & Laidlaw, A. (2014). Behavior and burnout in medical students. *Medical Education Online*, *25209*(19). doi:10.3402/meo.v19.25209 PMID:25160716

Census India. (2011) Office of the Registrar General and Census Commissioner, India. Retrieved from http://www.censusindia.gov.in/2011census

Center for Advancement of Interprofessional Education. (2016). *The definition and principles of interprofessional education*. Retrieved from http://caipe.org.uk/about-us/the-definition-and-principles-of-interprofessional-education/

Centers for Disease Control and Prevention CDC. (2009). Flu Information Sheet. Retrieved from http://www.cdc.gov/flu/weekly/weeklyarchives2008-2009/weekly39.htm

Centers for Disease Control and Prevention- CDC. (2012). Heart Disease Facts. Retrieved from http://www.cdc.gov/heartdisease/facts.htm

Centers for Disease Control and Prevention- CDC. (2015). Mental health data and statistics. Retrieved from http://www.cdc.gov/mentalhealth/data-stats.htm

Centers for Disease Control and Prevention, National Center for Health Statistics. (2015). Underlying Cause of Death 1999-2013.

Centers for Disease Control and Prevention. (2000). *Measuring healthy days: Population assessment of health-related quality of life*. Atlanta, GA: Centers for Disease Control and Prevention.

Centers for Disease Control and Prevention. (2013). *Collaborative practice agreements and pharmacists' patient care services: A resource for pharmacists*. Retrieved from http://www.cdc.gov/dhdsp/pubs/docs/Translational_Tools_Pharmacists.pdf

Centers for Disease Control and Prevention. (2013). Death and Mortality. NCHS FastStats Web Site. Retrieved from: http://www.cdc.gov/nchs/fastats/deaths.htm

Centers for Medicare & Medicaid Services. (2016a). *Community-based care transitions program*. Retrieved from https://innovation.cms.gov/initiatives/CCTP/index.html SG – change from 2016 to this.

Centers for Medicare & Medicaid Services. (2016b). *Readmissions reduction program (HRRP)*. Retrieved from https://www.cms.gov/Medicare/Medicare-Fee-for-Service-Payment/AcuteInpatientPPS/Readmissions-Reduction-Program.html

Centre for the Advancement of Interprofessional Education. (2002). *Defining IPE*. Retrieved from http://caipe.org.uk/resources/defining-ipe/

Centre for the Advancement of Interprofessional Education. (2016). *Welcome to CAIPE*. Retrieved from http://caipe.org.uk/

Chapman, B. P., Hampson, S., & Clarkin, J. (2014). Personality-informed interventions for healthy aging: Conclusions from a National Institute on Aging work group. *Developmental Psychology*, *50*(5), 1426–1441. doi:10.1037/a0034135 PMID:23978300

Chapman, J. D., & Aspin, D. N. (1997). *The school, the community, and lifelong learning*. London, UK: Cassell.

Charnetski, C. J., Riggers, S., & Brennan, F. X. (2004). Effect of petting a dog on immune system function. *Psychological Reports*, *95*(3, Pt. 2), 1087–1091. PMID:15762389

Charon, R. (2006). *Narrative medicine: honoring the stories of illness*. New York, NY: Oxford University Press.

Chatterjee, H., Vreeland, S., & Noble, G. (2009). Museopathy: Exploring the healing potential of handling museum objects. *Museum & Society*, *7*(3), 164–177.

Checker, M. (2011). Wiped out by the Greenwave: Environmental gentrification and the paradoxical politics of urban sustainability. *City and Society*, *23*(2), 210–229. doi:10.1111/j.1548-744X.2011.01063.x

Chen, L.-C., Wang, T.-F., Shih, Y.-N., & Wu, L.-J. (2013). Fifteen-minute music intervention reduces pre-radiotherapy anxiety in oncology patients. *European Journal of Oncology Nursing*, *17*(4), 436–441. doi:10.1016/j.ejon.2012.11.002 PMID:23218591

Childre, D., & Rozman, D. (2007). *Transforming depression. The HeartMath® solution to feeling overwhelmed, sad, and stressed.* Oakland, CA: New Harbinger.

Children's Museum of Cleveland. (2015). House and hospital. Retrieved from http://www.clevelandchildrensmuseum.org/exhibit/house-and-hospital/

Chilton, G. (2007). Altered books in art therapy with adolescents. *Art Therapy: Journal of the American Art Therapy Association*, *24*(2), 59–63. doi:10.1080/07421656.2007.10129588

Chirmulay, D., & Gupte, A. (1997). Factors Affecting Health Seeking and Utilization of Curative Healthcare, Pune: Bharatiya Agro Industries Foundation (BAIF) Development and Research Foundation.

Chopin, K. (1981). *The awakening*. New York, NY: Bantam. (Original work published 1899).

Christakis, D. A., & Feudtner, C. (1997). Temporary matters. The ethical consequences of transient social relationships in medical training. *Journal of the American Medical Association*, *278*(9), 739–743. Retrieved from http://jama.jamanetwork.com/journal.aspx doi:10.1001/jama.1997.03550090063034 PMID:9286834

Christian, H., Zubrick, S. R., Foster, S., Giles-Corti, B., Bull, F., Wood, L., & Boruff, B. et al. (2015). The influence of the neighborhood physical environment on early child health and development: A review and call for research. *Health & Place*, *33*, 25–36. doi:10.1016/j.healthplace.2015.01.005 PMID:25744220

Clandinin, D. J., & Connelly, F. M. (2000). *Narrative inquiry*. San Francisco, CA: Jossey-Bass.

Clark, D. (1987). The concept of community education. In A. Garth, J. Bastiani, I. Martin, & K. Richards (Eds.), *Community education: An agenda for educational reform*. Philadelphia, PA: Open University Press.

Clutton-Brock, J. (2006). Origins of the dog: Domestication and early history. In J. Serpell (Ed.), *The domestic dog: Its evolution, behaviour and interactions with people* (pp. 7–20). New York: Cambridge University Press.

Cohen, P. (2009). Training for expertise: The Harvard Medical School Cambridge integrated clerkship tutorial. *The Clinical Teacher*, *6*(1), 28–33. doi:10.1111/j.1743-498X.2008.00260.x

Cole, M., & Wertsch, J. V. (1996). Beyond the individual-social antinomy in discussions of Piaget and Vygotsky. *Human Development*, *39*(5), 250–256. doi:10.1159/000278475

Coleman, E. A., & Boult, C. E. (2003). Improving the quality of transitional care for persons with complex care needs. *Journal of the American Geriatrics Society*, *51*(4), 556–557. doi:10.1046/j.1532-5415.2003.51186.x PMID:12657079

Colligan, T. W., & Higgins, E. M. (2005). Workplace stress: Etiology and consequences. *Journal of Workplace Behavioral Health*, *21*(2), 89–97. doi:10.1300/J490v21n02_07

Collins, J., & Porras, J. (1991). Organizational vision and visionary organizations. *California Management Review*, *34*(1), 30–51. doi:10.2307/41166682

Commission office of the Prime Minister. (1999). *National Education Act of BE 2542.* Retrieved from http://planipolis.iiep.unesco.org/upload/Thailand/Thailand_Education_Act_1999.pdf

Connelly, F. M., & Clandinin, D. J. (1988). *Teachers as curriculum planners*. New York, NY: Teachers College.

Conner, J. (2008). *Writing down your soul*. San Francisco, CA: Conari.

Constantino, M. I., Molyneaux, L., Limacher-Gisler, F., Al-Saeed, A., Luo, C., Wu, T., & Wong, J. et al. (2013). Long-term complications and mortality in young-onset diabetes: Type 2 diabetes is more hazardous and lethal than type 1 diabetes. *Diabetes Care*, *36*(12), 3863–3869. doi:10.2337/dc12-2455 PMID:23846814

Cooke, M., Irby, D., & O'Brien, B. (2010). *Educating physicians: A call for reform of medical school and residency*. San Francisco, CA: Jossey-Bass.

Coombs, P. H., & Ahmed, M. (1974). *Attacking rural poverty: How nonformal education can help*. Baltimore, MD: Johns Hopkins University Press.

Cooperative Program Centers for Disease Control and Prevention. (2016). *Self-management education. CDC- recommended programs. Chronic Disease Self-Management Program (CDSMP)*. Atlanta, GA: Centers for Disease Control and Prevention.

Corbin, J., & Strauss, A. (1988). *Unending work and care: Managing chronic illness at home*. San Francisco: Jossey-Bass.

Corson, S. A., & Corson, O. E. (1980). Pet animals as nonverbal communication mediators in psychotherapy in institutional settings. In S. A. Corson & E. O. Corson (Eds.), *Ethology and nonverbal communication in mental health* (pp. 83–110). Oxford: Pergamon Press.

Cosma, D., & Gilceava, S. A. (2014). How important is money as an incentive to motivate employees in the higher education sector? *Analele Universitatii Constantin Brancusi din Targu Jiu. Seria Economie*, *2*(2), 116–122.

Coulehan, J., & Williams, P.C. (2001). Vanquishing virtue: The impact of medical education. *Academic Medicine, 76*(6), 598–605. Retrieved from:10.1097/00001888-200106000-00008

Covey, S. M. R. (2010). How can workplace learning and performance professionals instill trust in an organization's leaders? *T+D, 64*(10), 10-11.

Cowherd, D. M., & Levine, D. I. (1992). Product quality and pay equity between lower-level employees and top management: An investigation of distributive justice theory. *Administrative Science Quarterly*, *37*(2), 302. doi:10.2307/2393226

Cowley, E., & Smith, S. (2014). Motivation and mission in the public sector: Evidence from the world values survey. *Theory and Decision*, *76*(2), 241–263. doi:10.1007/s11238-013-9371-6

Cox, J. H. (2009). *Humane education: A guide on methodology for educators*. Prepared for the Humane Education Trust of South Africa. Retrieved from http://www.worldanimal.net/docs/HET%20Humane%20Education%20Methodology.pdf

Cramer, H., Lange, S., Klose, P., Paul, A., & Dobos, G. (2012a). Yoga for breast cancer patients and survivors: A systematic review and meta-analysis. *BMC Cancer*, *12*(1), 412. doi:10.1186/1471-2407-12-412 PMID:22988934

Cramer, H., Lauche, R., Haller, H., & Dobos, G. (2013a). A Systematic review and meta- analysis of yoga for low back pain. *The Clinical Journal of Pain*, *29*(5), 450–460. doi:10.1097/AJP.0b013e31825e1492 PMID:23246998

Cramer, H., Lauche, R., Klose, P., Langhorst, J., & Dobos, G. (2013b). Yoga for schizophrenia: A systematic review and meta-analysis. *BMC Psychiatry*, *13*(1), 32. doi:10.1186/1471-244X-13-32 PMID:23327116

Cramer, H., Lauche, R., Paul, A., & Dobos, G. (2012b). Mindfulness-based stress reduction for breast cancer-a systematic review and meta-analysis. *Current Oncology (Toronto, Ont.)*, *19*(5), e343–e352. doi:10.3747/co.19.1016 PMID:23144582

Crawford, E. K., Worsham, N. L., & Swinehart, E. R. (2006). Benefits derived from companion animals, and the use of the term "attachment". *Anthrozoos*, *19*(2), 98–112. doi:10.2752/089279306785593757

Creer, T., Renne, C., & Christian, W. (1976). Behavioral contributions to rehabilitation and childhood asthma. *Rehabilitation Literature*, *37*, 226–232, 247. PMID:959645

Cross-Durrant, A. (2001). Basil Yeaxlee and the origins of lifelong education. In P. Jarvis (Ed.), *Twentieth century thinkers in adult education* (pp. 31–48). London, UK: Croom Helm.

Curtis, J. E. (1979). *Recreation: Theory and practice*. St. Louis, MO: Mosby.

Curtis, P. A., Alexander, G., & Lunghofer, L. A. (2001, October). A literature review comparing the outcomes of residential group care and therapeutic Foster care. *Child & Adolescent Social Work Journal*, *18*(5), 5. doi:10.1023/A:1012507407702

Cusack, O. (2014). *Pets and mental health*. Routledge.

Cutt, H., Giles-Corti, B., & Knuiman, M. (2008). Encouraging physical activity through dog walking: Why don't some owners walk with their dog? *Preventive Medicine*, *46*(2), 120–126. doi:10.1016/j.ypmed.2007.08.015 PMID:17942146

Cyber Laws in India and Technology Laws and Regulations in India. (2014). Retrieved from http://perry4law.org/cyberlawsinindia

Czamanski-Cohen, J. (2012). The use of art in the medical decision-making process of oncology patients. *Art Therapy: Journal of the American Art Therapy Association*, *29*(2), 60–67. doi:10.1080/07421656.2012.680049

D'Haee, S., De Meester, F., Cardon, G., De Bourdeaudhuij, I., Deforche, B., & Van Dyck, D. (2015). Changes in the perceived neighborhood environment in relation to changes in physical activity: A longitudinal study from childhood into adolescence. *Health & Place*, *33*, 132–141. doi:10.1016/j.healthplace.2015.03.004 PMID:25840351

Dacin, M. T., Goodstein, J., & Scott, W. R. (2002). Institutional theory and institutional change: Introduction to the special research forum. *Academy of Management Journal*, *45*(1), 45–56. doi:10.5465/AMJ.2002.6283388

Dai, D. Y., & Sternberg, R. J. (2004). *Motivation, Emotion, and Cognition*. Mahwah, New York: Lawrence Erlbaum Associates.

Davenport, N., Schwartz, R. D., & Elliott, G. P. (2005). *Mobbing: Emotional abuse in the American workplace*. Ames, IA: Civil Society.

David, I. R., & Ilusorio, S. (1995). Tuberculosis: Art therapy with patients in isolation. *Art Therapy: Journal of the American Art Therapy Association*, *12*(1), 24–31. doi:10.1080/07421656.1995.10759120

Davidson, R. A., & Waddell, R. (2005). A historical overview of interdisciplinary family health: A community-based interprofessional health professions course. *Academic Medicine*, *80*(4), 334–338. doi:10.1097/00001888-200504000-00005 PMID:15793015

Davies, R. A. (2012). The value of prevention. In *IOM (Institute of Medicine) & NRC (National Research Council), Social and economic costs of violence: Workshop summary*. Washington, DC: The National Academies Press.

Daykin, N., Byrne, E., Souteriou, T., & O'Connor, S. (2008). Review: The impact of art, design and environment in mental healthcare: a systematic review of the literature. *Perspectives in Public Health*, *128*(2), 85–94. PMID:18402179

Deane, K., Fitch, M., & Carman, M. (2000a). An innovative art therapy program for cancer patients. *Canadian Oncology Nursing Journal*, *10*(4), 147–151, 152–157. doi:10.5737/1181912x104147151 PMID:11894321

Deane, K., Fitch, M., & Carman, M. (2000b). The cancer journey: Bridging art therapy and museum education. *Canadian Oncology Nursing Journal*, *10*(4), 140–142, 143–146. doi:10.5737/1181912x104140142 PMID:11894320

DeBecker, G. (1997). *The gift of fear*. Boston, MA: Little, Brown and Company.

Deming, W. E. (1986). *Out of the crisis*. Cambridge, MA: Massachusetts Institute of Technology.

Deng, G., & Cassileth, B. R. (2014). *Integrative oncology: An overview. American Society of Clinical Oncology Education Book* (pp. 233–242). New York: Integrative Medicine Service, Memorial Sloan Kettering Cancer Center.

Denver Art Museum. (2012). *Denver Art Museum and Children's Hospital Colorado team up to focus on the restorative and transformational powers of art*. Retrieved from http://denverartmuseum.org/article/press-release/denver-art-museum-and-children-s-hospital-colorado-team-focus-restorative-and

Deogaonkar, M. (2004). Socio-economic inequality and its effect on healthcare delivery in India: Inequality and health-care. *Electronic Journal of Sociology*, 8(1). Retrieved from http://www.sociology.org/content/vol8.1/deogaonkar.html

Developmental Goals, S. A. A. R. C. India Country Report (2013), Central Statistics Office Ministry of Statistics and Programme Implementation. Government of India.

Dickerson, S., & Kemeny, M. (2004). Acute stressors and cortisol responses: A theoretical integration and synthesis of laboratory research. *Psychological Bulletin*, *130*(3), 355–391. doi:10.1037/0033-2909.130.3.355 PMID:15122924

Dickinson, H. O., Mason, J. M., Nicolson, D. J., Campbell, F., Beyer, F. R., Cook, J. V., & Ford, G. A. et al. (2006). Lifestyle interventions to reduced raised blood pressure: A systematic review of randomized control trials. *Journal of Hypertension*, *24*(2), 215–233. doi:10.1097/01.hjh.0000199800.72563.26 PMID:16508562

Digby, A. (1984). The changing profile of a nineteenth-century asylum: The york retreat. *Psychological Medicine*, *14*(4), 739. doi:10.1017/S003329170001970X PMID:6400132

DiMeglio, L. (2013). Help yourself form healthy habits. Alexndria, VA: American Diabetes Association. Retrieved from http://www.diabetesforecast.org/2013/jul/help-yourself-form-healthy-habits.html

Dimitrius, J. (1998). *Reading people*. New York, NY: Ballantine.

Dissanayake, E. (1992). *Homoaesthetics: Where art comes from and why*. New York: Macmillan Inc.

Dobbs, J. M. (2014). *The relationship between perceived toxic leadership styles, leader effectiveness, and organizational cynicism* (Doctoral dissertation).

Dotson, M. J., & Hyatt, E. M. (2008, May). Understanding dog-human companionship. *Journal of Business Research*, *61*(5), 457–466. doi:10.1016/j.jbusres.2007.07.019

Doty, J., & Fenlason, J. (2013). Narcissism and toxic leaders. *Military Review*, *93*(1), 55–60.

Drais-Parrillo, A. (2005). The Odyssey Project: A descriptive and prospective study of children and youth in residential group care and therapeutic foster care. *Child Welfare League of America*. Retrieved from http://www.cwla.org/programs/research/odysseyfinalreport.pdf4

Drake, J. E., & Winner, E. (2012). Confronting sadness through art-making: Distraction is more beneficial than venting. *Psychology of Aesthetics, Creativity, and the Arts*, *6*(3), 255–261. doi:10.1037/a0026909

Drazkiewicz, A., Challies, E., & Newig, J. (2015). Public participation and local environmental planning: Testing factors influencing decision quality and implementation in four case studies from Germany. *Land Use Policy*, *46*, 211–222. doi:10.1016/j.landusepol.2015.02.010

Drucker, P. (1998). *Managing and leadership*. Retrieved from http://web.mit.edu/mbarker/www/ideas/drucker.html

Druss, B. G., Zhao, L., von Esenwein, S. A., Bona, J. R., Fricks, L., Jenkins-Tucker, S., & Lorig, K. et al. (2010). The health and recovery peer (HARP) program: A peer-led intervention to improve medical self-management for persons with serious mental illness. *Schizophrenia Research*, *118*(1-2), 264–270. doi:10.1016/j.schres.2010.01.026 PMID:20185272

Duffy, M., & Sperry, L. (2014). *Overcoming mobbing: A recovery guide for workplace aggression and bullying*. New York, NY: Oxford University Press.

DuMaurier, D. (1938). Rebecca. New York, NY: Avon.

Dunbar, J. (2015). Qigong Therapy. Magic Tortoise Taichiquan School. Retrieved from: http://www.magictortoise.com/qigong_therapy.htm

Dustin, D., Mckenney, A., Hibbler, D., & Blitzer, L. (2004). Thinking outside the box: Placing park and recreation professionals in K-12 schools. *Journal of Physical Education, Recreation & Dance*, *75*(1), 51–54. doi:10.1080/07303084.2004.10608542

Dweck, C. (2006). *Mindset*. New York, NY: Ballantine.

Eagleman, D. (2011). *Incognito: The Secret lives of the brain*. New York, NY: Pantheon Books.

Educational Testing Service. (2014, October 10). ETS to host experts for innovative assessment of collaboration. Retrieved from https://www.ets.org/newsroom/news_releases/ets_host_experts

Edwards, B. D., Franco-Watkins, A., Cullen, K. L., Howell, J. W., & Acuff, R. E. Jr. (2014). Unifying the challenge-hindrance and sociocognitive models of stress. *International Journal of Stress Management*, *21*(2), 162–185. doi:10.1037/a0034730

Edwards, K., Radcliffe, S., Patchell, B., Broussard, K., Wood, E., & Ogans, J. (2009). Outcomes: The recruitment enhancement cultural affirmation project. *Journal of Cultural Diversity*, *16*(2), 64–67.

Einstein Healthcare. (2013, July 11). Moss Rehab's art therapy program with Philadelphia museum of art receives award. Retrieved from http://www.einstein.edu/news/mossrehab%E2%80%99s-art-therapy-program-with-philadelphia-museum-of-art-receives-award/

Elias, M. J. (2011). The character of schools, the character of individuals, and the character of society: Creating educational policy to reflect inextricable interconnection. *KEDI Journal of Educational Policy*, 2011, 141-149.

Elkis-Abuhoff, D., Gaydos, M., Goldblatt, R., Chen, M., & Rose, S. (2009). Mandala drawings as an assessment tool for women with breast cancer. *The Arts in Psychotherapy*, *36*(4), 231–238. doi:10.1016/j.aip.2009.04.004

Elmer, P. J., Obarzanek, E., Vollmer, W. M., Simons-Morton, D., Stevens, V. J., Young, D. R., & Svetkey, L. P. et al. (2006). Effects of Comprehensive lifestyle modification on diet, weight, physical fitness, and blood pressure control: 18-month results of a randomized trial. *Annals of Internal Medicine*, *144*(7), 485–495. doi:10.7326/0003-4819-144-7-200604040-00007 PMID:16585662

Enayati, A. (2015). *Seeking serenity*. New York, NY: New American Library.

Ernst, J., Berger, S., Weißflog, G., Schröder, C., Körner, A., Niederwieser, D., & Singer, S. (2013). Patient participation in the medical decision-making process in haemato-oncology—A qualitative study. *European Journal of Cancer Care*, *22*(5), 684–690. doi:10.1111/ecc.12077 PMID:23731258

Esch, T., Fricchione, G. L., & Stefano, G. B. (2003). The therapeutic use of the relaxation response in stress-related diseases. *Medical Science Monitor*, *9*, RA23–RA34. PMID:12601303

European Commission. (2007). *Making a European Area of Lifelong Learning a Reality*. Retrieved from http://eurlex.europa.eu/LexUriServ/LexUriServ.do?uri=COM:2001:0678:FIN:EN:PDF

European Interprofessional Education Network. (n. d.). *Our history*. Retrieved from http://www.eipen.eu/geschiedenis_9.html

Everett, B., Salamonson, Y., & Davidson, P.M. (2009). Bandura's exercise self-efficacy scale: Validation in an Austrian cardiac rehabilitation setting. *Int. J. Nurs. Stud., 46*(6), 824-829.

Ezzo, J., Vickers, A., & Richardson, M. A. (2005). Acupuncture-point stimulation for chemotherapy-induced nausea and vomiting. *Journal of Clinical Oncology*, *23*(28), 7188–7198. doi:10.1200/JCO.2005.06.028 PMID:16192603

Fan, Y., & Chen, Q. (2012). Family functioning as a mediator between neighborhood conditions and children's health: Evidence from a national survey in the United States. *Social Science & Medicine*, *74*(12), 1939–1947. doi:10.1016/j.socscimed.2012.01.039 PMID:22465381

FAO/WHO. (1998). Carbohydrates in human nutrition. *FAO Food and Nutrition Paper*, 1998, 66.

Fawcett, N. R., & Gullone, E. (2001). Cute and cuddly and a whole lot more? A call for empirical investigation into the therapeutic benefits of human-animal interaction for children. *Behaviour Change*, *18*(2), 124–133. doi:10.1375/bech.18.2.124

Federal Interagency Forum on Aging-Related Statistics. (2012). *Older Americans 2012: Key indicators of well-being*. Washington, D.C.: U.S. Government Printing Office.

Feeney, B. C., & Collins, N. L. (2003). Motivations for caregiving in adult intimate relationships: Influences on caregiving behavior and relationship functioning. *Personality and Social Psychology Bulletin*, *29*(8), 950–968. doi:10.1177/0146167203252807 PMID:15189615

Feudtner, C., Christakis, D.A., & Christakis, N.A. (1994). Do clinical clerks suffer ethical erosion? Students' perceptions of their ethical environment and personal development. *Academic Medicine, 69*(8), 670-679. doi:10.1097/00001888-199408000-00017

Fincher, S. (2010). *Creating mandalas for insight, healing and self-expression*. Boston, MA: Shambhala Publications, Inc.

Fincher, S. F. (2007). Mandalas and the gestalt of self. *International Gestalt Journal*, *30*(2), 65–78.

Fitzgerald, F. S. (1925). *The great Gatsby*. New York, NY: Scribner.

Florida Atlantic University. (2012). *Christine E. Lynn College of Nursing philosophy*. Retrieved http://nursing.fau.edu/index.php?main=1&nav=635

Florida Atlantic University. (2014). *Owls care health promotion*. Retrieved from http://www.fau.edu/owlscare/

Florida Atlantic University. (2016). *Office of Interprofessional Education*. Retrieved http://fau.edu/provost/academic-affairs/interprofessional-education.php

Flum, H. (2015). Relationships and career development: An integrative approach. In P. J. Hartung, M. L. Savickas, & W. B. Walsh (Eds.), *APA handbook for career intervention* (pp. 145–158)., doi:10.1037/14438-009

Forman, S. G. (2015). *Leadership for implementation and change. Implementation of mental health programs in schools: A change agent's guide* (pp. 55–69). Washington, DC: American Psychological Association; doi:10.1037/14597-005

Forzoni, S., Perez, M., Martignetti, A., & Crispino, S. (2010). Art therapy with cancer patients during chemotherapy sessions: An analysis of the patients' perception of helpfulness. *Palliative & Supportive Care*, *8*(1), 41–48. doi:10.1017/S1478951509990691 PMID:20163759

Foster, A. J., Murff, H. J., Peterson, J. F., Gandhi, T. K., & Bates, D. W. (2003). The incidence and severity of adverse events affecting patients after discharge from the hospital. *Annals of Internal Medicine*, *138*(3), 161–167. doi:10.7326/0003-4819-138-3-200302040-00007 PMID:12558354

Foster, C., Hillsdon, M., Thorogood, M., Kaur, A., & Wedatilake, T. (2005). Interventions for promoting physical activity. *Cochrane Database of Systematic Reviews*, (1): CD003180. PMID:15674903

Foster, M. T. (1992). Experiencing a "creative high.". *The Journal of Creative Behavior*, *26*(1), 29–39. doi:10.1002/j.2162-6057.1992.tb01154.x

Fox, K. R. (1999). The influence of physical activity on mental well-being. *Public Health Nutrition*, *2*(3a3A), 411–418. doi:10.1017/S1368980099000567 PMID:10610081

Fraley, R., Garner, J., & Shaver, P. (2000). Adult attachment and the defensive regulation of attention and memory: Examining the role of preemptive and postemptive defensive processes. *Journal of Personality and Social Psychology*, *79*(5), 816–826. doi:10.1037/0022-3514.79.5.816 PMID:11079243

Fraley, R., Niedenthal, P., Marks, M., Brumbaugh, C., & Vicary, A. (2006). Adult attachment and the perception of emotional expressions: Probing the hyperactivating strategies underlying anxious attachment. *Journal of Personality*, *74*(4), 1163–1182. doi:10.1111/j.1467-6494.2006.00406.x PMID:16787432

Francis, L. E. (2003). Feeling good, feeling well: Identity, emotion and health. In Advances in identity theory and research (pp. 123-134). Springer US.

Frank, L., Kerr, J., Chapman, J., & Sallis, J. (2007). Urban form relationships with walk trip frequency and distance among youth. *American Journal of Health Promotion*, *21*(4), 305–311. doi:10.4278/0890-1171-21.4s.305 PMID:17465175

Friedmann, E., Katcher, A. H., Thomas, S. A., Lynch, J. J., & Messent, P. R. (1983). Social interaction and blood pressure: The influence of animal companions. *The Journal of Nervous and Mental Disease*, *171*(8), 461–465. doi:10.1097/00005053-198308000-00002 PMID:6875529

Fulton-Kehoe, D., Hamman, R. F., Baxter, J., & Marshall, J. (2001). A case-control study of physical activity and non-insulin dependent diabetes mellitus (NIDDM). The San Luis Valley Diabetes Study. *Annals of Epidemiology*, *11*(5), 320–327. doi:10.1016/S1047-2797(01)00218-6 PMID:11399446

Gabriel, B., Bromberg, E., Vandenbovenkamp, J., Walka, P., Kornblith, A. B., & Luzzatto, P. (2001). Art therapy with adult bone marrow transplant patients in isolation: A pilot study. *Psycho-Oncology*, *10*(2), 114–123. doi:10.1002/pon.498 PMID:11268138

Gagne, J., & Deci, E. L. (2005). Self-determination theory and work motivation. *Journal of Organizational Behavior*, *26*(4), 331–362. doi:10.1002/job.322

Galindo, J. personal communication, December 5, 2015

Galvin, J. A., Benson, H., Deckro, G. R., Fricchione, G. L., & Dusek, J. A. (2006). The relaxation response: Reducing stress and improving cognition in healthy aging adults. *Complementary Therapies in Clinical Practice*, *12*(3), 186–191. doi:10.1016/j.ctcp.2006.02.004 PMID:16835029

Gardner-Nix, J. (2009). The mindfulness solution to pain: Step-by-step techniques for chronic pain management. Oakland, CA: New Harbinger Publications; Retrieved from http://search.proquest.com/docview/622056475?accountid=4840

Garfield, C. (1992). *Second to none: How our smartest companies put people first*. Homewood, IL: Business One Irwin.

Garvin, D. A., Edmondson, A. C., & Gino, F. (2008). Is yours a learning organization? *Harvard Business Review*, *86*(3), 1–11. Retrieved from http://mfi.caifos.com/wp-content/uploads /2013/03/Is-Yours-a-Learning-Organization.pdf PMID:18411968

Gaufberg, E., Shtasel, D., Hirsh, D., Ogur, B., & Bor, D. (2008). The Harvard Medical School Cambridge integrated clerkship: Challenges of longitudinal integrated training. *Clinical Teacher, 5*(2), 78-82. doi:10.1111/j.1743-498x.2008.00209.x

Gender Tests. (2006), Actions Sought Against 35 Doctors, The Hindu (Delhi), May 14, 2006.

General Pharmaceutical Council. (2016). *What does a pharmacist do?* Retrieved from https://www.pharmacyregulation.org/raising-concerns/raising-concerns-about-pharmacy-professional/what-expect-your-pharmacy/what-does-0

Germain, C. B. (1991). *Human behavior in the social environment: An ecological view*. New York, NY: Columbia University Press.

Germer, C. K. (2009). *The Mindful path to self-compassion*. New York, NY: Guilford.

Gerteis, J., Izrael, D., Deitz, D., LeRoy, L., Ricciardi, R., Miller, T., & Basu, J. (2014). *Multiple chronic condition chartbook: 2010 medical expenditure panel survey data*. Rockville, MD: Agency for Healthcare Research and Quality.

Gilbert, E. (2015). *Big magic: creative living beyond fear*. New York, NY: Riverhead Books.

Gilbert, J. (2011). The millennials: A new generation of employees, a new set of engagement policies. *Ivey Business Journal*, *75*(5), 26–28.

Gilbert, J. A., Carr-Ruffin, N., Ivancevich, J. M., & Konopaske, R. (2012). Toxic versus cooperative behaviors at work: The role of organizational culture and leadership in creating community-centered organizations. *International Journal of Leadership Studies*, *7*(1), 24–46.

Giovannucci, E., Ascherio, A., Rimm, E. B., Colditz, G. A., Stampfer, M. J., & Willett, W. C. (1995). Physical activity, obesity, and risk for colon cancer and adenoma in men. *Annals of Internal Medicine*, *122*(5), 327–334. doi:10.7326/0003-4819-122-5-199503010-00002 PMID:7847643

Glass, K. E., Wills, C. E., Holloman, C., Olson, J., Hechmer, C., Miller, C. K., & Duchemin, A. M. (2012). Shared decision making and other variables as correlates of satisfaction with health care decisions in a United States national survey. *Patient Education and Counseling*, *88*(1), 100–105. doi:10.1016/j.pec.2012.02.010 PMID:22410642

Godbey, G. (2009). Outdoor recreation, health, and wellness: Understanding and enhancing the relationship.

Goffee, R., & Jones, G. (2006). *Why should anyone be led by you? Harvard Business Review*. Boston, MA: Harvard Business School Press.

Goldberg, N. (1986). *Writing down the bones*. Boston, MA: Shambhala.

Goldberg, N. (1990). *Wild mind*. New York, NY: Bantam.

Goldberg, N. (2000). *Thunder and lightning*. New York, NY: Bantam.

Goldberg, N. (2007). *Old friend from far away*. New York, NY: Free Press.

Goldberg, N. (2013). *The true secret of writing*. New York, NY: Atria.

Goldberg, N. (2016). *The great spring*. Boulder, CO: Shambhala.

Goldstein, J. (2012). *Play in children's development, health and well-being*. Brussels: Toy Industries of Europe.

Goldstein, N. J., Martin, S. J., & Cialdini, R. B. (2008). *Yes!: 50 scientifically proven ways to be persuasive*. New York: Free Press.

Golechha, M. (2015). Health agenda for Indian government. *The Indian Journal of Medical Research*, *141*(2), 151–153. doi:10.4103/0971-5916.155541 PMID:25900948

Goleman, D. (1995). *Emotional Intelligence*. New York, NY: Free Press.

Goleman, D. (2004). *What makes a leader? Harvard Business Review*. Boston, MA: Harvard Business School Press.

Good, M., Anderson, G. C., Stanton-Hicks, M., Grass, J. A., & Makii, M. (2002). Relaxation and music reduce pain after gynecologic surgery. *Pain Management Nursing*, *3*(2), 61–70. doi:10.1053/jpmn.2002.123846 PMID:12050837

Good, M., & Zauszniewski, J. A. (2014). Biofeedback. In R. Lindquist, M. Snyder, & M. F. Tracy (Eds.), *Complementary & alternative therapies in nursing* (pp. 153–166). New York, NY: Springer Publishing Company.

Goodman, R., Williams, K., Agell, G., & Gantt, L. (1998). Talk, talk, talk, when do we draw? *American Journal of Art Therapy*, *37*(2), 39.

Gorelick, P. B., Sacco, R. L., Smith, D. B., Alberts, M., Mustone-Alexander, L., Rader, D., & Rhew, D. C. et al. (1999). Prevention of a first stroke: A review of guidelines and a multidisciplinary consensus statement from the National Stroke Association. *Journal of the American Medical Association*, *281*(12), 1112–1120. doi:10.1001/jama.281.12.1112 PMID:10188663

Gorman, J. M., & Sloan, R. P. (2000). Heart rate variability in depressive and anxiety disorders. *American Heart Journal*, *140*(4Suppl.), 77–83. doi:10.1067/mhj.2000.109981 PMID:11011352

Graham, S., & Weiner, B. (1996). Theories and principles of motivation. In D. C. Berliner & R. C. Calfee (Eds.), *Handbook of educational psychology* (pp. 63–84). New York, NY: Macmillan.

Gray, P. (2010). The decline in play and rise in children's mental disorders. *Psychology Today, Blog*. Retrieved from https://www.psychologytoday.com/blog/freedom-learn/201001/the-decline-play-and-rise-in-childrens-mental-disorders

Green, A. (2002). The many faces of lifelong learning: Recent education policy trends in Europe. *Journal of Education Policy*, *17*(6), 611–626. doi:10.1080/0268093022000032274

Greene, M. (1995). *Releasing the imagination: Essays on education, the arts, and social change*. New York: Wiley.

Greene, M. (2001). *Variations on a blue guitar: The Lincoln Center Institute lectures on aesthetic education*. New York: Teachers College Press.

Greenleaf, R. K. (1970). *The servant as leader*. Indianapolis, IN: Greenleaf Center.

Gregory, B., Harris, S., Armenakis, A., & Shook, C. (2009). Organizational culture and effectiveness: A study of values, attitudes, and organizational outcomes. *Journal of Business Research*, *62*(7), 673–679. doi:10.1016/j.jbusres.2008.05.021

Grey, M., Schulman-Green, D., Knafl, K., & Reynolds, N. R. (2015). A revised self-and family management framework. *Nursing Outlook*, *63*(2), 162–170. doi:10.1016/j.outlook.2014.10.003 PMID:25771190

Groopman, J. (2007). *How doctors think*. New York, NY: Mariner Books.

Gross, R. (1999). *Peak Learning*. New York, NY: Penguin Putnam Inc.

Gruwell, E. (2007). Teach with your heart. New York, NY: Broadway.

Gruwell, E., & the The Freedom Writers. (1999). The Freedom Writers diary. New York, NY: Broadway.

Guillén, M., Ferrero, I., & Hoffman, W. M. (2015). The neglected ethical and spiritual motivations in the workplace. *Journal of Business Ethics*, *128*(4), 803–816. doi:10.1007/s10551-013-1985-7

Gururaj, G. (2006). Road traffic injury prevention in India. National Institute of Mental Health and Neuro Sciences, Bangalore, Publication No. 56.

Guttmann, J., & Regev, D. (2004). The phenomenological approach to art therapy. *Journal of Contemporary Psychotherapy*, *34*(2), 153–162. doi:10.1023/B:JOCP.0000022314.69354.41

Haas, B. W., Anderson, I. W., & Filkowski, M. M. (2015). Interpersonal reactivity and the attribution of emotional reactions. *Emotion (Washington, D.C.)*, *15*(3), 390–398. doi:10.1037/emo0000053 PMID:25706827

Hafferty, F.W. (1998). Beyond curriculum reform: Confronting medicine's hidden curriculum. *Academic Medicine*, *73*(4), 403-437. doi:10.1097/00001888-199804000-00013

Hale, M. (2013). *The single woman*. Nashville, TN: Thomas Nelson.

Hale, M. (2015). *Beautiful uncertainty*. Nashville, TN: Thomas Nelson.

Halkett, G. K. B., Arbon, P., Scutter, S. D., & Borg, M. (2007). The phenomenon of making decisions during the experience of early breast cancer. *European Journal of Cancer Care*, *16*(4), 322–330. doi:10.1111/j.1365-2354.2007.00778.x PMID:17587355

Hall, G. E., & Hord, S. M. (2015). *Implementing change: Patterns, principles, and potholes* (4th ed.). Upper Saddle River, NJ: Prentice-Hall.

Halm, M. A. (2009). Relaxation: A self-care healing modality reduces harmful effects of anxiety. *American Journal of Critical Care*, *18*(2), 169–172. doi:10.4037/ajcc2009867 PMID:19255107

Hamilton, S. S., & Armando, J. (2008). Oppositional Defiant Disorder. *American Family Physician*, *78*, 861–867. PMID:18841736

Handler, J. (2013). *Braving the fire*. New York, NY: St. Martin's Griffin.

Hare, B., & Woods, V. (2013). *The genius of dogs: how dogs are smarter than you think*. Penguin.

Harrison, M. D. (2002). *Narrative based evaluation*. New York, NY: Peter Lang Publishing.

Hart, K. E., Turner, S. H., & Cardozo, S. R. (1987). Ongoing research. Stress, personality, coping and well-being: A four-wave longitudinal process study. *Personality and Individual Differences*, *8*(4), 591–593. doi:10.1016/0191-8869(87)90226-1

Haub, C., & Sharma, O. P. (2006). India's Population Reality: Reconciling Change and Tradition. *Population Bulletin*, 61(3), 8. Retrieved from http://www.prb.org/pdf06/61.3indiaspopulationreality_eng.pdf

Haugk, K. C. (2000). *When and how to use mental health resources*. St. Louis, MO: Stephen Ministries.

Hawthorne Effect. (n.d.). *Harvard Business School Baker Library Collections.* Retrieved from http://www.library.hbs.edu/hc/hawthorne/09.html

Hazan, C., & Shaver, P. (1987). Romantic love conceptualized as an attachment process. *Journal of Personality and Social Psychology, 52*(3), 511–524. doi:10.1037/0022-3514.52.3.511 PMID:3572722

Headey, B., Na, F., & Zheng, R. (2008). Pet dogs benefit owners' health: A 'natural experiment' in china. *Social Indicators Research, 87*(3), 481–493. doi:10.1007/s11205-007-9142-2

Health Resources and Services Administration. (2016). *Health literacy.* Retrieved from http://www.hrsa.gov/publichealth/healthliteracy/

Healthy People 2020. (n. d.). Physical activity. Washington, D.C.: U.S. Department of Health & Human Services.

Heard, G. (1995). *Writing toward home.* Portsmouth, NH: Heinemann.

Heard, G. (1999). *Awakening the heart.* Portsmouth, NH: Heinemann.

HeartMath® Institute. (2016). *HeartMath Institute's mission and vision.* Retrieved from https://www.heartmath.org/about-us/hmi-mission/

Helldorfer, M., & Moss, T. (2007). *Healing with heart.* Orinda, CA: Moss Communications.

Hendrickson, R., Lane, J., Harris, J., & Dorman, R. (2013). *Academic leadership and governance of higher education.* Sterling, VA: Stylus.

Herzberg, F. (2003). One more time: How do you motivate employees? Retrieved from https://hbr.org/2003/01/one-more-time-how-do-you-motivate-employees

Hibbler, D. K., & Scott, L. (2015). Role of leisure in humanizing learning cities. In L. Scott (Ed.), *Learning cities for adult learners* (pp. 73–82). San Francisco, CA: Jossey-Bass. doi:10.1002/ace.20124

Hillen, M. A., de Haes, H. C. J. M., Stalpers, L. J. A., Klinkenbijl, J. H. G., Eddes, E., Verdam, M. G. E., & Smets, E. M. A. (2014). How attachment style and locus of control influence patients' trust in their oncologist. *Journal of Psychosomatic Research, 76*(3), 221–226. doi:10.1016/j.jpsychores.2013.11.014 PMID:24529041

Hilterbrand, E. U. (1999). Coping with Cancer through image manipulation. In C. A. Malchiodi (Ed.), *Medical art therapy with adults* (pp. 113–135). London: Jessica Kingsley.

Hirsh, D., Gaufberg, E., Ogur, B., Cohen, P., Krupat, E., Cox, M., . . . Bor, D. (2012). Educational outcomes of the Harvard Medical School Cambridge integrated clerkship: A way forward for medical education? *Academic Medicine, 87*(5), 643-650. doi:10.1097/acm.0b013e31824d9821

Hirsh, D., Walters, L., & Poncelet, A.N. (2012). Better learning, better doctors, better delivery system: Possibilities from a case study of longitudinal integrated clerkships. *Medical Teacher, 34*(7), 548–554. doi:10.3109/0142159x.2012.696745

Hirsh, D.A., Ogur, B., Thibault, G.E., & Cox, M. (2007). "Continuity" as an organizing principle for clinical education reform. *New England Journal of Medicine, 356*(8), 858-866. doi:10.1056/nejmsb061660

Hodges, K., & Winstanley, S. (2012). Effects of optimism, social support, fighting spirit, cancer worry and internal health locus of control on positive affect in cancer survivors: A path analysis. *Stress and Health: Journal of the International Society for the Investigation of Stress, 28*(5), 408–415. doi:10.1002/smi.2471 PMID:23129560

Hodgkinson, G. P., Sadler-Smith, E., Burke, L. A., Claxton, G., & Sparrow, P. R. (2009). Intuition in organizations: Implications for strategic management. *Long Range Planning, 42*(3), 277-297. doi:10.1016/j.lrp.2009.05.003

Hogan, P., Dall, T., & Nikolov, P. (2003). Economic costs of diabetes in the US in 2002. *Diabetes Care*, *26*(3), 917–932. doi:10.2337/diacare.26.3.917 PMID:12610059

Hojat, M., Vergare, M.J., Maxwell, K., Brainard, G., Herrine, S., Isenberg, G.A., . . . Gonnella, J.S. (2009). The devil is in the third year: A longitudinal study of erosion of empathy in medical school. *Academic Medicine*, *84*(9), 1182-1191. doi:10.1097/acm.0b013e3181b17e55

Horton, A. I. (1989). *The Highlander folk school: A history of its major programs, 1932-1961.* New York, NY: Carlson Publishing.

Howard, D. Z. (2003). *Stress@work: An exploration of the impact of information and communication technology on Canadian workers* [Master's thesis]. Concordia University, Montreal, Quebec, Canada.

Howard, J., Howard, D., & Dotson, E. (2015). A connected history of health and education: Learning together toward a better city. In L. Scott (Ed.), *Learning cities for adult learners* (pp. 57–72). San Francisco, CA: Jossey-Bass. doi:10.1002/ace.20123

Hsiao, W. (2003). *What Is A Health System? Why Should We Care?* Cambridge, MA: Harvard School of Public Health.

Huang, T. Y. (2012). Intuition and emotion: Examining two nonrational approaches in complex decision making (Unpublished doctoral dissertation). London, England: City University; Retrieved from http://openaccess.city.ac.uk/2072/1/Huang,_Tori_Yu-Wen.pdf

Huang, E. S., Basu, A., O'Grady, M., & Capretta, J. C. (2009). Projecting the future diabetes population: Size and related costs for the U.S. *Diabetes Care*, *32*(12), 2225–2229. doi:10.2337/dc09-0459 PMID:19940225

Huesmann, L. R. (2012). The contagion of violence: The extent, the processes, and the outcomes. In *IOM (Institute of Medicine) & NRC (National Research Council), Social and economic costs of violence: Workshop summary*. Washington, DC: The National Academies Press.

Hu, F. B., Manson, J. E., Stampfer, M. J., Colditz, G., Liu, S., Solomon, C. G., & Willett, W. C. (2001). Diet, lifestyle, and the risk of type 2 diabetes mellitus in women. *The New England Journal of Medicine*, *345*(11), 790–797. doi:10.1056/NEJMoa010492 PMID:11556298

Hu, F. B., Stampfer, M. J., Colditz, G. A., Ascherio, A., Rexrode, K. M., Willett, W. C., & Manson, J. E. (2000). Physical activity and risk of stroke in women. *Journal of the American Medical Association*, *283*(22), 2961–2967. doi:10.1001/jama.283.22.2961 PMID:10865274

Huitt, W. (2007). Maslow's hierarchy of needs, educational psychology interactive. Retrieved from http://www.edpsycinteractive.org/topics/cponation/maslow.html

Human Resources, U. C. S. F. (n.d.). Chapter 14: Team building. Retrieved from http://ucsfhr.ucsf.edu/index.php/pubs/hrguidearticle/chapter-14-team-building/

Humane education for kids. (2015). Retrieved from http://www.safehavenhumane.org/humane-education-kids

Humane Society of the United States (HSUS). Declawing Cats: More Than Just a Manicure, Retrieved from http://www.hsus.org/pets/pet_care/cat_care/declawing_cats_more_than_just_a_manicure/

Hunt, C. (2005). Community education. In L. English (Ed.), *International encyclopedia of adult education* (pp. 131–136). New York, NY: Palgrave Macmillan.

Ibsen, H. (1958). A doll's house. In *Four great plays*. New York, NY: Bantam. (Original work published 1879)

India's Population. (2015). Retrieved from http://www.indiaonlinepages.com/population/india-current-population.html

Institute for Healthcare Improvement. (2016). *IHI triple aim initiative*. Retrieved from http://www.ihi.org/engage/initiatives/TripleAim/Pages/default.aspx

Institute for Humane Education. (2008). What is humane education? Retrieved from http://humaneeducation.org/sections/view/what_is_humane_education

Institute of HeartMath®. (2014). *The resilience advantage: Skills for personal and professional effectiveness*. Boulder Creek, CA: Institute of HeartMath®.

Institute of Medicine (IOM) & National Research Council. (NRC). (2012). Social and economic costs of violence: Workshop summary. Washington, DC: The National Academies Press.

Institute of Medicine. (1972). *Educating for the health team*. Retrieved from https://nexusipe-resource-exchange.s3.amazonaws.com/Educating_for_the_Health_Team_IOM_1972.pdf

Institute of Medicine. (2001). Crossing the quality chasm: A new health system for the 21st century. Retrieved from http://iom.nationalacademies.org/~/media/Files/Report%20Files/2001/Crossing-the-Quality-Chasm/Quality%20Chasm%202001%20%20report%20brief.pdf

Interprofessional Education Collaborative. (2011). *Core competencies for interprofessional collaborative practice: Report of an expert panel*. Retrieved from http://www.aacn.nche.edu/education-resources/ipecreport.pdf

Interprofessional Education Collaborative. (2016). *Resources*. Retrieved from https://ipecollaborative.org/Resources.html

Iwasaki, Y., & Schneider, I. E. (2003). Leisure, stress, and coping: An evolving area of inquiry. *Leisure Sciences*, *25*(2-3), 107–113. doi:10.1080/01490400306567

Jackson, R. J., Dannenberg, A. L., & Frumkin, H. (2013). Health and the built environment: 10 years after. *American Journal of Public Health*, *103*(9), 1542–1544. doi:10.2105/AJPH.2013.301482 PMID:23865699

Jacobson, S., & Samdahl, D. M. (1998). Leisure in the lives of old lesbians: Experiences with and responses to discrimination. *Journal of Leisure Research*, *30*(2), 233–255.

Jacomino, M., Bamdas, J. M., Keller, K., Hamlin, E., Hawkins, M., Gordon, S., & Ouslander, J. (2015). An innovative interprofessional education program for university medical, nursing, and social work students learning in teams during sessions and visits with geriatric mentors. *Journal of Interprofessional Education & Practice*, *1*(3-4), 100–103. doi:10.1016/j.xjep.2015.10.003

Jaglal, S. B., Kreiger, N., & Darlington, G. (1993). Past and recent physical activity and risk of hip fracture. *American Journal of Epidemiology*, *138*, 107–118. PMID:8342529

Jain, A. (Ed.), (1998). Do Population Policies Matter? Fertility and Policies in Egypt, India, Kenya, and Mexico. New York: Population Council.

Jaramillo, F., Locander, W. B., Spector, P. E., & Harris, E. G. (2007). Getting the job done: The moderating role of initiative on the relationship between intrinsic motivation and adaptive selling. *Journal of Personal Selling & Sales Management, 27*, 59-74. doi:10.2753/PSS0885-3134270104

Jarvis, P. (2004). *Adult education and lifelong learning: Theory and practice* (3rd ed.). New York, NY: RoutledgeFalmer.

Jarvis, P. (Ed.). (2001). *Twentieth century thinkers in adult education* (2nd ed.). London, UK: Croom Helm.

Jencks, S. F., Williams, M. V., & Coleman, E. A. (2009). Rehospitalizations among patients in the Medicare fee-for-service program. *The New England Journal of Medicine*, *360*(14), 1418–1428. doi:10.1056/NEJMsa0803563 PMID:19339721

Johnson, L. (1998). *Two parts textbook, one part love*. New York, NY: Hyperion.

John, T. J., Dandona, L., Sharma, V. P., & Kakkar, M. (2011). Continuing challenge of infectious diseases in India. *Lancet*, *377*(9761), 252–269. doi:10.1016/S0140-6736(10)61265-2 PMID:21227500

Jones, S. M. (2005). Attachment style differences and similarities in evaluations of affective communication skills and person-centered comforting messages. *Western Journal of Communication*, *69*(3), 233–249. doi:10.1080/10570310500202405

Joseph, J., & Krishnan, A. (2004), Hospital Waste Management in the Union Territory of Pondicherry: An exploration. Retrieved from www.pon.nic.in/citizen/science/ppcc-new/joe.pdf

Joshi, R., Cardona, M., Iyengar, S., Sukumar, A., Raju, C. R., Raju, K. R., & Neal, B. et al. (2006). Chronic diseases now a leading cause of death in rural India: Mortality data from the Andhra Pradesh Rural Health Initiative. *International Journal of Epidemiology*, *35*(6), 1522–1529. doi:10.1093/ije/dyl168 PMID:16997852

Joumard, I., & Kumar, A. (2015). *"Improving health outcomes and health care in India", OECD economics department working papers, No. 1184*. OECD Publishing. Doi:10.1787/5js7t9ptcr26-en

Juli, T. (2011). *Leadership principles for project success*. New York, NY: CRC Press.

Jung, C. (1972). *Mandala symbolism*. Princeton, NJ: Princeton University Press.

Kacchap, N. M. (2015). Budget 2015: In search of an effective healthcare system. Retrieved from http://www.financialexpress.com/article/healthcare/cover-story-healthcare/budget-2015-in-search-of-an-effective-healthcare-system/62145/

Kaczynski, A. T., & Henderson, K. A. (2007). Environmental correlates of physical activity: A review of evidence about parks and recreation. *Leisure Sciences*, *29*(4), 315–354. doi:10.1080/01490400701394865

Kallio, P., Kolehmainen, M., Laaksonen, D. E., Kekäläinen, J., Salopuro, T., Sivenius, K., & Uusitupa, M. et al. (2007). Dietary carbohydrate modification induces alterations in gene expression in abdominal subcutaneous adipose tissue in persons with the metabolic syndrome: The FUNGENUT Study. *The American Journal of Clinical Nutrition*, *85*, 1417–1427. PMID:17490981

Kane, H., Jaremka, L., Guichard, A., Ford, M., Collins, N., & Feeney, B. (2007). Feeling supported and feeling satisfied: How one partner's attachment style predicts the other partner's relationship experiences. *Journal of Social and Personal Relationships*, *24*(4), 535–555. doi:10.1177/0265407507079245

Kapilashrami, M. C. (2000). Review of the present health status of India, emerging, health problems and their Solutions. *Health and Population; Perspectives and Issues*, *23*(1), 1–10.

Karadag, F., Ozcan, H., Eskin, M., Karul, A. B., Ceylan, E., Tufek, Y., & Cildag, O. (2008). Psychological distress in chronic obstructive pulmonary disease patients. *Stress and Health*, *24*(2), 115–122. doi:10.1002/smi.1178

Katsapis, C. C. A. (2008). *Incidence and types of occupational role stress among university research administrators* [Doctoral dissertation].

Katz, J. (2003). *The New Work of Dogs: Tending to Life, Love, and Family*. New York, NY: Random House Trade Paperbacks.

Katz, J., & Joiner, T. (2002). Being known, intimate, and valued: Global self-verification and dyadic adjustment in couples and roommates. *Journal of Personality*, *70*(1), 33–58. doi:10.1111/1467-6494.00177 PMID:11908534

Kelley, G. A., & Kelley, K. S. (2015). Meditative movement therapies and health-related quality- of-life in adults: A systematic review of meta-analyses. *PLoS ONE*, *10*(6), e129181. doi:10.1371/journal.pone.0129181 PMID:26053053

Kelly, J. R., & Godbey, G. (1992). *The sociology of leisure*. State College, PA: Venture.

Kendall-Tackett, K., & Marshall, R. (1999). Victimization and diabetes: An exploratory study. *Child Abuse & Neglect*, *23*(6), 593–596. doi:10.1016/S0145-2134(99)00033-2 PMID:10391516

Kern-Pilch, K. (1980). Art therapy with a terminally ill patient. *American Journal of Art Therapy*, *20*(1), 3–11. PMID:10251680

Kerr, J., Frank, L., Sallis, J., & Chapman, J. (2007). Urban form correlates of pedestrian travel in youth: Differences by gender, race-ethnicity and household attributes. *Transportation Research Part D, Transport and Environment*, *12*(3), 177–182. doi:10.1016/j.trd.2007.01.006

Kickbusch, I. (1994). Tell me a story. In A. Pedersen et al (Eds.), Introduction to Health Promotion in Canada (pp. 8-17). Provincial, National and International Perspectives Canada, WB Saunders.

Kiecolt-Glaser, J. K., Christian, L., Preston, H., Houts, C. R., Malarkey, W. B., Emery, C. F., & Glaser, R. (2010). Stress, inflammation, and yoga practice. *Psychosomatic Medicine*, *72*(2), 113–121. doi:10.1097/PSY.0b013e3181cb9377 PMID:20064902

Kilcup, M., Schultz, D., Carlson, J., & Wilson, B. (2003). Postdischarge pharmacist medication reconciliation: Impact on readmission rates and financial savings. *Journal of the Journal of the American Pharmacists Association*, *53*(1), 78–84. doi:10.1331/JAPhA.2013.11250 PMID:23636160

Kim, C. H., & Scullion, H. (2013). The effect of corporate social responsibility on employee motivation: A cross-national study. The Poznan University of Economics Review, 13(2), 5-30.

Kirkland, B. J. (1996, May). Psychological adjustment to breast cancer: Congruence of locus of control and information and decision making participation. *Dissertation Abstracts International: Section B: The Sciences and Engineering*.

Knowles, M. J. (1973). *The modern practice of adult education: From pedagogy to andragogy*. New York, NY: Cambridge Book Company.

Kodeih, F., & Greenwood, R. (2014). Complexity: The Role of identity. *Organization Studies*, *35*(1), 7–39. doi:10.1177/0170840613495333

Kohn, L. T., Corrigan, J. M., & Donaldson, M. S. (Eds.). (2000). *Institute of medicine: To err is human: Building a safer health system*. Washington, DC: National Academies Press.

Kohrt, W. M., Snead, D. B., Slatopolsky, E., & Birge, S. J. Jr. (1995). Additive effects of weight- bearing exercise and estrogen on bone mineral density in older women. *Journal of Bone and Mineral Research*, *10*(9), 1303–1311. doi:10.1002/jbmr.5650100906 PMID:7502701

Koohsari, M. J., Badland, H., & Giles-Corti, B. (2013). (Re) Designing the built environment to support physical activity: Bringing public health back into urban design and planning. *Cities (London, England)*, *35*, 294–298. doi:10.1016/j.cities.2013.07.001

Koohsari, M. J., Mavoa, S., Villianueva, K., Sugiyama, T., Badland, H., Kaczynski, A. T., & Giles-Corti, B. (2015). Public open space, physical activity, urban design and public health: Concepts, methods and research agenda. *Health & Place*, *33*, 75–82. doi:10.1016/j.healthplace.2015.02.009 PMID:25779691

Kreitler, S., Oppenheim, D., & Segev-Shoham, E. (2012). *Fantasy, art therapies, and other expressive and creative psychosocial interventions*. Somerset, NJ: Wiley-Blackwell. doi:10.1002/9781119941033.ch13

Krishna, V., & Marquardt, M. J. (2007). *A framework for the development of organizational commitment using action learning.*

Krumholz, H. M. (2010). Informed consent to promote patient- centered care. *Journal of the American Medical Association*, *303*(12), 1190–1191. doi:10.1001/jama.2010.309 PMID:20332406

Kubler –Ross. E. & Kessler, D. (2015). On Grief & Grieving: Finding the meaning of grief through the five stages of loss. New York, NY: Simon and Schuster.

Kumpakaite, V. K. (2008). Human resource development in learning organization. *Journal of Business Economics and Management*, *9*(1), 25–31. doi:10.3846/1611-1699.2008.9.25-31

Laaksonen, D. E., Toppinen, L. K., Juntunen, K. S., Autio, K., Liukkonen, K. H., Poutanen, K. S., & Mykkänen, H. M. et al. (2005). Dietary carbohydrate modification enhances insulin secretion in persons with the metabolic syndrome. *The American Journal of Clinical Nutrition*, *82*, 1218–1227. PMID:16332654

Lakshminarayanan, S. (2011). Role of government in public health: Current scenario in India and future scope. *J. Family Community Med.*, *18*(1), 26–30. doi:10.4103/1319-1683.78635 PMID:21694957

Lalley, H. (2012, May 13). Chicago civic groups contribute art to Ann and Robert H. Lurie Children's Hospital. Retrieved from https://www.luriechildrens.org/en-us/our-home/Pages/community-partner-spaces.aspx

Lamott, A. (1994). *Bird by bird.* New York: Anchor Books.

Lawton, R. B. (2014a). A System Perspective on India's Healthcare Industry, Global economy, Healthcare Reform, India, World Development. *The World Financial Review*. Retrieved from http://www.worldfinancialreview.com/?p=2604

Lawton, R. B. (2014b). A system perspective on India's healthcare delivery, Industry, Global economy, Healthcare Reform, India, World Development. *The World Financial Review*. Retrieved from http://www.worldfinancialreview.com/?p=2604

Lazarus, J. (2000). *Stress relief & relaxation techniques*. Los Angeles, CA: Keats.

Lazarus, R. S. (1966). *Psychological stress and the coping process*. New York, NY: McGraw-Hill.

Le Roux, M. C., Swartz, L., & Swart, E. (2014, May30). The Effect of an animal-assisted reading program on the reading rate, accuracy, and comprehension of grade 3 students: A randomized control study. *Child and Youth Care Forum*, *43*(1), 655–673. doi:10.1007/s10566-014-9262-1

Leaf, C. (2013). *Switch on your brain*. Grand Rapids, Michigan: Baker Books.

Ledesma, D., & Kumano, H. (2009). Mindfulness-based stress reduction and cancer: A meta- analysis. *Psychooncology, 18,* 571-579. Leeds, A.R. (1979). The dietary management of diabetes in adults. *The Proceedings of the Nutrition Society*, *98*, 365–371.

Lee-Chai, A. Y., & Bargh, J. A. (2001). *The use and abuse of power: Multiple perspectives on the causes of corruption*. Philadelphia, PA: Taylor & Francis Group.

Lejsted, M., & Johannes, N. (2006, December). Art created by psychiatric patients. *Lancet*, *368*, S10–S11. doi:10.1016/S0140-6736(06)69906-6

Lemaire, J. B., Wallace, J. E., Lewin, A. M., de Grood, J., & Schaefer, J. P. (2011). The effect of a biofeedback-based stress management tool on physician stress: A randomized controlled clinical trial. *Open Medicine*, *5*(4), E154–E163. PMID:22567069

Lencioni, P. (2002). *The five dysfunctions of a team: A leadership fable*. San Francisco, CA: Jossey-Bass.

Lenker, S. L., Lorig, K., & Gallagher, G. (1984). Reasons for the lack of association between changes in health behavior and improved health status: An exploratory study. *Patient Education and Counseling*, *6*(2), 69–72. doi:10.1016/0738-3991(84)90036-3 PMID:10268098

Liao-Troth, M., & Dunn, C. P. (1999). Social constructs and human service: Managerial sensemaking of volunteer motivation. *Voluntas, 10*(4), 345-361. doi:10.1023/A:1021486408619

Lifelong Learning. (n.d.). In *Macmillan Online Dictionary*. Retrieved from http://www.macmillandictionary.com/dictionary/british/lifelong-learning

Linden, T. C., Jackson, C., Rutledge, S., Nath, C., & Lof, L. N. (2010). The heart of Grinnell: A community–wide rural health wellness initiative: A pilot observational study and a prospective study design. *The Journal of Alternative Therapies*, *16*(4), 46–49. PMID:20653295

Lindh, D. (2013). *Workplace stress, Mindfulness Based Stress Reduction (MBSR) and Gas Discharge Visualization (GDV): Innovative practical measurements in Organization Development (OD) and employee wellness* [Doctoral dissertation].

Lin, K. Y., Hu, Y. T., Chang, K. J., Lin, H. F., & Tsauo, J. Y. (2011). Effects of yoga on psychological health, quality of life, and physical health of patients with cancer: A meta- analysis. *Evidence-Based Complementary and Alternative Medicine*. PMID:21437197

Livingston, D. W. (2002). Lifelong learning and underemployment in the knowledge society: A North American perspective. In R. Edwards, N. Miller, N. Small, & A. Tait (Eds.), *Supporting lifelong learning* (Vol. 3, pp. 50–75). New York, NY: RoutledgeFalmer.

Lloyd, A., Brett, D., & Wesnes, K. (2010). Coherence training in children with attention-deficit hyperactivity disorder: Cognitive functions and behavioral changes. *Alternatives Therapies*, *16*(4), 34–42. PMID:20653294

Locke, E. A., & Latham, G. P. (2002). Building a practically useful theory of goal setting and task motivation: A 35-year odyssey. *The American Psychologist*, *57*(9), 705–717. doi:10.1037/0003-066X.57.9.705 PMID:12237980

Loeser, J. (2014). Values, character, & moral education.

Long, J. K. (2004). Medical art therapy: Using imagery and visual expression in healing. In P. M. Camic & S. J. Knight (Eds.), *Clinical handbook of health psychology; a practical guide to effective interventions* (2nd ed., pp. 315–342). Portland, OR: Ringgold Inc.

Longworth, N. (1999). *Making lifelong work: Learning cities for a learning century*. Sterling, VA: Kogan Page.

Lopez, A. D., Mathers, C. D., Ezzatti, M., Jamison, D. T., & Murray, C. J. L. (2006). Global and regional burden of disease and risk factors, 2001: Systematic analysis of population health data. *Lancet*, *367*(9524), 1747–1757. doi:10.1016/S0140-6736(06)68770-9 PMID:16731270

Lopez, A. D., Shibuya, K., & Rao, C. (2006). Chronic obstructive pulmonary disease: Current burden and future projections. *The European Respiratory Journal*, *27*(2), 397–412. doi:10.1183/09031936.06.00025805 PMID:16452599

Lorig, K. R., Chastain, R. L., Ung, E., Shoor, E., & Holtman, H. R. (1989). Development and evaluation of a scale to measure perceived self-efficacy in people with arthritis. *Arthritis and Rheumatism*, *32*(1), 37–44. doi:10.1002/anr.1780320107 PMID:2912463

Lorig, K. R., & Holman, R. H. (2003). Self-management education: History, definition, outcomes, and mechanisms. *Annals of Behavioral Medicine*, *26*(1), 1–7. doi:10.1207/S15324796ABM2601_01 PMID:12867348

Lorig, K. R., Sobel, D. S., Stewart, A. L., Brown, B. W. Jr, Ritter, P. L., González, V. M., & Holman, H. R. et al. (1999). Evidence suggesting that a chronic disease self- management program can improve health status while reducing utilization and costs: A randomized trial. *Medical Care*, *37*(1), 5–14. doi:10.1097/00005650-199901000-00003 PMID:10413387

Lorig, K. R., Stewart, A. L., Gonzalez, V. M., Laurent, D. D., & Lynch, J. (1996). *Outcome Measures for Health Education and Other Health Care Interventions*. Thousand Oaks, CA: Sage Publications.

Lott, D. (1988). Feeding wild animals: The urge, the interaction, and the consequences. *Anthrozoos*, *1*(4), 255–257. doi:10.2752/089279388787058326

Louv, R. (2008). *Last child in the woods: Saving our children from nature-deficit disorder*. Chapel Hill, NC: Algonquin Books.

Lumeng, J., Appugliese, D., Cabral, H. J., Bradley, R. H., & Zuckerman, B. (2006). Neighborhood safety and overweight status in children. *Archives of Pediatrics & Adolescent Medicine*, *160*(1), 25–31. doi:10.1001/archpedi.160.1.25 PMID:16389207

Luthans, F., & Avolio, B. J. (2003). Authentic leadership: A positive developmental approach. In K. S. Cameron, J. E. Dutton, & R. E. Quinn (Eds.), *Positive organizational scholarship* (pp. 241–261). San Francisco: Barrett-Koehler.

Maas, J., Verheij, R. A., Groenewegen, P. P., De Vries, S., & Spreeuwenberg, P. (2006). Green space, urbanity, and health: How strong is the relation? *Journal of Epidemiology and Community Health*, *60*(7), 587–592. doi:10.1136/jech.2005.043125 PMID:16790830

Madigan, S. (2011). *Narrative therapy*. Washington, DC: American Psychological Association.

Magee Rehabilitation. (2013). Maggee rehabilitation art therapy program becomes a community partner of Philadelphia museum of art. Retrieved from: http://www.mageerehab.org/page.php?id=1420

Magidson, J. F., Roberts, B. W., Collado-Rodriguez, A., & Lejuez, C. W. (2014). Theory driven intervention for changing personality: Expectancy value theory, behavioral activation, and conscientiousness. *Developmental Psychology*, *50*(5), 1442–1450. doi:10.1037/a0030583 PMID:23106844

Magnusson, D. (1996). Interactionism and the person approach in developmental psychology. *European Child & Adolescent Psychiatry*, *5*(S1), 18–22. doi:10.1007/BF00538538 PMID:9010658

Malchiodi, C. (1999). Art therapy, arts medicine, and arts in healthcare: A vision for collaboration in the next millennium. *International Journal of Arts Medicine*, *6*(2), 13–16.

Malchiodi, C. A. (Ed.), (2013). *Art therapy and health care*. New York: Guilford Press.

Mann, D. (2010). *Gestalt therapy: 100 key points & techniques* (1st ed.). New York: Routledge.

Marquardt, M. J. (2011). *Building the learning organization: Achieving strategic advantage through a commitment to learning* (3rd ed.). Boston, MA: Nicholas Brealey.

Martimiianakis, M.A., Michalec, B., Lam, J., Cartmill, C., Taylor, J.S., & Hafferty, F.W. (2015). Humanism, the hidden curriculum, and educational reform: A scoping review and thematic analysis. *Academic Medicine,* 90(11), S5-S13. doi:10.1097/ACM.0000000000000894

Martin, F., & Farnum, J.Martin & Farnum. (2002, October). Animal-assisted therapy for children with pervasive developmental disorders. *Western Journal of Nursing Research, 24*(6), 657–670. doi:10.1177/019394502320555403 PMID:12365766

Maslow, A. (1954). *Motivation and personality*. New York, NY: Harper.

Maslow, A. H. (1943). A theory of human motivation. *Psychological Review, 50*(4), 370–396. doi:10.1037/h0054346

Mathieu, R.A., Powell-Wiley, T.M., Ayers, C., McGuire, D.K., Khera, A., & Das, S.R., & Lakoski, S. G. (2012). Physical activity participation, health perceptions, and cardiovascular disease mortality in a multiethnic population: The Dallas Heart Study. *American Heart Journal, 163*(6), 1037–1040. doi:10.1016/j.ahj.2012.03.005 PMID:22709758

Mazotti, L., O'Brien, B., Tong, L., & Hauer, K.E. (2011). Perceptions of evaluation in longitudinal versus traditional clerkships. *Medical Education, 45*(5), 464-470. doi:10.1111/j.1365-2923.2010.03904.x

McCain, J. (1999). *Faith of my fathers*. New York, NY: Random House.

McClelland, D. C. (1961). *The achieving society*. Princeton, NJ: D Van Nostrand; doi:10.1037/14359-000

McCleskey, J. (2013). The dark side of leadership: Measurement, assessment, and intervention. *Business Renaissance Quarterly, 8*(2), 35–53.

McConnachie, M. M., & Shackleton, C. M. (2010). Public green space inequality in small towns in South Africa. *Habitat International, 34*(2), 244–248. doi:10.1016/j.habitatint.2009.09.009

McCown, D., & Reibel, D. (2010). Mindfulness and mindfulness-based stress reduction. Integrative psychiatry (pp. 289–338). New York, NY: Oxford University Press. Retrieved from http://search.proquest.com/docview/622134155?accountid=4840

McCraty, R., Atkinson, M., & Tomasino, D. (2003). Impact of a workplace stress reduction program on blood pressure and emotional health in hypertensive employees. *Journal of Alternative and Complementary Medicine, 9*(3), 355–369. doi:10.1089/107555303765551589 PMID:12816624

McCraty, R., & Childre, D. (2010). Coherence: Bridging personal, social and global health. *The Journal of Alternative Therapies, 16*(4), 10–22. PMID:20653292

McCraty, R., & Zayas, M. A. (2014). Cardiac coherence, self-regulation, autonomic stability, and psychosocial well-being. *Frontiers in Psychology, 5*, 1–12. doi:10.3389/fpsyg.2014.01090 PMID:25324802

McDaniel, A., & Robertson, K. (1995). Interdisciplinary professional education: A collaborative clinical teaching project. *American Journal of Pharmaceutical Education, 59*(2), 131–136.

McDermott, M. S., & While, A. E. (2013). Maximizing the healthcare environment: A systematic review exploring the potential of computer technology to promote self-management of chronic illness in healthcare settings. *Patient Education and Counseling, 92*(1), 13–22. doi:10.1016/j.pec.2013.02.014 PMID:23566427

McDowell, G. R. (2001). *Land grant universities and extension into the 21st Century: Renegotiating or abandoning a social contract*. Hoboken, NJ: Wiley-Blackwell.

McEwen, B. S. (2005). Stressed or stressed out: What is the difference? *Journal of Psychiatry & Neuroscience*, *30*(5), 315–318. PMID:16151535

McNutt, J. V. (2013). Art therapy as a form of visual narrative in oncology care. In C. A. Malchiodi (Ed.), *Art therapy and health care* (pp. 127–135). New York: Guilford Press.

McVicar, M. (2015). Decisions in crisis - An examination. *Comparative Strategy*, *34*(1), 14–43. doi:10.1080/01495933.2015.994403

Mehta, M. (2012). Situational leadership and personal effectiveness: Managers in Indian development organizations. *Foundation for Organizational Research & Education*, *30*(1), 23–34.

Melchior, M. A., Seff, L. R., Albatineh, A. N., McCoy, H. V., Page, T. F., & Palmer, R. C. (2014). Intermediate outcomes of chronic disease self-management program offered by members of the Healthy Aging Regional Collaborative in South Florida. *Research on Aging*, *36*(4), 431–449. doi:10.1177/0164027513500054 PMID:25651315

Melson, G. F. (1991). Children's attachment to their pets: Links to socioemotional development. *Children's Environments Quarterly*, *82*, 55–65.

Melson, G. F. (2003). Child development and the human-companion animal bond. *The American Behavioral Scientist*, *47*(31), 31–39. doi:10.1177/0002764203255210

Memorandum on Lifelong Learning. (2007). *European society of association executives.* Retrieved from http://www.esae.org/articles/2007_08_005.pdf

Memorial Sloan Kettering Cancer Center (MSKCC) Bendheim Integrative Medicine Center. (2015). Nutritional and dietary-supplement counseling. Retrieved from: https://www.mskcc.org/locations/bendheim-integrative-medicine

Memorial Sloan Kettering Cancer Center (MSKCC) Integrative Medicine. (2015). About herbs, botanicals, and other products. Retrieved from https://www.mskcc.org/cancer-care/treatments/symptom-management/integrative-medicine/expertise

Menasche, D. (2013). *The priority list*. New York, NY: Touchstone.

Mentgen, J. (2002). Healing touch. *The Nursing Clinics of North America*, *36*(1), 143–157.

Merrifield, J. (2012). *Ecologies of learning: How culture and context impact outcomes of workplace literacy and essential skills*. Montreal, QC, Canada: Centre for Literacy of Quebec.

Messent, P. R. (1983). Social facilitation of contact with other people with pet dogs. In A. H. B. Katcher & M. Alan (Eds.), *New perspectives on our lives with companion animals* (pp. 351–359). Philadelphia: University of Pennsylvania Press.

Metcalf, J. A. (2014). *The challenges of replicating human resource (HR) practices in a global environment: A qualitative study of HR leaders in a manufacturing company* (Order No. AAI3602346).

Meyer, H.E., Tverdal, A., & Falch, J.A. (1993). Risk factors for hip fracture in middle-aged Norwegian women and men. *American Journal of Epidemiology*, *137*, 1203–1211.

Michel, A., Bosch, C., & Rexroth, M. (2014). Mindfulness as a cognitive-emotional segmentation strategy: An intervention promoting work-life balance. *Journal of Occupational and Organizational Psychology*, *87*(4), 733–754. doi:10.1111/joop.12072

Michele, L. (2015). *You first: journal your way to your best life*. New York, NY: Crown Archetype.

Mikulciner, M., Florian, V., Cowan, P. A., & Cowan, C. P. (2002). Attachment security in couple relationships: A systematic model and its implications for family dynamics. *Family Process*, *41*(3), 405–434. doi:10.1111/j.1545-5300.2002.41309.x PMID:12395567

Mikulincer, M. (1998). Attachment working models and the sense of trust: An exploration of interaction goals and affect regulation. *Journal of Personality and Social Psychology*, *74*(5), 1209–1224. doi:10.1037/0022-3514.74.5.1209

Millan, R. O. (2008). *Examining emotional intelligence differences among nursing students at a college in South Texas* (Doctoral dissertation).

Miller, W. R., & Rollnick, S. (2002). *Motivational interviewing* (2nd ed.). New York, NY: The Guilford Press.

Miner, W. (2007). Training massage therapists to work in oncology. *Journal of the Society for Integrative Oncology*, *5*(4), 163–166. doi:10.2310/7200.2007.015 PMID:19087760

Ministry of Health & Family Welfare (MoHFW). (1983c). *National Health Policy*. New Delhi: Government of India.

Ministry of Health & Family Welfare (MoHFW). (2004b). *Integrated Disease Surveillance Project: Project Implementation Plan 2004–09*. New Delhi: Government of India.

Ministry of Health & Family Welfare (MoHFW). (2014a). Draft National Health Policy, 2015, Government of India, New Delhi.

Ministry of Health & Family Welfare (MoHFW). (2014d). *Draft National Health Policy, 2015*. New Delhi: Government of India.

Mink, M. (2012, October 17). Gain the right direction. *Investor's Business Daily*.

Mirmiran, P., Bahadoran, Z., & Azizi, F. (2014). Functional foods-based diet as a novel dietary approach for management of type 2 diabetes and its complications: A review. *World J. Diabetes*, *5*(3), 267–281. doi:10.4239/wjd.v5.i3.267 PMID:24936248

Moadel, A. (2010). Einstein on Cancer: Dr. Alyson Moadel. Psychosocial oncology: Coping with cancer. Bronx, NY: Albert Einstein College of Medicine. Retrieved from http://www.einstein.yu.edu/video/?VID=259#top

Moadel, A. B., Shah, C., & Sisco, R. (2009). Description of the Yoga-based Cancer Rehabilitation Program of the Montefiore-Einstein Cancer Center. Retrieved from: https://www.einstein.yu.edu/docs/faculty/profiles/479-alyson-moadel/integral-hatha-yoga-protocol-description-MECC-rehab-ca-pgm.pdf

Moberg, C. R., & Leasher, M. (2011). Examining the differences in salesperson motivation among different cultures. *American Journal of Business*, *26*(2), 145–160. doi:10.1108/19355181111174525

Monti, D. A., Peterson, C., Kunkel, E. J. S., Hauck, W. W., Pequignot, E., Rhodes, L., & Brainard, G. C. (2006). A randomized, controlled trial of mindfulness-based art therapy (MBAT) for women with cancer. *Psycho-Oncology*, *15*(5), 363–373. doi:10.1002/pon.988 PMID:16288447

Moss Rehab. (2012). Art therapy program. Retrieved from http://www.mossrehab.com/special-services/mossrehab-outpatient-art-therapy-program.html

Mroczek, D. (2014). Personality plasticity, healthy aging, and interventions. *Developmental Psychology*, *50*(5), 1470–1474. doi:10.1037/a0036028 PMID:24773109

Mudur, G. (2004). Inadequate Regulations Undermine India's Healthcare. British Medical Journal (BMJ), 2004, 124, 328.

Muo, I. (2013). Motivating and managing knowledge workers: Evidences from diverse industries and cultures. *Journal of Management and Sustainability, 3*(2), 119-131. doi:10.5539/jms.v3n2p119

Murray, C. J. L., & Lopez, A. D. (1997). Alternative projections of mortality and disability by cause 1990-2020; Global Burden of Disease Study. *Lancet, 349*(9064), 1498–1504. doi:10.1016/S0140-6736(96)07492-2 PMID:9167458

Muscalu, E., & Muntean, S. (2013). Motivation a stimulating factor for increasing human resource management performance. *Review of International Comparative Management, 14*(2), 303–309.

Museum of Fine Arts Boston. (2015). Artful healing. Retrieved from http://www.mfa.org/programs/community-programs/artful-healing

Nagengast, S. L., Baun, M. M., Megel, M., & Leibowitz, J. (1997). The effects of the presence of a companion animal on physiological arousal and behavioral distress in children during a physical examination. *Journal of Pediatric Nursing, 12*(6), 323–330. doi:10.1016/S0882-5963(97)80058-9 PMID:9420370

Nainis, N. A. (2008). Approaches to art therapy for cancer inpatients: Research and practice Considerations. *Journal of the American Art Therapy Association, 25*(3), 115–121. doi:10.1080/07421656.2008.10129597

Nainis, N., Paice, J. A., Ratner, J., Wirth, J. H., Lai, J., & Shott, S. (2006). Relieving symptoms in cancer: Innovative use of art therapy. *Journal of Pain and Symptom Management, 31*(2), 162–169. doi:10.1016/j.jpainsymman.2005.07.006 PMID:16488349

Namie, G., & Namie, R. (2003). *The bully at work: What you can do to stop the hurt and reclaim your dignity on the job.* Naperville, IL: Sourcebooks.

Nandan, D., & Agarwal, D. (2012). Human resources for health in India: Urgent need for reforms. *Indian Journal of Community Medicine, 37*(4), 205–206. doi:10.4103/0970-0218.103464 PMID:23293430

Narayan, D., Patel, R., Schafft, K., Rademacher, A., & Koch-Schulte, S. (2000). Changing gender relations in the household. In *Voices of the Poor: Can Anyone Hear Us?* New York, NY: Oxford University Press. doi:10.1596/0-1952-1601-6

National Alliance on Mental Illness- NAMI. (2015). Mental health by the numbers. Retrieved from https://www.nami.org/Learn-More/Mental-Health-By-the-Numbers

National Center for Education Statistics. (n. d.). *What is NAAL?* Retrieved from https://nces.ed.gov/naal/

National Center for Interprofessional Practice and Education. (2015). *About the national center.* Retrieved from https://nexusipe.org/informing/about-national-center

National Coordinating Council for Medication Error and Prevention. (2016). *About medication errors.* Retrieved from http://www.nccmerp.org/about-medication-errors

National Heart, Lung, and Blood Institute. (2015). Description of the DASH eating plan. National Institutes of Health. U.S. Department of Health & Human Services. Retrieved from http://www.nhlbi.nih.gov/health/health-topics/topics/dash/

National Institute on Drug Abuse (NIDA). (2015). *DrugFacts: Prescription and over-the-counter medications.* Washington, D.C.: National Institute of Health.

National Population Policy. (2000). National Health Portal, Government of India, New Delhi. Retrieved from http://www.nhp.gov.in/national-population-policy-2000_pg

National Sample Survey Organization (NSSO), Department of Statistics: Government of India, 42nd round (1986-87).

National Sample Survey Organization (NSSO), Department of Statistics: Government of India, 52nd round (1995-96).

Naylor, M. D., & Keating, S. K. (2008). Transitional care: Movement from one care setting to another. *The American Journal of Nursing*, *108*(S9), 58–63. doi:10.1097/01.NAJ.0000336420.34946.3a PMID:18797231

Neelam, R. (2006, March 29). Sex Selection is High-Volume, Low-Risk Biz. *The Times of India* (New Delhi).

Neff, K. (2011). *Self compassion: the proven power of being kind to yourself.* New York, NY: HarperCollins.

Neithercott, T. (2014). A Mediterranean food plan can protect health. Diabetes Forecast: The Healthy Living Magazine. Alexandria, VA: American Diabetes Association. Retrieved from http://www.diabetesforecast.org/2014/08-aug/a-mediterranean-food-plan-can.html?loc=ymal

Nelson, C., Fox, N., & Zeanah, C. (2013). The Anguish of the abandoned Child. Retrieved from http://www.adoption-policy.org/sad0413Nels3pRV.pdf

Něměčková, I. (2012). Education as employee motivation and retention factor of the companies operating in the Czech Republic. *Central European Business Review*, *1*(1), 33–37. doi:10.18267/j.cebr.6

New Economic Foundation. (2012, November). *Well being patterns uncovered* [Report]. London, UK: New Economic Foundation.

Newton, B.W., Barber, L., Clardy, J., Cleveland, E., & O'Sullivan, P. (2008). Is there hardening of the heart during medical school? *Academic Medicine, 83*(3), 244-249. doi:10.1097/acm.0b013e3181637837

Norris, T.E., Schaad, D.C., DeWitt, D., Ogur, B., Hunt, D.D., & Consortium of Longitudinal Integrated Clerkships. (2009). Longitudinal integrated clerkships for medical students: An innovation adopted by medical schools in Australia, Canada, South Africa, and the United States. *Academic Medicine, 84*(7), 902-907. doi:10.1097/acm.0b013e3181a85776

Northouse, P. G. (2012). *Introduction to leadership: Concepts and practice*. Los Angeles, CA: Sage.

O'Brien, T. (1990). *The things they carried.* New York, NY: Broadway Books.

O'Connell, T., Rasanathan, K., & Chopra, M. (2014). What does universal health coverage mean? *Lancet*, *383*(9913), 277–279. doi:10.1016/S0140-6736(13)60955-1 PMID:23953765

Odendaal, J. S. J. (2000). Animal-assisted therapy -- magic or medicine? *Journal of Psychosomatic Research*, *49*(4), 275–280. doi:10.1016/S0022-3999(00)00183-5 PMID:11119784

Office of the National Education Commission. (1999). *National Education act BE 2542. office of the prime minister Kingdom of Thailand.* Retrieved from http://www.onesqa.or.th/en/publication/nation_edbook.pdf

Ogden, C. L., Carroll, M. D., Kit, B. K., & Flegal, K. M. (2014). Prevalence of Childhood and Adult Obesity in the United States, 2011-2012. *Journal of the American Medical Association*, *311*(8), 806–814. doi:10.1001/jama.2014.732 PMID:24570244

Ogur, B., Hirsh, D., Krupat, E., & Bor, D. (2007). The Harvard Medical School-Cambridge integrated clerkship: An innovative model of clinical education. *Academic Medicine, 82*(4), 397-404. Retrieved from: 10.1097/acm.0b013e31803338f0

Olson, P. N. (2002). The modern working dog: A call for interdisciplinary collaboration. *Journal of the American Medical Association*, *221*(3), 352–355. doi:10.2460/javma.2002.221.352 PMID:12164529

Omachonu, V.K. & Einspruch, N.G., (2010), Innovation in Healthcare Delivery Systems: A Conceptual Framework. The Innovation Journal: The Public Sector Innovation Journal, Volume 15(1), Article 2

Ortiz, A. (2015, February). Humane liberation: Incorporating animal rights into critical pedagogy. *The Vermont Connection*, *32*, 67–77.

Ory, M. G., Anh, S. N., Jiang, L., Lorig, K., Ritter, P., Laurent, D. D., & Smith, M. L. et al. (2013). National Study of Chronic Disease Self-Management: Six-Month Outcome Findings. *Journal of Aging and Health*, *25*(7), 1258–1274. doi:10.1177/0898264313502531 PMID:24029414

Öster, I., Egberg Thyme, K., Sundin, E. C., & Lindh, J. (2009). Individual brief art therapy can be helpful for women with breast cancer. *Palliative & Supportive Care*, *7*(1), 87–95. doi:10.1017/S147895150900011X PMID:19619378

Panda, A., Arjona, A., Sapey, E., Bai, F., Fikrig, E., Montgomery, R. R., & Shaw, A. C. et al. (2009). Human innate immunosenescence: Causes and consequences for immunity in old age. *Trends in Immunology*, *30*(7), 325–333. doi:10.1016/j.it.2009.05.004 PMID:19541535

Panksepp, J. (2007). Can PLAY Diminish ADHD and Facilitate the Construction of the Social Brain? *Journal of the Canadian Academy of Child and Adolescent Psychiatry*, *16*(2), 57–66. PMID:18392153

Pan, L., Yan, J., Guo, Y., & Yan, J. (2013). Effects of Tai Chi training on exercise capacity an quality of life in patients with chronic heart failure: A meta-analysis. *European Journal of Heart Failure*, *15*(3), 316–323. PMID:23099355

Parents and teachers. (2015). Retrieved from http://www.paws.org/kids/parents-and-teachers/

Parker, R. (2000). Health literacy: A challenge for American patients and their healthcare providers. *Health Promotion International*, *15*(4), 277–283. doi:10.1093/heapro/15.4.277

Parks, J., & Svedsen, D. (2006). *Morbidity and mortality in people with serious mental illness*. Alexandria, VA: National Association of State Mental Health Program Directors.

Patel, V., Chatterji, S., Chisholm, D., Shah, E., Gopalakrishna, G., Mathers, C., & Reddy, K. S. et al. (2011). Chronic diseases and injuries in India. *Lancet*, *377*, 413–428. doi:10.1016/S0140-6736(10)61188-9 PMID:21227486

Patient Protection and Affordable Care Act, 42 U.S.C. § 18001 (2010).

Patricelli, K., & Dombeck, M. (Eds.). (2015). Grief is a normal and natural process. *Making a difference in your community every day*. Aroostook, ME: Aroostook Mental Health Center (AMHC). Retrieved from http://www.amhc.org/58-grief-bereavement-issues/article/8442-grief-is-a-normal-and-natural-process

Patricelli, K., & Dombeck, M. (Eds.). (2015). Introduction to grief and bereavement issues. *Making a difference in your community every day*. Aroostook, ME: Aroostook Mental Health Center (AMHC). Retrieved from http://www.amhc.org/58-grief-bereavement-issues/article/8441-introduction-to-grief-and-bereavement-issues

Paul, G., Elam, B., & Vehulst, S. (2007). A longitudinal study of student's perceptions of using deep breathing meditation to reduce testing stress. *Teaching and Learning in Medicine: An International Journal*, *19*(3), 287–292. doi:10.1080/10401330701366754 PMID:17594225

Pauwels, R. A., Buist, A. S., Calverley, P. M. A., Jenkins, C. R., & Hurd, S. S. (2001). Global strategy for the diagnosis, management, and prevention of chronic obstructive pulmonary disease: National Heart Lung and Blood Institute and World Health Organization Global Initiative for Chronic Obstructive Lung Disease (GOLD): executive summary. *Respiratory Care*, *46*(8), 798–825. PMID:11463370

Payne, R. A., & Avery, A. J. (2011). Polypharmacy: One of the greatest prescribing challenges in general practice. *The British Journal of General Practice*, *61*(583), 83–84. doi:10.3399/bjgp11X556146 PMID:21276330

Pennebaker, J. W. (1997). *Opening up: the healing power of expressing emotions*. New York, NY: The Guilford Press.

Pennebaker, J. W., & Evans, J. F. (2014). *Expressive writing: words that heal*. Enumclaw, WA: Idyll Arbor.

Peters, J. M., & Bell, B. (2001). Horton of Highlander. In P. Jarvis (Ed.), *Twentieth century thinkers in adult education* (pp. 242–257). New York, NY: Croom Helm. doi:10.3998/mpub.16549

Peters, R. K., Benson, H., & Peters, J. M. (1977). Daily relaxation response breaks in a working population: 2. Blood pressure. *American Journal of Public Health*, *67*(10), 954–959. doi:10.2105/AJPH.67.10.954 PMID:333958

Pfohl, M., & Schatz, H. (2001). Strategies for the prevention of type 2 diabetes. *Experimental and Clinical Endocrinology & Diabetes*, *109*(Suppl. 2), S240–S249. doi:10.1055/s-2001-18585 PMID:11460574

Philipp, S. F. (1995). Race and leisure constraints. *Leisure Sciences*, *17*(2), 109–120. doi:10.1080/01490409509513247

Philipp, S. F. (1997). Race, gender, and leisure benefits. *Leisure Sciences*, *19*(3), 191–207. doi:10.1080/01490409709512249

Pieterse, A. H., Baas-Thijssen, M. C. M., Marijnen, C. A. M., & Stiggelbout, A. M. (2008). Clinician and cancer patient views on patient participation in treatment decision-making: A quantitative and qualitative exploration. *British Journal of Cancer*, *99*(6), 875–882. doi:10.1038/sj.bjc.6604611 PMID:18781148

Piet, J., Wurtzen, H., & Zachariae, R. (2012). The effect of mindfulness-based therapy on symptoms of anxiety and depression in adult cancer patients and survivors: A systematic review and meta-analysis. *Journal of Consulting and Clinical Psychology*, *80*(6), 1007–1020. doi:10.1037/a0028329 PMID:22563637

Pimouguet, C., LeGoff, M., Thiebaut, R., Dartigues, J.F., & Helmer, C. (2011). Effectiveness of disease-management programs for improving diabetes care: A meta-analysis. *Canadian Medical Association Journal, 183(2)*, E115.

Pink, D. (2009). *Drive*. New York, NY: Riverhead Books.

Pink, D. H. (2009). *Drive: The surprising truth about what motivates us*. New York, NY: Riverhead Books.

Pinquart, M., & Sorensen, S. (2003). Differences between caregivers and noncaregivers in psychological health and physical health: A meta-analysis. *Psychology and Aging*, *18*(2), 250–267. doi:10.1037/0882-7974.18.2.250 PMID:12825775

Planning Commission of India. (2011). High level expert group report on universal health coverage for India. Retrieved from http://planningcommission.nic.in/reports/genrep/rep_uhc0812.pdf

Plichta, S. B. (2004). Intimate partner violence and physical health consequences: Policy and practice implications. *Journal of Interpersonal Violence*, *19*(11), 1296–1323. doi:10.1177/0886260504269685 PMID:15534333

Poggi, E. (2006). Beyond traditional treatment: Establishing art as therapy. *Healthcare Design*, *6*(7), 23–25.

Poncelet, A., Bokser, S., Calton, B., Hauer, K.E., Kirsch, H., Jones, T., . . . Robertson, P. (2011). Development of a longitudinal integrated clerkship at an academic medical center. *Medical Education Online, 16*. doi:10.3402/meo.v16i0.5939

Poncelet, A.N., Mazotti, L.A., Blumberg, B., Wamsley, M.A., Grennan, T., & Shore, W.B. (2014). Creating a longitudinal integrated clerkship with mutual benefits for an academic medical center and a community health system. *Permanente Journal*, 18(2), 50–56. doi:10.7812/tpp/13-137

Ponde, P. M., & Santana, S. V. (2000). Participation in leisure activities: Is it a protective factor for women's mental health? *Journal of Leisure Research*, *32*(4), 457–472.

Prakash, I. J. (1997). Women and Ageing. *The Indian Journal of Medical Research*, *106*, 396–408. PMID:9361474

Prasad, K., Sharma, V., Lackore, K., Sarah, M., Jenkins, S. M., Prasad, A., & Sood, A. (2010). Use of complementary therapies in cardiovascular disease. *The American Journal of Cardiology*, *111*(3), 339–345. doi:10.1016/j.amjcard.2012.10.010 PMID:23186602

Prevention Institute. (2007). *The California Endowment: Reducing health care costs through prevention*. Oakland, CA: The Prevention Institute.

Prevention Institute. (2010). *Addressing the intersection: Preventing violence and promoting healthy eating and active living*. Oakland, CA: The Prevention Institute.

Prevention Institute. (2011). *Unity fact sheet: Violence and chronic illness*. Retrieved from www.preventioninstitute.org/unity

Prideaux, D., Worley, P., & Bligh, J. (2007). Symbiosis: A new model for clinical education. *Clinical Teacher, 4*(4), 209-212. doi:10.1111/j.1743-498x.2007.00188.x

Pritchett, L., & Natrajan, G. (2015), Putting the 'Universal in Healthcare' Retrieved from http://indianexpress.com/article/opinion/columns/putting-the-universal-in-healthcare/

Project RED. (2014). *Project RED (re-engineered discharge)*. Retrieved from http://www.bu.edu/fammed/projectred/

Puig, A., Lee, S. M., Goodwin, L., & Sherrard, P. A. D. (2006). The efficacy of creative arts therapies to enhance emotional expression, spirituality, and psychological well-being of newly diagnosed stage I and stage II breast cancer patients: A preliminary study. *The Arts in Psychotherapy*, *33*(3), 218–228. doi:10.1016/j.aip.2006.02.004

Quindlen, A. (2004). *Loud and clear*. New York, NY: Ballentine Books.

Racine, E., Troyer, J. L., Warren-Findlow, J., & McCauley, W. J. (2011). The effect of medical nutrition therapy on changes in dietary knowledge and DASH diet adherence in older adults with cardiovascular disease. *The Journal of Nutrition, Health & Aging*, *15*(10), 868–876. doi:10.1007/s12603-011-0102-9 PMID:22159775

Ramachandran, R. (2015, October 16). For private plunder. Frontline, 16-20.

Rankin, L. (2013). *Mind over medicine*. Carlsbad, CA: Hay House.

Rankin, L. (2015a). *The fear cure*. Carlsbad, CA: Hay House.

Rankin, L. (2015b). *The anatomy of a calling*. New York, NY: Rodale.

Ratanasiripong, P., Ratanasiripong, N., & Kathalae, D. (2012). Biofeedback intervention for stress and anxiety among nursing students: A randomized controlled study. *International Scholarly Research Network*. Retrieved from http://www.heartmath.com/wp-content/uploads/2014/04/biofeedback_intervention_stress_nursing_students.pdf

Ratanasiripong, P., Sverduk, K., Prince, J., & Hayashino, D. (2012). Biofeedback and counseling for stress and anxiety among college students. *Journal of College Student Development*, *53*(5), 742–749. doi:10.1353/csd.2012.0070

Ratey, J. (2013). *Spark*. Boston, MA: Little, Brown and Company.

Raye, J. (2014). Fractal organisation theory. *Organisational Transformation and Social Change*, *11*(1), 50–68. doi:10.1179/1477963313Z.00000000025

Reading to dogs: A library's guide to getting started. (2015). Retrieved from http://readingtodogs.weebly.com/research.html

Reig-Ferrer, A., Ferrer-Cascales, R., Santos-Ruiz, A., Campos-Ferrer, A., Prieto-Seva, A., Velasco-Ruiz, I., & Albaladejo-Blazquez, N. et al. (2014). A relaxation techniques enhances psychological well-being and immune parameters in elderly people from a nursing home: A randomized controlled study. *BMC Complementary and Alternative Medicine*, *14*(1), 311. doi:10.1186/1472-6882-14-311 PMID:25151398

Research Starters. (2010). *The mutt-i-grees curriculum*. Port Washington, New York: The Petsavers Foundation.

Rhondali, W., Rhondali, W., & Lasserre. (2013). Art therapy among palliative care inpatients with advanced cancer. *Palliative Medicine, 27*(6), 571; 571-572; 572.

Riaz, M. N., Riaz, M. A., & Batool, N. (2014). Managerial decision making styles as predictors of personal and organizational outcomes of in-service employees. *Journal of Behavioural Science*, *24*(2), 100–116.

Riddick, C. C., & Stewart, D. G. (1994). An examination of the life satisfaction and importance of older female retirees: A comparison of blacks to whites. *Journal of Leisure Research*, *26*(1), 75–87.

Risely-Curtiss, C. (2010). Social work practitioners and the human-companion animal bond: A national study. *Social Work*, *55*(1), 38–46. doi:10.1093/sw/55.1.38 PMID:20069939

Robbins, S. P., DeCenzo, D. A., & Wolter, R. (2013). *Supervision today?* (7th ed.). Upper Saddle River, NJ: Pearson.

Robertson, B. J. (1994). An investigation of leisure in the lives of adolescents who engage in delinquent behavior for fun, thrills, and excitement. *Dissertation Abstracts International. A, The Humanities and Social Sciences*, *54*(12-A), 4587.

Robertson, B. J. (1999). Leisure and family: Perspectives of male adolescents who engage in delinquent activity as leisure. *Journal of Leisure Research*, *31*(4), 335.

Roberts, S., Camic, P. M., & Springham, N. (2011). New roles for art galleries: Art-viewing as a community intervention for family carers of people with mental health problems. *Arts & Health: An International Journal for Research. Policy & Practice*, *3*(2), 146–159.

Rogers, A. (1992). Adults Learning for Development. Cassell Educational Limited, 387 Park Avenue South, New York, NY.

Rohrer, J. E., Arif, A. A., Pierce, J. R. Jr, & Blackburn, C. (2004). Unsafe neighborhoods, social group activity, and self-rated health. *Journal of Public Health Management and Practice*, *10*(2), 124–129. doi:10.1097/00124784-200403000-00006 PMID:14967979

Rollnick, S., Miller, W. R., & Butler, C. C. (2008). *Motivational interviewing in health care: helping patients change behavior*. New York, NY: The Guilford Press.

Romano, T. (1987). *Clearing the way*. Portsmouth, NH: Heinemann.

Romano, T. (1995). *Writing with passion*. Portsmouth, NH: Heinemann.

Romano, T. (2000). *Blending genre, altering style*. Portsmouth, NH: Heinemann.

Romano, T. (2004). *Crafting authentic voice*. Portsmouth, NH: Heinemann.

Romano, T. (2008). *Zigzag*. Portsmouth, NH: Heinemann.

Romano, T. (2013). *Fearless writing*. Portsmouth, NH: Heinemann.

Rosenbach, W. E., Taylor, R. L., & Youndt, M. A. (2012). *Contemporary issues in leadership*. Boulder, CO: Westview Press.

Rosenblatt, B. (2014). Museum education and art therapy: Promoting wellness in older adults. *Journal of Museum Education*, *39*(3), 293–301. doi:10.1080/10598650.2014.11510821

Rosén, L. A., Silva, L. O., Andersson, U. K., Holm, C., Ostman, E. M., & Björck, I. M. (2009). Endosperm and whole grain rye breads are characterized by low post-prandial insulin response and a beneficial blood glucose profile. *Nutrition Journal*, *8*(1), 42. doi:10.1186/1475-2891-8-42 PMID:19781071

Ross, D. B., Matteson, R., & Exposito, J. A. (2014, December). Servant leadership to toxic leadership: Power of influence over power of control. *Paper presented at the Fifth Annual Virtual Conference on Moral Leadership: Narcissism and Toxic Leadership*, Regent University. Paper retrieved from http://www.regent.edu/acad /global/conferences/virtual/2014/papers/2014_Moral_Leadership_Conference _Ross_Matteson_Exposito.pdf

Rostand, E. (1950). *Cyrano de Bergerac*. New York, NY: Bantam. (Original work published 1898).

Rozich, J. D., & Resar, R. K. (2001). Medication safety: One organization's approach to the challenge. *Journal of Clinical Outcomes Management*, *8*(10), 27–34.

Rubert, R., Long, D. L., & Hutchinson, M. L. (2007). Creating a healing environment in the ICU. In R. Kaplow & S. R. Hardin (Eds.), *Critical care nursing; synergy for optimal outcomes (2007)* (pp. 27–39). Portland, OR: Ringold, Inc.

Rubin, J. (2001). *Approaches to art therapy: Theory and technique* (2nd ed.). New York: Brunner-Routledge.

Ruiz-Mercader, J., Merono-Cerdan, A. L., & Sabater-Sanchez, R. (2006). Informational technology and learning: Their relationship and impact on organizational performance in small businesses. Retrieved from papers.ssrn.com/sol3/papers.cfm?abstract_id=1501588

Russack, N. (2000). *Animal guides: In life, myth and dreams*. Toronto, Ontario, Canada: Inner City Books.

Russell, L. M. (2014). An empirical investigation of high-risk occupations. *Management Research Review*, *37*(4), 367–384. doi:10.1108/MRR-10-2012-0227

Russell, R. (1996). *Pastimes: The context of contemporary Leisure*. Madison, WI: Brown & Benchmark.

Ruvolo, A. P., & Brennan, C. J. (1997). What's love got to do with it? Close relationships and perceived growth. *Personality and Social Psychology Bulletin*, *23*(8), 814–823. doi:10.1177/0146167297238003

Ryan, R. M., & Deci, E. L. (2000). Self-determination theory and the facilitation of intrinsic motivation, social development, and well-being. *The American Psychologist*, *55*(1), 68–68. doi:10.1037/0003-066X.55.1.68 PMID:11392867

Rzeznik, J. (1998). Iris [Recorded by Goo Goo Dolls]. On City of angels soundtrack [CD]. Burbank, CA: Warner Brothers.

Sable, P. (2007, December). Accentuating the positive in adult attachments. *Attachment & Human Development*, *9*(4), 361–374. doi:10.1080/14616730701711573 PMID:18049933

Sahrawat, R., & Rao, D. K. (2011). Insured yet vulnerable: Out-of pocket payments and India's poor. *Health Policy and Planning*, 2011, 1–9.

Salamon, E., Bernstein, S. R., Kim, S. A., Kim, M., & Stefano, G. B. (2003). The effects of auditory perception and musical preference on anxiety in naïve human subjects. *Medical Science Monitor*, *9*, R396–CR399. PMID:12960929

Sallis, J. F., Owen, N., & Fisher, E. B. (2008). Ecological models of health behavior. *Health behavior and health education: Theory, research, and practice, 4*, 465-486.

Sallis, J. F., Cervero, R. B., Ascher, W., Henderson, K. A., Kraft, M. K., & Kerr, J. (2006). An ecological approach to creating active living communities. *Annual Review of Public Health*, *27*(1), 297–322. doi:10.1146/annurev.publhealth.27.021405.102100 PMID:16533119

Sandberg, S. (2013). *Lean in*. New York, NY: Alfred A. Knopf.

Santaguida, P. L., Balion, C., Hunt, D., Morrison, K., Gerstein, H., Raina, P., & Yazdi, H. et al. (2005). Diagnosis, prognosis, and treatment of impaired glucose tolerance and impaired fasting glucose. *Evidence Report/Technology Assessment (Summary)*, 128,1–11. PMID:16194123

Schachner, D., Shaver, P., & Mikulincer, M. (2005). Patterns of nonverbal behavior and sensitivity in the contest of attachment relationships. *Journal of Nonverbal Behavior*, *29*(3), 141–169. doi:10.1007/s10919-005-4847-x

Schaefer, K. (2002, January). Human-animal interactions as a therapeutic intervention. *Counseling and Human Development*, *34*(5), 1–18.

Schaffer, C. B. (2009, Winter). Animals connecting people to people: Insights into animal-assisted therapy and animal-assisted activities. *Reflections: The SoL Journal*, *15*(1), 42–45.

Scheier, M., Matthews, J., Owens, J., Magovern, G., Lefebvre, R., Abbott, R., & Carver, C. (1989). Dispositional optimism and recovery from coronary artery bypass surgery: The beneficial effects on physical and psychological well-being. *Journal of Personality and Social Psychology*, *57*(6), 1024–1040. doi:10.1037/0022-3514.57.6.1024 PMID:2614656

Schigelone, A., White, C., & Krupat, E. (2005). *Medical students' attitudes toward the doctor-patient relationship: a cross-sectional study*. Madison, WI: Association of American Medical Colleges Central Group on Educational Affairs.

Schmidt, A. A. (2014). *An examination of toxic leadership, job outcomes, and the impact of military deployment.*

Schultz, J. R. (2014). Creating a culture of empowerment fosters the flexibility to change. *Global Business and Organizational Excellence*, *34*(1), 41–50. doi:10.1002/joe.21583

Schulz, R., Newsom, J., Mittelmark, M., Burton, L., Hirsch, C., & Jackson, S. (1997). Health effects of caregiving: The caregiver health effects study: An ancillary study of the cardiovascular health study. *Annals of Behavioral Medicine*, *19*(2), 110–116. doi:10.1007/BF02883327 PMID:9603685

Schumacher, D. J., Englander, R., & Carraccio, C. (2013). Developing the master learner: Applying learning theory to the learner, the teacher and the learning environment. *Academic Medicine*, *88*(11), 1635–1645. doi:10.1097/ACM.0b013e3182a6e8f8 PMID:24072107

Schvaneveldt, P. L., Young, M. H., Schvaneveldt, J. D., & Kivett, V. R. (2001). Interaction of people and pets in the family setting: A life course perspective. *Journal of Teaching in Marriage & Family*, *1*(2), 34–52. doi:10.1300/J226v01n02_03

Scott, L. (Ed.). (2015). *Learning cities for adult learners. New Directions for Adult and Continuing Education, 145.* San Francisco, CA: Jossey-Bass.

Scott, W. R. (2003). *Organizations*. Upper Saddle River, NJ: Prentice Hall Press.

Script Your Future. (2014). *Script your future program*. Retrieved from http://www.scriptyourfuture.org/wp-content/uploads/2014/11/lessons_learned.pdf

Script Your Future. (2016). *Tools*. Retrieved from http://www.scriptyourfuture.org/tools/

Sebaaly, J., Parsons, L. B., Pilch, N. A., Bullington, W., Hayes, G. L., & Easterling, H. (2015). Clinical and financial impact of pharmacist involvement in discharge medication reconciliation at an academic medical center: A prospective pilot study. *Hospital Pharmacy*, *50*(6), 505–513. doi:10.1310/hpj5006-505 PMID:26405342

Seligman, M. E. P. (2015). Authentic happiness. University of Pennsylvania Positive Psychology Center. Retrieved from https://www.authentichappiness.sas.upenn.edu/content/about-us

Seligman, M. E. P. (2011). *Flourish: A visionary new understanding of happiness and well- being*. New York: Simon and Schuster.

Seligman, M. E. P., & Csikszentmihalyi, M. (2000). Positive psychology: An introduction. *The American Psychologist*, *55*(1), 5–14. doi:10.1037/0003-066X.55.1.5 PMID:11392865

Senge, P. (2006). *The fifth discipline: The art and practice of the learning organization*. New York, NY: Currency Doubleday.

Sensory Processing Disorder Foundation SPDF. (2015). About sensory processing disorder. Retrieved from http://www.spdfoundation.net/about-sensory-processing-disorder/

SEO Services. (2011). *Residential Treatment Center*. Retrieved from http://www.residentialtreatmentcenter.net/

Sepucha, K. R., Belkora, J. K., Mutchnick, S., & Esserman, L. J. (2002). Consultation planning to help breast cancer patients prepare for medical consultations: Effect on communication and satisfaction for patients and physicians. *Journal of Clinical Oncology*, *20*(11), 2695–2700. doi:10.1200/JCO.2002.10.068 PMID:12039932

Sesso, H. D., Paffenbarger, R. S. Jr, & Lee, I. M. (2000). Physical activity and coronary heart disease in men: The Harvard Alumni Health Study. *Circulation*, *102*(9), 975–980. doi:10.1161/01.CIR.102.9.975 PMID:10961960

Shaffer, A. (2002). *The persistence of L.A.'s grocery gap: The need for a new food policy and approach to market development*. Los Angeles, CA: Center for Food and Justice, Urban and Environmental Policy Institute.

Shakespeare, W. (1602/1623). Twelfth Night, Act 1, scene 1, 1-3. First Folio. British Library.

Shambrook, J. (2007). Results from the 2007 research administrator stress perception survey. *Research Management Review*, *15*(2), 12.

Sharp, C. (2000). *A writer's workshop*. New York: St. Martin's Press.

Shashtri, A. D. (Ed.), (2007). *Sushruta Samhita*. Varanasi: Chaukambha Sanskrit Sansthan.

Shennan, C., Payne, S., & Fenlon, D. (2011). What is the evidence for the use of mindfulness- based interventions in cancer care? A review. *Psycho-Oncology*, *20*(7), 681–697. doi:10.1002/pon.1819 PMID:20690112

Shen, R. L., Cai, F. L., Dong, J. L., & Hu, X. Z. (2011). Hypoglycemic effects and biochemical mechanisms of oat products on streptozotocin-induced diabetic mice. *Journal of Agricultural and Food Chemistry*, *59*(16), 8895–8900. doi:10.1021/jf200678q PMID:21749041

Shetty, P. S. (2000). Diet and life-style and chronic non-communicable diseases: what determines the epidemic in developing societies? In K. Krishnaswami (Ed.), *Nutrition Research: Current Scenario and Future Trends. New Delhi* (pp. 153–167). Oxford: IBH Publishing Co.

Shiloh, S., Sorek, G., & Terkel, J. (2003). Reduction of state-anxiety by petting animals in a controlled laboratory experiment. *Anxiety, Stress, and Coping*, *16*(4), 387–395. doi:10.1080/1061580031000091582

Shinew, K. J., Floyd, M. F., McGuire, F. A., & Noe, F. P. (1995). Gender, race, and subjective social class and their association with leisure preferences. *Leisure Sciences*, *17*(2), 75–89. doi:10.1080/01490409509513245

Shinew, K. J., Floyd, M. F., McGuire, F. A., & Noe, F. P. (1996). Class polarization and leisure activity preferences of African-Americans: Intragroup comparisons. *Journal of Leisure Research*, *28*(4), 219–232.

Shinew, K. J., & Parry, D. C. (2005). Examining college students' participation in the leisure pursuits of drinking and illegal drug use. *Journal of Leisure Research*, *37*(3), 364.

Shneerson, C., Taskila, T., Gale, N., Greenfield, S., & Chen, Y. F. (2013). The effect of complementary and alternative medicine on the quality of life of cancer survivors: A systematic review and meta-analyses. *Complementary Therapies in Medicine*, *21*(4), 417–429. doi:10.1016/j.ctim.2013.05.003 PMID:23876573

Shores, K. A., Scott, D., & Floyd, M. F. (2007). Constraints to outdoor recreation: A multiple hierarchy stratification perspective. *Leisure Sciences*, *29*(3), 227–246. doi:10.1080/01490400701257948

Silo Mentality. (2016). In *Business Dictionary.com*. Retrieved from http://www.businessdictionary.com/definition/silo-mentality.html#ixzz3yZpAGcrA

Singh, K., & Ghosh, P. (2015). *Aarogya Bharat India Healthcare Roadmap for 2025*. New Delhi: Bain and Company.

Smith, L.L., Lake, N.H., Simmons, L.A., Perlman, A., Wroth, S., & Wolever, R.Q. (2013). Integrative health coach training: a model for shifting the paradigm toward patient-centricity and meeting new national prevention goals. *Global advances in health and medicine, 2*(3), 66-74.

Smith, M. K. (2009). Jean Lave, Etienne Wenger and communities of practice: The encyclopedia of informal education. Retrieved from www.infed.org/biblio/communities_of _practice.htm

Snyder, C. R., & Lopez, S. J. (2007). *Positive Psychology*. Thousand Oaks, CA: Sage Publications.

Society of Hospital Medicine. (2015). *Project BOOST® mentored implementation program*. Retrieved from http://www.hospitalmedicine.org/BOOST/

Sokal, J., Dickerson, F. B., Kreyenbuhl, J., Brown, C. H., Goldberg, R. W., & Dixon, L. B. (2004). Comorbidity of medical illnesses among adults with serious mental illness who are receiving community psychiatric services. *The Journal of Nervous and Mental Disease*, *192*(6), 421–427. doi:10.1097/01.nmd.0000130135.78017.96 PMID:15167405

Sousa, L. A. (2002). The medium is the message: The costs and benefits of writing, talking aloud, and thinking about lifes triumphs and defeats. *Dissertation abstracts International: Section B. The Sciences and Engineering*, 62(7-B), 3397.

Southard, S. (1993). *Total quality management (team building and cross training): From business to academe and back again to business.*

SPD Foundation. (2015). About Sensory Processing Disorder. Retrieved from: http://www.spdfoundation.net/about-sensory-processing-disorder/

Spurlock, M. (Writer & Dir.). (2004). *Supersize Me.*

Sreenu, N. (2011). A study of healthcare infrastructure financing and economic growth in India. In A. S. Lather & D. Gakhar (Eds.), *Contemporary issues in corporate finance* (p. 164). New Delhi: Excel Books.

St. Louis Children's Hospital. (2015). The magic house, St. Louis children's museum. Retrieved from http://www.stlouischildrens.org/health-resources/community-education/community-partnerships/the-magic-house-st-louis-childrens-museum

Stallings, J. (in press). Collage as expressive medium in art therapy. In D. Gussak and M. Rosal's (Eds). The Wiley-Blackwell Handbook of Art Therapy. Oxford England: Wiley Blackwell Publishing. doi:10.1002/9781118306543.ch16

Stamps, S. M., & Stamps, M. B. (1985). Race, class and leisure activities of urban residents. *Journal of Leisure Research, 17*(1), 40–56.

Stanczyk, M. M. (2011). Music therapy in supportive cancer care. *Reports of Practical Oncology and Radiotherapy, 16*(5), 170–172. doi:10.1016/j.rpor.2011.04.005 PMID:24376975

Stanton, A., Revenson, T., & Tennen, H. (2007). Health psychology: Psychological adjustment to chronic disease. *Annual Review of Psychology, 58*(1), 565–592. doi:10.1146/annurev.psych.58.110405.085615 PMID:16930096

Stanton, M. P., & Lammon, C. A. (2008). The "wins" of change: Evaluating the impact of predicted changes on case management practice. *Professional Case Management, 13*(3), 161–168. doi:10.1097/01.PCAMA.0000319970.61358.9a PMID:18562911

Starr, B., & Sacks, R. (2010). *Improving outcomes for patients with chronic disease: The medication adherence project (MAP).* Retrieved from http://www.nyc.gov/html/doh/downloads/pdf/cardio/cardio-map-tools-manual.pdf

Starratt, R. J. (1993). *The drama of leadership.* London, England: The Falmer Press.

Step, M. M., Rose, J. H., Albert, J. M., Cheruvu, V. K., & Siminoff, L. A. (2009). Modeling patient-centered communication: Oncologist relational communication and patient communication involvement in breast cancer adjuvant therapy decision-making. *Patient Education and Counseling, 77*(3), 369–378. doi:10.1016/j.pec.2009.09.010 PMID:19811883

Stevens, C.D., Wilkerson, L., & Uijtdehaage, S. (2014). Longitudinal continuity experiences can repair disconnects in the core clerkships for medical students. *Academic Medicine, 89*(2), 205–207. doi:10.1097/acm.0000000000000108

Strang, D., & Macy, M. W. (2001). In search of excellence: Fads, success stories, and adaptive emulation. *American Journal of Sociology, 107*(1), 147–182. doi:10.1086/323039

Strasser, R., & Hirsh, D. (2011). Longitudinal integrated clerkships: Transforming medical education worldwide? *Medical Education*, 45(5), 436-437. doi:10.1111/j.1365-2923.2011.03939.x

Stubblefield, H. W., & Keane, P. (1994). *Adult education in the American experience: From the colonial period to the present.* San Francisco, CA: Jossey-Bass.

Sturm, R., Ringel, J. S., Stein, B. D., & Kapur, K. (2001). Mental health care for youth who gets it? How much does it cost? Who pays? Where does the money go? *Rand.* Retrieved from http://www.rand.org/pubs/research_briefs/RB4541/index1.html

Sugiyama, T., Neuhaus, M., Cole, R., Giles-Corti, B., & Owen, N. (2012). *Destination and route attributes associated with adults' walking: a review* [Doctoral dissertation]. American College of Sports Medicine.

Svensk, A. C., Oster, I., Thyme, K. E., Magnusson, E., Sjodin, M., Eisemann, M., & Lindh, J. et al. (2009). Art therapy improves experienced quality of life among women undergoing treatment for breast cancer: A randomized controlled study. *European Journal of Cancer Care, 18*(1), 69–77. doi:10.1111/j.1365-2354.2008.00952.x PMID:19473224

Swabe, J. (2000). Veterinary dilemmas: ambiguity and ambivalence in human-animal interaction. In A.L. Podberscek, E.S. Paul, & J.A. Serpell (Eds.), Companion Animals and Us: Exploring the relationships between people and pets. Cambridge: Cambridge University Press.

Syrus, P. (42BC). Found in *Familiar quotations.*

Tam, V. C., Knowles, S. R., Cornish, P. L., Fine, N., Marchesano, R., & Etchells, E. E. (2005). Frequency, type and clinical importance of medication history errors at admission to hospital: A systematic review. *Canadian Medical Association Journal, 173*(5), 510–515. doi:10.1503/cmaj.045311 PMID:16129874

Tannen, D. (2004). Talking the dog: Framing Pets as interactional resources in family discourse. *Research on Language and Social Interaction, 37*(4), 399–420. doi:10.1207/s15327973rlsi3704_1

Teherani, A., O'Brien, B.C., Masters, D.E., Poncelet, A.N., Robertson, P.A., & Hauer, K.E. (2009). Burden, responsibility, and reward: Preceptor experiences with the continuity of teaching in a longitudinal integrated clerkship. *Academic Medicine, 84*(10), S50-S53. doi:10.1097/acm.0b013e3181b38b01

The Big Book Online (4th ed.). (2001). Retrieved from http://www.aa.org/bigbookonline

The Joint Commission. (2016). *National patient safety goals effective January 1, 2016.* Retrieved from http://www.jointcommission.org/assets/1/6/2016_NPSG_AHC.pdf

The Joint Commission. Joint Commission Center for Transforming Healthcare, & Joint Commission Resources. (n. d.). *Transitions of care: The need for a more effective approach to continuing patient care.* Retrieved from http://www.jointcommission.org/assets/1/18/Hot_Topics_Transitions_of_Care.pdf

The Need for humane education. (2014). Retrieved from http://worldanimal.net/our-programs/humane-education/the-need-for-humane-education

The University of Texas at Austin. (n. d.). *Physician role.* Retrieved from http://www.healthipe.org/healthcare-roles/physician

The World Bank working for world free of poverty, (2015). Retrieved from http://data.worldbank.org/indicator

Think Florida. (n. d.). *Home page.* Retrieved from http://think-florida.org

Thomas, J. R., & Holley, R. P. (2012). Management versus repetitive tasks-avoiding "working for the weekend". *New Library World, 113*(9), 462-473. doi:10.1108 /03074801211273939

Thomas, S. C., & Beirne, P. (2002). Humane education and humanistic philosophy: Toward a new curriculum. *The Journal of Humanistic Counseling, Education and Development, 41*(2), 190–199. http://www.c-ahead.com/publications.htm doi:10.1002/j.2164-490X.2002.tb00142.x

Thompson, H. L. (2007). Catastrophic leadership failure: An overview. Retrieved from https://www.hpsys.com/PDFs/CatastrophicLeadershipFailureOverviewv2_18SEP2007 .pdf

Thompson, H. L. (2010). *The stress effect: Why smart leaders made dumb decisions and what to do about it* (1st ed.). San Francisco, CA: Jossey-Bass.

Thorpe, K. E., Florence, C. S., & Joski, P. (2004). Which medical conditions account for the rise in health care spending? *Health Affairs, 23*(5), W437–W445. PMID:15451978

Thurber, M. R., Bodenhamer-Davis, E., Johnson, M., Chesky, K., & Chandler, C. (2010). Effects of heart rate variability coherence biofeedback training and emotional management techniques to decrease music performance anxiety. *Biofeedback, 38*(1), 28–39. doi:10.5298/1081-5937-38.1.28

Tindle, H. (2013). *Up: How positive outlook can transform our health and aging.* New York, NY: Hudson Street Press.

Tokuhama-Espinosa, T. (2011). *Mind, brain, and education science: A comprehensive guide to the new brain-based teaching*. WW Norton & Company.

Tough, A. M. (1979). *The adult's learning projects: A fresh approach to theory and practice in adult learning*. Toronto, Canada: Ontario Institute for Studies in Education.

Treadon, C. B., Rosal, M., & Wylder, V. D. T. (2006). Opening the doors of art museums for therapeutic processes. *The Arts in Psychotherapy*, *33*(4), 288–301. doi:10.1016/j.aip.2006.03.003

Tripathi, B. N. (Ed.). (1983). *Charaka Samhita*. Varanasi: Nidana Sthana, Chaukhambha Surbharti Prakashana.

Trivedi, L., & Perl, J. (1995). Animal Facilitated Counseling in the Elementary School: A Literature Review and Practical Considerations. *Elementary School Guidance & Counseling*, *29*(3), 223–234.

Trovato, F. (2009). *Canada's Population in a Global Context: An Introduction to Social Demography*. Oxford University Press Canada.

U.S. Census Bureau. (2010). Facts for features: Older Americans month. May 2010. Retrieved from http://www.census.gov/newsroom/releases/pdf/cb10-ff06.pdf

UAMS. (2015). Spiritual Wellness. Retrieved from http://medicine.uams.edu/faculty/current-faculty/faculty-wellness-program/spiritual-wellness/

United Nations. (2001). World Population Monitoring, Population, Environment, and Development (ESA/P/WP.164). Population Division, Department of Economic and Social Affairs, New York, United Nations.

University of Alabama Department of Radiology. (2014). *Department of Radiology Mission, Vision & Values Statement*. Retrieved from https://www.uab.edu/medicine/radiology/about/mission-vision-values

University of Hawai'i at Hilo. (2012). *College of pharmacy awarded $14.3 million to develop system to save healthcare costs* [News release]. Retrieved from http://hilo.hawaii.edu/news/press/release/1196

University of Washington. (2016). *Center for health sciences interprofessional education, research, and practice*. Retrieved from http://collaborate.uw.edu/about/about-us.html

Unti, B., & DeRosa, B. (2003). Humane education: Past, present, and future. In D. J. Salem & A. N. Rowan (Eds.), *The state of the animals II: 2003*. Washington, DC: Humane Society Press.

Urist, J. (2014, September 23). The healing power of art: Can hospital collections help? Retrieved from http://www.nbcnews.com/health/health-news/healing-power-art-can-hospital-collections-help-n208966

Valentine, D. P., Kiddoo, M., & LaFleur, B. (1993). Psychosocial implications of service dog ownership for people who have mobility or hearing impairments. *Social Work in Health Care*, *19*(1), 109–125. doi:10.1300/J010v19n01_07 PMID:8296220

van den Bosch, M. A., Mudu, P., Uscila, V., Barrdahl, M., Kulinkina, A., Staatsen, B., & Egorov, A. I. (2015). Development of an urban green space indicator and the public health rationale. *Scandinavian Journal of Public Health*.

Veevers, J. E. (1985). The social meanings of pets: Alternative roles for companion animals. In M. B. Sussman (Ed.), *Pets and the family* (pp. 11–30). New York: Haworth Press. doi:10.1300/J002v08n03_03

Velde, B. P., Cipriani, J., & Fisher, G. (2005). Resident and therapist views of animal- assisted therapy: Implications for occupational therapy practice. *Australian Occupational Therapy Journal*, *52*(1), 43–50. doi:10.1111/j.1440-1630.2004.00442.x

Venn, B. J., & Mann, J. I. (2004). Review: Cereal grains, legumes, and diabetes. *European Journal of Clinical Nutrition*, *58*(11), 1443–1451. doi:10.1038/sj.ejcn.1601995 PMID:15162131

Verghese, A. (2008). Spirituality and mental health. *Indian Journal of Psychiatry*, *50*(4), 233–237. doi:10.4103/0019-5545.44742 PMID:19823605

Verner, J. M., Babar, M. A., Cerpa, N., Hall, T., & Beecham, S. (2014). Factors that motivate software engineering teams: A four country empirical study. *Journal of Systems and Software*, *92*, 115–127. doi:10.1016/j.jss.2014.01.008

Verwey, R., van der Weegen, S., Spreeuwenberg, M., Tange, H., van der Weijden, T., & de Witte, L. (2014a). A monitoring and feedback tool embedded in a counseling protocol to increase physical activity of patients with COPD or type 2 diabetes in primary care: Study protocol of a three-arm cluster randomized controlled trial. *BMC Family Practice*, *15*(1), 93. doi:10.1186/1471-2296-15-93 PMID:24885096

Verwey, R., van der Weegen, S., Tange, H., Spreeuwenberg, M., van der Weijden, T., & de Witte, L. (2014b). A pilot study of a tool to stimulate physical activity in patients with COPD or type 2 diabetes in primary care. *Journal of Telemedicine and Telecare*, *20*(1), 29–34. doi:10.1177/1357633X13519057 PMID:24414397

Vickers, A. J., Cronin, A. M., Maschino, A. C., Lewith, G., MacPherson, H., Foster, N. E., & Linde, K. et al. (2012). Acupuncture for chronic pain: Individual patient data meta-analysis. *Archives of Internal Medicine*, *172*(19), 1444–1453. doi:10.1001/archinternmed.2012.3654 PMID:22965186

Vickers, A. J., & Linde, K. (2014). Acupuncture for chronic pain. *Journal of the American Medical Association*, *311*(9), 955–956. doi:10.1001/jama.2013.285478 PMID:24595780

Villarreal, J. (2014). Addressing narcissistic leadership through organizational leadership and systematic implementations. *Paper presented at the Fifth Annual Virtual Conference on Moral Leadership: Narcissism and Toxic Leadership*, Regent University. Paper retrieved from http://www.regent.edu/acad/global/conferences/virtual/2014/papers/2014_Moral_Leadership_Conference_Villarreal.pdf

Virago, M., & Dunkley, M. (2008, March). A journey past the sun and back: Using art psychotherapy to investigate the connection between immunological and psychosocial function following a diagnosis of melanoma. *Psycho-Oncology*, *17*(3), S27–S28.

Volpato, E., Banfi, P., Rogers, S. M., & Pagnini, F. (2015). Relaxation techniques for people with chronic obstructive pulmonary disease: A systematic review and a meta-analysis. *Evidence-Based Complementary and Alternative Medicine*, *2015*, 1–22. doi:10.1155/2015/628365 PMID:26339268

Vranova, S. (2012). Identifying the specifics of motivating different groups of employees. *Journal of Global Science and Technology Forum*, *2*(2), 98–104. doi:10.5176/2010-4804_2.2.188

Wahbeh, H., Calabrese, C., & Zwickey, H. (2007). Binaural Beat Technology in Humans: A Pilot Study To Assess Psychologic and Physiologic Effects. *Journal of Alternative and Complementary Medicine (New York, N.Y.)*, *13*(1), 25–32. doi:10.1089/acm.2006.6196 PMID:17309374

Walsh, F. (2009). Human-animal bonds II: The role of pets in family systems and family therapy. *Family Process*, *48*(4), 481–499. doi:10.1111/j.1545-5300.2009.01297.x PMID:19930434

Wang, F., Man, J. K., Lee, E. K., Wu, T., Benson, H., & Fricchione, G. L. (2013). The effects of qigong on anxiety, depression, and psychological well-being: A systematic review and meta-analysis. *Evidence-Based Complementary and Alternative Medicine*. PMID:23401706

Wang, Y., Ph, D., Yang, C., Ph, D., Wang, K., & Ph, D. (2012). Comparing public and private employees' job satisfaction and turnover. *Public Personnel Management*, *41*(3), 557–573. doi:10.1177/009102601204100310

Wannamethee, S. G., & Shaper, A. G. (1999). Physical activity and the prevention of stroke. *Journal of Cardiovascular Risk*, *6*(4), 213–216. doi:10.1177/204748739900600404 PMID:10501271

Wannamethee, S. G., & Shaper, A. G. (2001). Physical activity in the prevention of cardiovascular disease: An epidemiological perspective. *Sports Medicine (Auckland, N.Z.)*, *31*(2), 101–114. doi:10.2165/00007256-200131020-00003 PMID:11227978

Ward, B. W., Schiller, J. S., & Goodman, R. A. (2014). Multiple chronic conditions among US adults: A 2012 update. *Preventing Chronic Disease*, 2014, 11. PMID:24742395

Wardell, D. W., & Weymouth, K. F. (2004). Review of studies of Healing Touch. *Journal of Nursing Scholarship*, *36*(2), 147–154. doi:10.1111/j.1547-5069.2004.04012.x PMID:15227762

Washburne, R. F. (1978). Black under-participation in wildland recreation: Alternative explanations. *Leisure Sciences*, *1*(2), 175–189. doi:10.1080/01490407809512880

Waters, E., Merrick, S., Treboux, D., Crowell, J., & Albersheim, L. (2000). Attachment security in infancy and early adulthood: A twenty-year longitudinal study. *Child Development*, *71*(3), 684–689. doi:10.1111/1467-8624.00176 PMID:10953934

Watson, R.T. (2003). Rediscovering the medical school. (2003). *Academic Medicine, 78*(7), 659-665. doi:10.1097/00001888-200307000-00002

Weeks, K. (2015). *University initiatives: FAU implements university-wide HeartMath training.* Retrieved from http://www.fau.edu/newsdesk/articles/university-wide-heartmath-training.php

Weil, Z. (2003). *Above all, be kind: Raising a humane child in challenging times*. Gabriola Island, BC: New Society.

Weiner-Davis, M. (1995). *Fire your shrink*. New York, NY: Simon & Schuster.

Weisenberger, J. (2014). Foods high in AGEs. Diabetes Forecast: The Healthy Living Magazine. Alexandria, VA: American Diabetes Association. Retrieved from http://www.diabetesforecast.org/2014/11-nov/foods-high-in-ages.html?loc=ymal

Welch, D. M. (2006). *Occupational stress, self-efficacy and symptom relationships among medical-surgical hospital nurses* [Doctoral dissertation].

Weldy, T. G., & Gillis, W. E. (2010). The learning organization: Variations at different organizational levels. *The Learning Organization, 17*(5), 455-470. doi:http://dx.doi.org.ezproxylocal.library.nova.edu/10.1108/09696471011059831

Weyerer, S. (1992). Physical inactivity and depression in the community. Evidence from the Upper Bavarian Field Study. *International Journal of Sports Medicine*, *13*(06), 492–496. doi:10.1055/s-2007-1021304 PMID:1428382

Wharton, E. (1920). *The age of innocence*. New York, NY: Collier.

Wheelan, C. (2013). *Naked statistics*. New York, NY: W.W. Norton.

Whitcomb, M.E. (2005). Redesigning clinical education: A major challenge for academic health centers. *Academic Medicine, 80*(7), 615-616. doi:10.1097/00001888-200507000-00001

White, C. (2011). Epilogue: continuing conversations. In M. White (Ed.), *Narrative practice* (pp. 157–179). New York, NY: W.W. Norton & Company.

White, M., & Epston, D. (1990). *Narrative means to therapeutic ends*. New York, NY: W.W. Norton & Company.

Wilenius, M. (2014). Leadership in the sixth wave-excursions into the new paradigm of the Kondratieff cycle 2010-2015. *Eur J Futures Res*, *2*(1), 36. doi:10.1007/s40309-014-0036-7

Wilkerson, L., & Irby, D. M. (1998). Strategies for improving teaching practices: A comprehensive approach to faculty development. *Academic Medicine*, *73*(4), 387–396. doi:10.1097/00001888-199804000-00011 PMID:9580715

Williams, P. (2013). *Happy. On Despicable Me 2 (Movie soundtrack)*. New York, NY: Columbia Record.

Williams, R. L. (1991). *The origins of federal support for higher education: George W. Atherton and the land-grant college movement*. University Park, PA: Penn State University Press.

Wisdom, J. P., Saedi, G. A., & Green, C. A. (2009). Another breed of "service" animals: Stars study findings about pet ownership and recovery from serious mental illness. *The American Journal of Orthopsychiatry*, *79*(3), 430–436. doi:10.1037/a0016812 PMID:19839680

Wolch, J. R., Byrne, J., & Newell, J. P. (2014). Urban green space, public health, and environmental justice: The challenge of making cities 'just green enough'. *Landscape and Urban Planning*, *125*, 234–244. doi:10.1016/j.landurbplan.2014.01.017

Wood, M. J. M., & Molassiotis, A. (2011). What research evidence is there for the use of art therapy in the management of symptoms in adults with cancer? A systematic review. *Psycho-Oncology, 20*(2), 135-145.

Woodard, M. D. (1988). Class, regionality, and leisure among urban Black Americans: The post-civil rights era. *Journal of Leisure Research*, *20*(2), 87–105.

Wood, L. J., Giles-Corti, B., Bulsara, M. K., & Bosch, D. A. (2007). More than a furry companion: The ripple effect of companion animals on neighborhood interactions and sense of community. *Society & Animals*, *15*(1), 43–56. doi:10.1163/156853007X169333

Wood, M. J. M., Low, J., Molassiotis, A., & Tookman, A. (2013). Art therapy's contribution to the psychological care of adults with cancer: A survey of therapists and service users in the UK. *International Journal of Art Therapy*, *18*(2), 42–53. doi:10.1080/17454832.2013.781657

World Health Organization (WHO). (1948a), Preamble to the Constitution of the World Health Organization as adopted by the International Health Conference, New York, 19-22 June, 1946; signed on 22 July 1946 by the representatives of 61 States (Official Records of the World Health Organization, no. 2, p. 100) and entered into force on 7 April 1948.

World Health Organization (WHO). (1996d). Creating Healthy Cities in the 21st Century Background Paper, *UN Conference on Human Settlements: Habitat II*, Istanbul

World Health Organization (WHO). (2000f). *Who Pays for the Health System? The World Health Report*. Geneva: WHO.

World Health Organization (WHO). (2001e). Private Sector Involvement in City Health Systems proceedings of a WHO conference meeting, Dunedin, New Zealand.

World Health Organization (WHO). (2001g). Making a Public-Private Partnership Work: An Insider's View. *Bulletin of the World Health Organization*, *79*(8), 795–796.

World Health Organization (WHO). (2007h). Everybody's business: strengthening health systems to improve health outcomes: WHO's framework for action. Geneva.

World Health Organization (WHO). (2008b). Closing the gap in a generation. Health equity through action on the social determinants of health. Geneva. Retrieved from http://apps.who.int/iris/bitstream/10665/43943/1/9789241563703_eng.pdf

World Health Organization (WHO). (2013c). Country cooperation strategy at a glance. Retrieved from http://www.who.int/countryfocus/cooperation_strategy/ccsbrief_ind_en.pdf

World Health Organization- WHO. (2009). Diarrheal Disease Factsheet. Retrieved from http://www.who.int/mediacentre/factsheets/fs330/en/index.html

World Health Organization. (2010). *Framework for interprofessional education and collaborative practice.* Retrieved from http://apps.who.int/iris/bitstream/10665/70185/1/WHO_HRH_HPN_10.3_eng.pdf?ua=1

World Health Organization. (2016). *Patients for patient safety.* Retrieved from http://www.who.int/patientsafety/patients_for_patient/en/

Yadav, S. (2014). The role of emotional intelligence in organization development. *ICFAI Journal of Knowledge Management, 12*(4), 49.

Yang, Y. C., Lu, F.-H., Wu, J.-S., Wu, C.-H., & Chang, C.-J. (2004). The protective effect of habitual tea consumption on hypertension. *Archives of Internal Medicine, 164*(14), 1534–1540. doi:10.1001/archinte.164.14.1534 PMID:15277285

Yorks, L., & Scott, L. (2013). Lifelong tools for the learner, educator, and worker. In V. C. X. Wang (Ed.), *Handbook of Research on Technologies for Improving the 21st Century Workforce: Tools for Lifelong Learning* (pp. 42–55)., doi:10.4018/978-1-4666-2181-7.ch004

Youssef, C. M., & Luthans, F. (2007). Positive organizational behavior in the workplace: The Impact of hope, optimism, and resilience. *Journal of Management, 33*(5), 774–800. doi:10.1177/0149206307305562

Zainal, N. Z., Booth, S., & Huppert, F. A. (2013). The efficacy of mindfulness-based stress reduction on mental health of breast cancer patients: A meta-analysis. *Psycho-Oncology, 22*(7), 1457–1465. doi:10.1002/pon.3171 PMID:22961994

Zeng, Y., Luo, T., Xie, H., Huang, M., & Cheng, A. S. (2014). Health benefits of qigong or tai chi for cancer patients: A systematic review and meta-analyses. *Complementary Therapies in Medicine, 22*(1), 173–186. doi:10.1016/j.ctim.2013.11.010 PMID:24559833

Zenk, S. N., Schulz, A. J., Israel, B. A., James, S. A., Bao, S. M., & Wilson, M. L. (2005). Neighborhood racial composition, neighborhood poverty, and the spatial accessibility of supermarkets in metropolitan. Detroit, MI. *American Journal of Public Health, 95*(4), 660–667. doi:10.2105/AJPH.2004.042150 PMID:15798127

Zhang, J., Yang, K. H., Tian, J. H., & Wang, C. M. (2012). Effects of yoga on psychologic function and quality of life in women with breast cancer: A meta-analysis of randomized controlled trials. *Journal of Alternative and Complementary Medicine, 18*(11), 994–1002. doi:10.1089/acm.2011.0514 PMID:22909345

Zhou, J., & Fischer, K. W. (2013). Culturally appropriate education: Insights from educational neuroscience. *Mind. Brain & Education, 7*(4), 225–231. doi:10.1111/mbe.12030

Zilcha-Mano, S., Mikulincer, M., & Shaver, P. R. (2012). Pets as safe havens and secure bases: The moderating role of pet attachment orientations. *Journal of Research in Personality, 46*(5), 571–580. doi:10.1016/j.jrp.2012.06.005

Zillich, A. J., Snyder, M. E., Frail, C. K., Lewis, J. L., Deshotels, D., Dunham, P., & Sutherland, J. M. et al. (2014). A randomized, controlled pragmatic trial of telephonic medication therapy management to reduce hospitalization in home health patients. *Health Services Research*, *49*(5), 1537–1554. doi:10.1111/1475-6773.12176 PMID:24712335

Zimmerman, L., Pozehl, B., Duncan, K., & Schmitz, R. (1989). Effects of music in patients who had chronic cancer pain. *Western Journal of Nursing Research*, *11*(3), 298–309. doi:10.1177/019394598901100304 PMID:2750142

Zimmermann, S. (2002). *Writing to heal the soul.* New York, NY: Three Rivers Press.

About the Contributors

Valerie C. Bryan is a Charles Stewart Mott Eminent Scholar and Professor in Educational Leadership & Research Methodology in Adult and Community Education at Florida Atlantic University. She will also receive the International Adult and Continuing Education Hall of Fame's (IACEHOF) Class of 2015 by the Board of Directors of the International Adult and Continuing Education in November, 2015. She also will be featured as one of "The 100 Women of Florida Atlantic University" in the Spring 2016. Other recognitions and awards include "woman of outstanding leadership" by The International Women's Leadership Association, 2013; an award for a research project with Homeland Security "Emergency Alert Technology for the Profoundly Deaf"; FAU's Unsung Hero Award for mentor roles, 2013; FAU's Outstanding Academic Advisor of the Year, 2012; Outstanding Virtual Presentation Award as a co-presenter at E-Learn 2011-2012--World Conference on E-Learning in Corporate, Government, Healthcare, and Higher Education, Honolulu, Hawaii; FAU Graduate Mentor Award, 2011; MacAWARD Exceptional Faculty for College of Education, 2009; FAU College of Education Distinguished Teacher of the Year, 2009; FAU's President's Award, 2006-2007; FAU College of Education's Distinguished Teacher of the Year, 2006; FAU College of Education Teacher of the Year, 2005-2006; Clemson University's President's Award, 1993; State of North Carolina's Individual of the Year, 1984, for the Mountain to the Sea Trail; and Co-Webmaster of One of Top Ten US Literacy Internet sites, 1998. At Florida Atlantic University, she teaches courses in adult learning, executive leadership, aging, integration of technology, and a host of other subjects (52 different courses), in multiple platforms. Her research areas focus on virtual learning communities, communities of practice, successful aging, and global learning. She has chaired over 90 dissertations while at FAU, received over $2 million in grants, and been asked to do 11 comprehensive evaluations of systems outside of FAU. She has served on two statewide assessments related to technology and online learning systems. She serves as a reviewer for the Journal of Applied Gerontology, has contributed to several blogs for Partnership for 21st Century Skills (P21); has abbreviated work in www.eddigest.com; has contributed the "information technology book chapter" for the National Recreation and Park Association's Management text, a required text for all parks and recreation programs nationwide (2016, 2010, 2005, 1999) and the accompanying Compendium (2016, 2010, 2005). She has contributed three books; 30 book chapters; reviews for 7 books; international, national and state journal articles (52 refereed; 11 non-refereed); international, national, state, regional and local presentations (84 refereed; 190 non-refereed); as well as international virtual presentations to Canada, Hawaii, Spain, and China. Her work is the highest cited on ResearchGate.net for her department.

Jennifer Lynne Bird teaches reading and writing classes for current and future teachers at Florida Atlantic University in Boca Raton, Florida. She received her Bachelor of Science in Education in Secondary English Education, Master of Education in Secondary English Education, and Doctor of Philosophy degrees from Miami University in Oxford, Ohio and her health coach certification from Duke University Integrative Medicine in Durham, North Carolina. Her research in writing and healing led to the publication of her book *Innovative Collaborative Practice and Reflection in Patient Education* (2015).

* * *

Chris Allison has worked in previous Residential Treatment Centers as a trainer in communication, verbal de-escalation skills, and mental illness healing. Chris currently works for Southwest Baptist University as the Director of the Meyer Wellness and Sport Center.

Krista Allison received her PhD in Educational Leadership from Florida Atlantic University in 2012. She currently works as faculty at the University of Phoenix.

Jo Ann M. Bamdas is the Director of Interprofessional Education (IPE) for the Office of the Provost at FAU. In this capacity she collaborates with the Associate Provost of Assessment and Programs and IPE Associate Directors as well as faculty and staff from the Charles E. Schmidt College of Medicine, Christine E. Lynn College of Nursing, and School of Social Work in the College for Design and Social Inquiry to plan, develop, implement, and administer the interprofessional education program for FAU's social work, nursing, and medical students. She holds a Ph.D. in Educational Leadership & Research Methodology. Her research interests include interprofessional education, health science, college level writing, and women's education and learning.

Charlotte D. Barry is a Professor in the Christine E. Lynn College of Nursing at Florida Atlantic University and a Fellow in the American Academy of Nursing. Dr, Barry teaches across the curriculum courses in caring, transcultural caring, community health, family theory, and policy. Her research areas of interest are caring for individuals and families across the lifespan, teaching/learning caring and the development of caring theories to guide nursing practice. She is also a certified HeartMath® trainer and has integrated this in her community practice.

Kimberly Bronner is a senior nursing student at Florida Atlantic University, Christine E. Lynn College of Nursing.

Susannah Brown is an Associate Professor of Art Education in the College of Education Department of Teaching and Learning since 2004. Prior to working at FAU, Dr. Brown taught at the University of North Carolina in Charlotte. She also worked for twelve years as an art teacher in the public school system, kindergarten through sixth grade. Her research includes the integration of the arts in school curriculum with a focus on literacy development and visual art for well-being. She has published several articles, chapters in edited books, and textbooks. She also presents at professional conferences around the world. She is a practicing artist and exhibits her work regularly.

Angelica Constanzo is first-year health system pharmacy administration resident of a two year residency at The University of Kansas Hospital.

Ebbin Dotson, PhD, MHSA, Associate Dean, Urban Health and Diversity Programs & Assistant Professor, Community Health Sciences at University of Illinois at Chicago (UIC). PhD, Health Services and Policy Analysis, University of California, Berkeley; MHSA, Health Management & Policy, University of Michigan-School of Public Health.

Joanna Lauren Drowos currently serves as an Assistant Professor of Clinical Biomedical Science in the Charles E. Schmidt College of Medicine at Florida Atlantic University. There she serves as the Interim Associate Chair of the Integrated Medical Science Department and the Director for the Clinical and Preventive Medicine Clerkship for the third year curriculum. Dr. Drowos earned her DO and Master of Public Health Degrees at Nova Southeastern University College of Osteopathic Medicine. She completed a Pediatrics tracked Internship at Palms West Hospital followed by a Preventive Medicine Residency with the Palm Beach County Health Department and a Family Practice Residency at Broward General Medical Center. She is board certified in Preventive Medicine, Family Medicine and Medical Quality. She earned her Master of Business Administration in Healthcare Administration from Florida Atlantic University in 2008.

Karethy A. Edwards, a family nurse practitioner, is an Associate Dean for Academic Programs and Professor for the Christine E. Lynn College of Nursing at Florida Atlantic University. Dr. Edwards, a certified HeartMath® Trainer, has used HeartMath® for over ten years and provided the leadership for the HeartMath Resilience Program initiative at Florida Atlantic University.

Linda Ellington currently serves as a Faculty Lead in Southern New Hampshire University. Previously she taught in the Graduate School of Leadership at Palm Beach Atlantic University which followed her 23 years working in IBM. Her passion and research is in strategic thinking and leadership, as well as helping children gain the tools to remove bullying from their lives. Linda conducted her doctoral research at the University of Oxford, in the UK, as she was fascinated as to how higher educational leaders continue to grow and flourish in such a university that has no known date of foundation but evidence of teaching as far back as 1096. From there her teaching and research has focused on teaching and leading in institutions of higher education. She is a peer reviewer for several academic organizations. She has written and co-authored chapters published in international journals, national journals, and textbooks. In addition to research and academic writing, she is involved in the Literacy Foundation, and is the author of seven children's book in the genre of bullying. She reads to children and parents at city libraries throughout the state of Florida.

Julie A. Exposito completed her Doctor of Education with a concentration in Higher Education Leadership and Organizational Leadership at Nova Southeastern University. She is completed a qualitative study using a phenomenological approach to explore and understand the experience of international students enrolled at a 4-year public American college. She has written articles on leadership, higher education, academic integrity, narcissism, simulation experiences, and the international student. Julie received a Master's in TESOL from Florida International University with a focus on language acquisition, skill and experiential based curriculum design, and international conflict resolution. She received a Bachelor of Science in Education and French from Skidmore College. Currently, she serves as the English Language Program Coordinator for the Florida Association of International Educators (FAIE). Her interest in international education 292 About the Contributors extends into the classroom of linguistically and culturally diverse adult learners with various learning styles and needs, and has served on the faculty at Miami Dade College and Broward College, teaching English for Academic Purposes in face-to-face classes with supplemental online lab and D2L platforms.

Jaclyn Nicole Falcone began working in the nonprofit, education arena in 2005, she has volunteered with the Crohn's and Colitis Foundation since 2010 and has received many awards including the Graduate Fellowship for Academic Excellence and the Newell Doctoral Award. She earned two bachelor's degrees from FSU in Psychology and Sociology and graduated from Vanderbilt University with a Master's in Organizational Leadership. She earned an Education Specialist from FAU and will receive her doctorate in 2017 with an emphasis on Adult & Community Education. Jaclyn is married to Nicholas who together with his brothers own NDM Hospitality and reside in south Florida near their families. They have a beautiful Cane Corso named Luna who lights up their lives. Jaclyn's research on humane education and pet safety is in memory of Gianni Falcone, their loving and energetic puppy whose life was taken too soon. She believes that education is the field with the most meaningful opportunity to shape minds and transform people's lives and is committed to reducing the number of preventable animal tragedies by providing pet owners with the education and training to save their pet's life.

Ashley Hartman is a PhD candidate specializing in Art Therapy at Florida State University. She holds a MS in Art Therapy, an M. Ed in Educational Psychology, and has seven years of teaching experience. Her research interests have been inspired by work in pediatric and oncology centers at the University of Washington, UF Health Shands, and the University of Alabama Medical Center Radiology Lab. She recently worked with an arts in healing collaborative program through the University of Alabama Medical Center, the Birmingham Museum of Art, and Florida State University's Graduate Program in Art Therapy.

Dan K. Hibbler, PhD, Associate Professor at DePaul University-School for New Learning. PhD, Leisure Behavior, University of Illinois at Urbana-Champaign.

Thomas D. Kennedy is an associate professor of research at Nova Southeastern University in Davie, Florida. He received his PhD in Counseling Psychology from the University of Miami and his MA in Clinical Psychology from Southern Methodist University. For 5 years, he has been a faculty member at NSU, where he has developed and taught research and statistic courses. He is the Institutional Review Board representative for the College of Education. His clinical experience consists of providing neuropsychological assessments, behavioral medicine interventions, and group therapy in inpatient and outpatient settings, including the following: the University of Texas Southwestern Medical Center, University of Miami Mailman Center for Child Development, Jackson Memorial Hospital, University of Miami Institute for Individual and Family Therapy, and the Dallas County Jail. His research interests include two convergent tracks, one focusing on at-risk children and adolescents and the other exploring biofeedback and other complementary and alternative medicine evaluations. He has received multiple grants and provides evaluation and grant writing services for various organizations in southern Florida.

He has published and presented in the areas of juvenile crime, psychophysiology, and research methodology. Dr. Kennedy is a licensed psychologist PY8307 and is certified through the Biofeedback Certification International Alliance in general biofeedback; he maintains a small private practice for children and adolescents.

Cassandra M. Kenski holds a M.Ed. from Florida Atlantic University and is currently working on a Ph.D. in Educational Leadership from Keiser University. Ms. Kenski currently resides in Wellington, FL. with her dog and cat. In addition to her work as a writer, Cassandra teaches at both the elementary and collegiate levels. Along with her passion for education and language arts, she works as a photographer and advocates for both animal and human rights. She attributes her impassioned humane education and animal rescue efforts to Bailey, the dog that "changed everything."

Beth M. King is an Assistant Professor of Nursing at Florida Atlantic University and teaches in the undergraduate and graduate programs. She is certified as an Adult Psychiatric & Mental Health Clinical Nurse Specialist and is a certified HeartMath® trainer. Dr. King's research focus is in the area of caring science and mental health related to affective symptomatology.

Prashant Mehta is consultant and accomplished Academic Professional with over 18 years of diverse working experience in academics and industry. Ph.D. Management, National Law University, Jodhpur 2010, MBA Marketing, Sikkim Manipal University, Sikkim 2011 Ph.D. Chemistry, Jai Narain Vyas University, Jodhpur 1996 M.SC. Chemistry, Jai Narain Vyas University, Jodhpur 1993 B.SC. SCIENCE, Lachoo Memorial College of Science, Jodhpur University, Jodhpur Publications: Books – 02, Research Papers - 24, Conferences Presentations - 24, Expert Lecture Delivered – 100, Online Articles - 12, Online Power Point Presentations – 53 Group Study Exchange Scholar, Rotary Foundation 2005.

David B. Ross has many years of experience in adult education, leadership, ethics, policy and curriculum development, and classroom instruction. In his present role as an Associate Professor at the Abraham S. Fischler College of Education, Nova Southeastern University, he teaches doctoral level courses in educational and organizational leadership to prepare today's practitioners who will assume leadership positions in any profession for current and future challenges. His courses focus on current trends and issues that impact society on both the national and global level. Learning from many perspectives and philosophies from mentors while attending Northern Illinois University, the University of Alabama, and Florida Atlantic University, it helps him guide students in the learning process. Dr. Ross earned his Doctorate in Educational Leadership, with an emphasis in Leadership, Research, Curriculum and Adult Education, and a Master of Justice Policy Management with a Professional Certificate in Public Administration at Florida Atlantic University. He earned his Bachelor of Science Degree in Computer Science at Northern Illinois University. Dr. Ross regularly speaks at conferences and provides consultation and training in the areas of leadership, policy issues, team building, professional development, academic writing, education, and behavior management. He has written articles on leadership, power, narcissism, plagiarism and fraud, policy development, professional development, and areas of homeland security. Dr. Ross is a dissertation chair and committee member of quantitative, qualitative, and mixed methods as well as an Institutional Review Board representative for the College of Education.

Leodis Scott, Ed.D., Adjunct Assistant Faculty, Columbia University-Teachers College; Faculty, DePaul University-School for New Learning; Cofounder at LearnLong Institute for Education and Learning Research. Ed.D., Adult Learning and Leadership from Columbia University-Teachers College.

Debra N. Weiss-Randall, EdD, MA, CHES teaches at the College of Education of Florida Atlantic University (FAU). She completed her Masters' degree (2007) and doctorate (2010) in health education at Teachers' College, Columbia University. Her Masters project was entitled "Get Smarter, Live Longer with Meditation" and was presented to executives at Time Inc. Her doctoral research was a statewide study of asthma management on NY college campuses. In 2013, the findings were replicated with a team from Texas State University and won a national award; the results were published in Respiratory Care in 2015. After completing her undergraduate degree at Columbia University in New York, she taught at the City University of New York for 15 years. Dr. Weiss-Randall became a certified online instructor in 2012. Since 2014, she has taught in the classroom and online at FAU. In Spring 2015 she completed an e-certification course for faculty in the design of online classes.

Sarah K. Wood, MD is the Senior Associate Dean for Medical Education at the Charles E. Schmidt College of Medicine at Florida Atlantic University. She leads the newly implemented innovative LICs at FAU for all 64 third year students with the help of dedicated and talented clerkship directors and community based preceptors throughout Palm Beach and Broward Counties.

Index

M

N

O

P

R

S

T

U

V

W

www.ingramcontent.com/pod-product-compliance
Lightning Source LLC
LaVergne TN
LVHW081251011026
849162LV00006BA/1428
* 9 7 8 1 5 2 2 5 0 6 4 0 9 *